Vedic Yoga: The Path of the Rishi

by Pandit Vamadeva Shastri
(Vedacharya David Frawley)

LOTUS PRESS

Twin Lakes, WI

DISCLAIMER

This book is not intended to treat, diagnose or prescribe. The information contained herein is in no way to be considered as a substitute for a consultation with a duly licensed health care professional.

Author: David Frawley

First Edition 2014

Printed in the United States of America

ISBN: 978-0-9406-7625-1

Library of Congress Control Number: 2014944858

LOTUS PRESS

Published by:
Lotus Press, P.O. Box 325, Twin Lakes, WI53181 USA
web:www.lotuspress.com
Email:lotuspress@lotuspress.com
800.824.6396

Credits

Cover Illustration – Hinduism Today

Line Drawings – Hinduism Today

Photographs

Kavyakantha Ganapati Muni, from Sampadananda Mishra

Brahmarshi Daivarata, from author's collection

Ramana Maharshi and Ganapati Muni, from K. Natesan

K. Natesan, from author's collection

Sri Aurobindo and the Mother, from Lotus Press

Kapali Shastri, from Lotus Press

MP Pandit, from Lotus Press

Sri Sadguru Sivananda Murty, from author's collection

Swami Veda Bharati, from Swami Rama Sadhaka Gram

Proofing and Copy editing – Vimala Rodgers

Table of Contents

Foreword by Swami Veda Bharati

Oṁ!
From the words of the poet,
"Men take what meanings please them, yet their last meaning points to Thee."

The above saying of the great poet Rabindranath Tagore is completely true in the case of the *Vedas*, ancient India's mantric books of Divine truth. As the *Atharvaveda* says about the *Veda*: "It has not left out anything that never dieth and never decays."

The most important point I wish to make is not about the interpretation of the *Vedas* but their source in the deepest states of meditation. We hear in the *Rigveda*:

> *Inspired wise poets (kavi), they of deep meditation, obtain the words and the highest state. Protecting it, the ever-undecaying one, in many ways, from the heart.*
>
> *Seeking to find they have seen the ocean and for these humans the sun revealed itself.*
>
> *Dirghatamas Auchatya, Rigveda 1.146.4*

There is a very detailed theory of such mantric revelation in the ancient Sanskrit philosophy of language. This revelation occurs in the depths of consciousness where from it pours having found the form of words. The words are a covering for the revealed reality, and only by unveiling it through meditation can one remove the word-covering and see the truth for what it is in all its glory. Thus only a Rishi can understand the language of the Rishi and otherwise we can only scratch the surface. If not fully a Rishi, we must be deep meditators in order for the true meaning to dawn on us.

There are the instances of later Rishis such as Ananda Tirtha, Swami Dayananda, and Sri Aurobindo who have seen the meanings of the *Vedas* and given spiritual translations of Vedic hymns. I have also come across a few lesser known figures.

Vamadeva mentions Maharshi Daivarata in his book. Two important Vedic works of Daivarata are available to us and other works of his, like *Yoga-Sudha*, lie unpublished. *Vak Sudha* is his versified commentary in over a thousand poetic verses, on select hymns and terms of the *Rigveda*. Unfortunately, no English translation is available. Daivarata's magnum opus *Chandodarshana* consists of four hundred and fifty revealed mantras from him in the Rigvedic language. These have been translated into English and include a Sanskrit commentary by his own great guru Sri Vasishtha Ganapati Muni, whose line of teachings goes back to Bhagavan Ramana Maharshi. The Muni created several new Vedic verses of his own as well, among his many other profound Sanskrit poetic and philosophical works of seer inspiration.

The foremost point in trying to understand the diction of the *Vedas*, as we have said at the beginning, is to reside in the same state of meditation in which the mantra was first revealed to the Rishi. The second most important point is to understand that all Vedic mantra meanings are multi-layered and cannot just be reduced to one level only.

In commenting on the revelations of Maharshi Daivarata, Sri Ganapati Vasishtha Muni has followed the second point. For example, in the first mantra of Daivarata, the Muni has explained the word *mitra* in six layers of the word and also cross-referenced these with other citations of the *Vedas*.

I was at one time preparing a dictionary of the *Vedas* from 1946, not completed and not published. *It was based on the principle that the Vedas themselves, and not grammar and etymologies, are the best source of Vedic interpretation.* I now look for scholars who will complete that work under my direction, also, if funding can be found. Ganapati Muni, to my delight, has also resorted to the same principle of understanding the *Veda* primarily through the *Veda*, as does Vamadeva in the current book. This kind of analysis of translations and interpretations by those who have the Vedic vision can take five decades or more and yet the depth of the Vedas will still not be fully fathomed.

Vamadeva mentions in this current book on the Vedic Yoga another contemporary teacher to whom Vedic mantras have been revealed, referring to my own work and writings. Swami Veda Bharati has so far published over three of these mantras (*Divo Duhita*, Chaukhamba, Delhi, 2013) and many more lie unpublished in addition to the ones that keep dawning on him from time to time. A translator/disciple is awaited to whom he may hand the keys to the interpretation of these mantras.

Here we render only a uni-layer translation of a randomly selected unpublished mantra from *Divo Duhita*:

> *As the words shine forth in splendour,*
> *The manifest and unmanifest ones, mixed and unmixed,*
> *Yoked in yoga together with the suns' horses,*
> *May we, entering within, becoming one with universal truths,*
> *Contemplate on these honeyed ones.*
> *Giving multi-layer meanings of the four*
> *lines could easily take dozens of pages.*

The secret of such Vedic revelation dwells in the depth of meditation. In the lab of his Ashram's Meditation Research Institute in Rishikesh, Swami Veda Bharati has demonstrated that in the depth of meditation he produces 101Hz gamma waves on one hand and on the other he produces below 0.5 Hz delta brain waves; this apparently has never been recorded before in the research of neurology on meditation.

As I read Vedacharya Vamadeva Shastri (David Frawley)'s book on the Vedic Yoga here, at every sentence my heart wants to nod and say, "yes, yes, indeed, yes!" Yes, it is so as he has indicated. Quite often when the two of us are together on the stage before students explaining the secrets of the *Vedas*, we find ourselves completing each other's sentences; so attuned are these two adherents of Vedic wisdom.

Every page of Vamadeva's work is an example of what the Vedic Rishis have extolled as *manīśa* (maneesha), the "mantra-bearing inspirational wisdom". Vamadeva is, as I would call him in Vedic language, *dhiyo yasya pracoditāḥ*, "one whose meditative wisdom has been impelled to manifest itself to the world."

Vamadeva would not have succeeded in obtaining these important insights if he had not been in contact with highest level guides in the lineages of the greatest yogis like Bhagavan Ramana Maharshi and Sri Aurobindo. The meditative unraveling of consciousness has awakened his *dhī* or "deeper intelligence," the higher faculty of knowing that Hindus have sought for thousands of years through the sacred Gayatri Mantra to the solar Self.

For those who have no direct access to the original language and the meditative depth of the *Vedas*, which is still limited to very few, Vamadeva's work provides the wide-open doorway. I hope and pray that one day he writes a full commentary on a few hymns of the *Vedas*, unveiling their multi-layer meanings.

Mahamandaleshvara Dr. Swami Veda Bharati
B.A. (Honours) London, M.A. (London), D. Litt. (Utrecht, Holland) Vedic scholar, meditation master, author, poet, international lecturer; chancellor of HIHT University, Dehradun, India; founder and spiritual guide to Swami Rama Sadhaka Grama, Rishikesh, India

Introductory Note by Sampadananda Mishra

The Vedic Yoga is the ancient system of integral Yoga shaped by the Vedic Rishis. These Rishis devoted to a life of the Spirit discovered a certain line of development beyond the range of sensory perception by means of their strength of self-discipline, and achieved a many-sided inner progress. Whatever they achieved by their *tapasya* (meditative concentration) they then cast into a veiled language that they called *Mantra*. It is through these Rishis that the secret words of the Vedas were revealed. The Rishis had the inner vision to see the light of truth (*ṛṣyaḥ mantradraṣṭaraḥ*) and the inner audition to hear the voice of the truth (*satyaśrutaḥ*). They possessed both great spiritual and occult knowledge, the complete inner wisdom. Each Rishi represented the ideal of a spiritual man who had realized in himself the integral spiritual consciousness that knows not only the highest truth of the Spirit but also the deepest truth of Life. He can view everything from above and from within. Since the Rishi has an integral vision of the past, present, and future he can create and recreate new teachings, new ideals, and new forms to make the humanity free from its limitations and elevate it to a higher state of being. The Rishis were considered to be the powerful authorities to guide the humanity towards its perfection.

To fulfill their vision, the Rishis of the Vedic age pursued the path of self-giving and surrender. They never shunned the world; never rejected any of the activities, powers, and enjoyments of the body, life, and mind in an ascetic withdrawal. Every aspect of life was offered to the Divine so that it could be illumined, purified, and transformed for the good of all. A complete spiritual transformation of the individual and collective life of humanity from the lowest material, vital, and mental, to the highest spiritual was the vision of the Rishis, reflected in the comprehensive Vedic system of Yoga.

I was fortunate enough to come into contact first with the writings of Sri Aurobindo and the Mother, which have since become an integral part of my sadhana. I regard Sri Aurobindo as the greatest among all the Rishis of modern times and feel the vibration of the mantric force in all his writings. Secondly, the writings of Vasishtha Ganapati Muni have also touched me deeply.

It was in the year 2002 that I came in contact with Sri Natesan, a senior disciple of Ganapati Muni. Until then I knew Vasishtha Ganapati Muni only as the author of *Uma Sahasram* and the guru of Sri Kapali Sastry, who later came and settled in Pondicherry as a disciple of Sri Aurobindo. I had also heard about the Muni as an *Ashtavadhani*, one who could simultaneously attend to eight different questioners and reply to them through extemporaneous Sanskrit poetry. But I had no idea about any other writings of the Muni. It was only when I came into close contact with Sri Natesan (who had preserved all the works of the Muni by copying them in his own personal notebooks) that I learnt about the many other writings of the Muni. I discovered that the Muni wrote extensively in Sanskrit on a wide range of topics from the *Vedas* to contemporary issues, including profound poetry and philosophy. His style, diction, language and use of various poetic devices are unique in the history of Sanskrit literature.

For Sri Natesan it was his dream and life's mission to see all the Sanskrit writings of the Muni in print. So he began to consider how to publish all the Muni's works. It was during this period that my initial contact with him took place. We then sat together and decided on the layout and format of the volumes. The work that he had started much before he met me began to take a definite shape. That is how editing and publishing the twelve volumes of the *Collected Works of Vasishtha Kavyakantha Ganapati Muni* took place. I was fortunate to be a part of this Divine work and it was an enriching experience for me to be the associate editor of the Collected Works of the Muni. One by one we worked on the volumes and eventually brought out the entire work in twelve volumes, including the Muni's important Vedic teachings.

Ganapati Muni was also an ardent adorer of Sri Aurobindo and the Mother. While going through the writings of Sri Aurobindo that appeared in the ashram journal *Arya*, he first developed an inner contact with the Master and the Mother. But he had not yet had any opportunity to experience their darshan. On August 15, 1928, Ganapati came to Pondicherry to participate in the birthday celebrations of Sri Aurobindo. After he saw the Master he had only one word to express from the deepest depths of his heart – *Divya Purusha*, the Divine personified. Later he told one of his disciples that he had witnessed a powerful spiritual radiance around Sri Aurobindo. He also exclaimed that Sri Aurobindo's face appeared to him as five hundred years old; there was so much of wisdom, so much of maturity, so much of ripeness in it.

Before Ganapati came to Pondicherry a copy of his magnum opus, *Uma Sahasram* (a thousand verses in Sanskrit praising goddess Uma) was sent to Sri Aurobindo. It was Sudhanva, a disciple of the Muni who settled in the Aurobindo Ashram, who gave this copy of *Umasahasram* to Sri Aurobindo. On examining the verses of this grand poem Sri Aurobindo had expressed that it was a "superhuman performance" and he would like to meet the author.

After having Sri Aurobindo's darshan, the Muni stayed in the Ashram for fifteen days at the residence of Sudhanva. On August 16 at 9 a.m. he saw the Mother with his disciple Kodandaraman. The Muni had three joint meditation sessions with the Mother during his stay at the Aurobindo Ashram. The Mother after the first session had remarked that the half an hour's meditation of the Muni was perfect, that it was a continuous, unbroken state, and that no sadhak with whom she meditated had yet done so for more than three to five minutes. On the other hand, the Muni also stated that during this meditation, he first felt a current emerging through his head, and then felt that an external current was very perceptibly falling on him from all sides. Then the Mother said to him that Sri Aurobindo and herself had recognized him as a man who could do their divine work.

It is interesting to note that even though the Muni did not know English, many of the higher Vedic teachings that Sri Aurobindo wrote about in his *Secret of the Veda* were reflected by the Muni in his own Sanskrit Vedic works. When Sri Aurobindo was asked how could this be possible, he said that when the great truths are ready to descend they are received and given expression by whoever is open to them. This was the secret of Vasistha Ganapati Muni – he was sufficiently open to receive vast truths descending from higher planes of consciousness about the whole of life.

This vision and ideal of the Rishis and the Vedic system of Yoga needs to be recovered today and given a new form suitable to the modern mind and the present challenging human situation. It is in this context that *Vedic Yoga – The Path of the Rishis* by Vedacharya David Frawley (Pandit Vamadeva Shastri) is a most brilliantly authored book that throws much light not just on the ways of the ancient Rishis, but on the whole of the Rishi tradition from ancient to modern periods – especially the roles of Ganapati Muni and Sri Aurobindo, both of whom he has been connected with for several decades. All the important aspects of the Vedic system of Yoga are well explained in the book and presented in a manner that is suitable to the contemporary world mentality and helpful to the spiritual needs of our current humanity – for whom the *Vedas* can offer a way forward to a new age of higher consciousness for all.

Sampadananda Mishra, Sri Aurobindo Society

Author's Preface

The *Rigveda* is the oldest and probably most important of the ancient texts of India, the spiritual motherland of humanity, and its great traditions of Yoga, mantra, and meditation. The *Rigveda* is the longest and most diverse of the ancient scriptures of the world that have survived to the present day. This makes the *Rigveda* a central part of our ancient global spiritual heritage filled with many secrets about our past and perhaps keys to our future. Yet the *Rigveda* remains probably the least understood of all the world's great scriptures, and the most in need of a new examination.

This situation of neglect is not surprising, as the *Rigveda* is composed in an ancient secret mantric code that is very difficult to decipher, the language of another *yuga* or world age, whose mentality and world view we no longer share, or even suspect. This means that a new examination of the *Rigveda* – particularly from a yogic standpoint – is essential for understanding our origins, as well as the place of religion, mysticism, and Yoga in human culture. A new study of the *Rigveda* is crucial today as we seek to understand our nature as a species and for developing a higher consciousness.

Looking into the *Rigveda* can provide us with a great adventure in historical studies, spiritual research, and meditation practice, widening our view of life and expanding our awareness on all levels. The *Rigveda* offers us the transformative vision of numerous ancient sages and Rishis in a special language of cosmic sound and symbol that is perhaps unparalleled and uniquely preserved in the world. It can help us create a global spiritual culture that honors the eternal truth in all of its forms and manifestations throughout nature and society.

In this book we will examine the core knowledge of the older Vedic Yoga that occurs in the *Rigveda*, and endeavor to make it accessible for our modern mind and its language. This Vedic Yoga is not only the possible origin of classical Yoga but of all the *dharmic* traditions of India's great civilization. Understanding the Vedic Yoga will help us to approach the *Rigveda* in its true depth and cosmic power.

In this book I approach the ancient Vedic knowledge from several angles, traditional and modern, both in terms of Indian thought and the new global culture arising today. Naturally a single book on such a vast topic as the *Vedas* cannot deal with everything and will raise many questions. Additional research will be necessary to bring out the Vedic vision in its full scope.

It is difficult to find accessible books in the English language on the Vedic Yoga, though many people may recognize the Vedas as the source of the Yoga tradition. Often the term "*Veda*" is used in a generic way to refer to later texts like the

Bhagavad Gita and *Upanishads*. There is little available in print on the *Rigveda* itself, the main Vedic text, apart from academic translations that are largely oblivious to the yogic meaning of the mantras, literalistic in their approach, and generally quite uninspiring. The current volume is meant to help fill that gap and to encourage a new yogic study throughout the Vedic field.

The purpose of this book is to teach the principles and practices of the Vedic Yoga, so that individuals today can take up its profound teachings as part of their own practice. The book does not look at the *Vedas* in isolation, but indicates how later Yoga, Tantra, Vedanta, and the Vedic Sciences can be found in seed form in the *Vedas*, and how these teachings represent different aspects of the older Vedic knowledge.

The book represents several decades of research and meditation, and reflects extensive previous work. I began studying the hymns of the *Rigveda* in 1970 and translating them in 1978, producing several volumes of Vedic translations up to 1984. After that time my focus was more on specialized studies of Yoga, Vedic sciences, and Vedic history. Now I wish to update that earlier work with a specific book on the Vedic Yoga, particularly the Yoga of the *Rigveda*, the primary Vedic text. While the other *Vedas* – *Yajur*, *Sama*, and *Atharva Veda* – have a yogic relevance, the current volume will emphasize the *Rigveda* in order to show how yogic teachings are integral to the oldest of the *Vedas*, not something new that developed over time.

I have drawn inspiration and support from a number of great modern Vedic teachers who I have studied and worked with. I hope that readers will examine these important teachers and their teachings. This book is also about the modern Vedic Yoga that has developed in India over the past two centuries and discusses its approaches, including how it has influenced India and the world as a whole.

Owing to limits of space, I have included only a small number of translations from Vedic hymns. An older book of mine can be consulted for these, *Wisdom of the Ancient Seers*, which contains translations of over eighty hymns of the *Rigveda* from a yogic and Vedantic perspective. I hope to bring out additional volumes of Vedic translations in the future that reflect what I have learned about the teachings since that earlier book.

I have not addressed in detail the historical implications and the new view of ancient India. That occurs in other published books of mine, notably *Gods, Sages and Kings: Vedic Secrets of Ancient Civilization*, and *Hidden Horizons: Unearthing Ten Thousand Years of Indian Culture*, as well as in the books of many other authors in the field.

Unless one has first gone deeply into the Vedic mantras and their profound and intricate symbolism, we cannot claim to know the origins of the ancient Yoga, nor can we claim to know our spiritual heritage as a species. For those who may be studying the *Vedas*, but who do not make the effort to examine the depths of Vedic symbolism, their studies may be limited in what they can reveal. It is time for this great global Vedic heritage to be reclaimed, and it will be of great benefit to the entire world. But this requires a new study and practice of the Vedic Yoga along with a better understanding of its connections with other yogic teachings, and with ancient spiritual teachings from throughout the world. For this endeavor, one needs a certain plasticity and adaptability of thought, for we are dealing with subtle energies rather than material structures. The Vedic view has several angles of approach and variable formulations that we must learn to appreciate.

I would like to thank the staff of Hinduism Today magazine for their help with this book and its illustrations as they have done in the past with other books of mine, particularly the Editor-in-Chief Paramacharya Sadasivanatha Swami. Vimala Rodgers was a special help in going over the text and making it more clear and readable. Todd Dearing and Pavan Kanwar added their important corrections as well.

I need to offer a most humble and special thanks to Swami Veda Bharati, who holds the living power of the *Vedas* in his mind and heart. He has provided not only a wonderful introduction to begin the book but a profound chapter to conclude, combining the most profound scholarship and the deepest meditative insight. His name means the voice (Bharati) of the Vedas. He is truly that. Such Rishis keep the *Vedas* alive not only in the outer world but in the Earth consciousness.

Finally I would like to dedicate this book to the main teachers who have inspired my research into the Vedic Yoga – K. Natesan, Kavyakantha Ganapati Muni, Brahmarshi Daivarata, M.P. Pandit, Sri Aurobindo, Kapali Shastry, Sivanananda Murty, and Swami Veda Bharati. May all humanity become receptive to the immortal Vedic wisdom!

Namaḥ Paramarṣibhyaḥ!
Reverence to the Supreme Seers!
Pandit Vamadeva Shastri (Vedacharya David Frawley)

Introductory Note Relative to Diacritical Marks and Sanskrit

For Sanskrit terms and book titles that are already in common usage in the English language like *Rigveda*, *Bhagavad Gita*, or Krishna, I have not used any transliteration.

For special terms and verses of the *Rigveda*, particularly in footnotes or in parenthesis, I have used diacritical marks. For readers not familiar with these marks I have included a special Sanskrit transliteration pronunciation guide in the Appendices.

The translations from the *Rigveda* and other Sanskrit texts are my own. I have emphasized verses from the *Rigveda* that relate to its primary deities of Indra, Agni, Surya, and Soma, with verses from all the ten books or mandalas of the text. This means that some better known hymns of the *Rigveda*, particularly from the tenth book, may not be highlighted.

I have added quotations and translations from the *Yajurveda, Upanishads, Yoga Sutras, Bhagavad Gita*, and *Mahabharata* in order to show the continuity of the Vedic teachings into later times. I have similarly added quotations and translations from the works of two modern Vedic gurus, Kavyakantha Ganapati Muni, the chief disciple of Bhagavan Ramana Maharshi, and Brahmarshi Daivarata, the chief disciple of Ganapati Muni. These are to show that the Vedic teachings continue to be alive, relevant, and vibrant today.

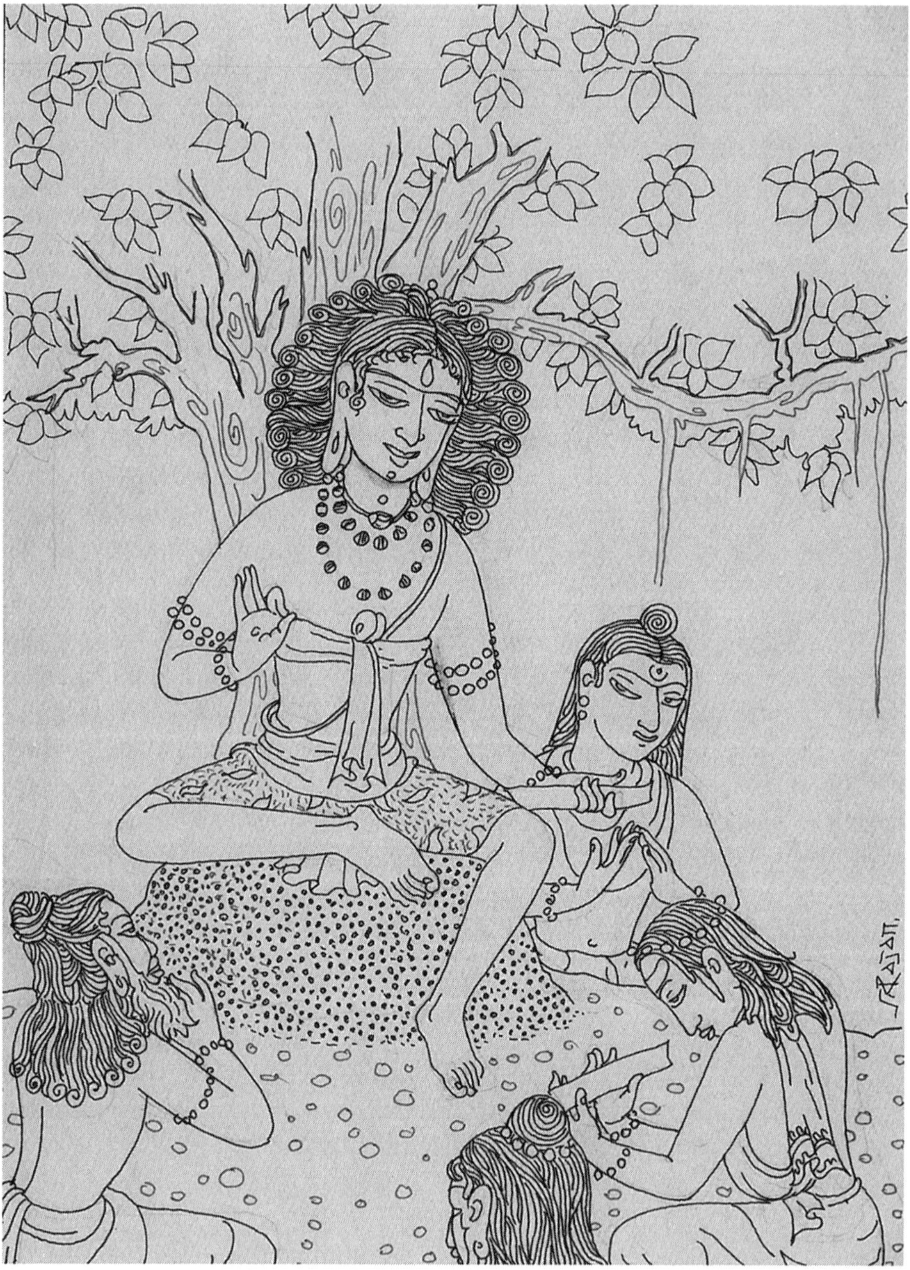

Shiva Dakshinamurti as the Supreme Guru of the Rishis

PART I

My Journey into the Vedic World

Oṁ Śrī Veda Puruṣāya Namah!

Oṁ, Reverence to the Vedic Purusha, the Soul of the Vedas!

Oṁ Agnaye Svāhā

Oṁ, Reverence to the Sacred Fire, the flame of Self-realization!

Oṁ Vāyave Svāhā

Oṁ, Reverence to the Sacred Wind, the spirit of the Absolute!

Oṁ Sūryāya Svāhā

Oṁ, Reverence to the Sun, the supreme light of Consciousness!

Oṁ Indrāya Svāhā

Oṁ, Reverence to the Supreme Self transcendent over all!

My Experience of the Vedic Yoga 1:

From Midwest America to the Ancient *Vedas*

We live in an era during which Yoga has spread globally and become popular throughout the world. Most of this popular Yoga is a modern physical Yoga that can seem quite removed from Yoga's ancient spiritual roots. Yet the search for the deeper Yoga of Self-realization remains behind all Yoga approaches as their ultimate aim. *Vedic Yoga* represents the ancient and primordial Yoga of the cosmic mind, the physical dimension of which is secondary.

In this book we will explore the ancient Yoga of the seers, the *Rishi Yoga* that is rooted in cosmic sound and reflects a communion with the whole of nature. This can help us understand both the origins of Yoga and its future, as Yoga helps us unfold our potential for higher awareness that is relevant for all time. The teachings of Yoga are based upon branches and lineages that take us back thousands of years to ancient Vedic teachings set in powerful but mysterious hymns and mantras. The influence of the Vedic Rishis remains in modern Yoga in the background, though in certain deeper Yogic teachings today, it is emerging back into the foreground as well.

Vedic Yoga is in many ways very different from modern Yoga. It is not a matter of a special asana style or a magical asana sequence. It is not centered on a special meditation technique or powerful *pranayama* method. Vedic Yoga contains many mantras but cannot be reduced to one set mantric formula. The Vedic Yoga is vast and many-sided. It requires adaptation at an individual level, and cannot be made into *en masse* formula. It contains all aspects of Yoga from lifestyle to devotion and deeper meditation. We can approach it both at a philosophical level and through mantra practices, and it can greatly enrich all that we do. Vedic Yoga rests upon reconnecting to the Divine and sacred presence that permeates and energizes all things. It returns us to the universal life, its deeper rhythms and transformational processes.

Yogic spiritual teachings exist in their own eternal dimension in the cosmic mind. They enter into human history at certain favorable points of time and culture, when a special possibility for their influence arises. They retreat back into their own higher domains, when the doors in the human mind shift and close. Today a new receptivity to the higher teachings is slowly emerging on the planet, as we gradually enter once more into ages of spiritual light. The *Vedas* contain an energy of renewal and transformation, and their power is rising once again, with a Vedic renaissance in India over the last two centuries that has recently become global. The purpose of the following narrative is to share a vision of this Vedic reemergence, and strengthen its presence in the dawning spiritual culture today.

Return to the *Vedas*

The *Vedas*, whether through books, teachers, or meditation, have been the most significant driving force and motivation that I have encountered in life. My life and thought has been rooted in the *Rigveda*, the oldest Vedic text, as the source of its primary inspiration and motivation. This began over forty years ago, when the vistas of the *Rigveda* first opened up for me – which was a life- and consciousness-transforming event.

All that I have written relative to yogic and Vedic teachings has its foundation in an earlier study of the *Rigveda*, an exploration of its mantras and a meditation on its deities. My writings on ancient India and the Vedic age have been based on my research into the *Rigveda* and correlating it with archaeological discoveries. Relative to my work as a whole, I feel that these teachings on the yogic meaning of the *Rigveda* are the most crucial, though perhaps more for the future.

Of course, it has been difficult to find a significant audience, particularly in the West, for the esoteric studies of the Vedic mantras necessary to open up the Vedic world for us. Vedic sciences like Ayurveda, Yoga, and Vedic astrology have more practical value to introduce us to Vedic thought and its profundity. Yet those who appreciate any Vedic discipline can benefit from an examination of the *Rigveda*. In doing so, they can access the core Vedic vision from which these later teachings arose and which holds their essence.

The *Rigveda* remains the book I most frequently read, study, and meditate upon as a key to both cosmic and Self-knowledge. The *Rigveda* provides a powerful tool to help one move into one's own deeper nature that is allied with the entire universe. I find it to be an inexhaustible source of wisdom, a key to all the workings of both the inner and outer worlds. While I first began my Vedic studies with translations of the *Rigveda*, I soon set these in the background for a direct examination of the original Sanskrit of the text, which has continually remained relevant in power, beauty, and profundity, even when looking at the same verse over again.

I have learned to perceive the *Rigveda* as the fountainhead of Yoga, mantra, and of the great philosophies of Self-realization that gained prominence in later India. The *Rigveda* provides the background for the dharmic approach that has come out of India in many names and forms over the millennia. The *Rigveda* holds the power of the ancient seers and sages such as once dwelled throughout the world. It is not just a doorway to India's ancient insights, but to similar traditions in other countries, including many that have not survived the onslaught of time.

The *Rigveda* has preserved the wisdom of the Rishis in their original language, allowing us to use it to listen to the voice of the ancient sages directly. The Rigveda is ever alive, deepening, challenging, and questioning us to a greater reality of Self and World – if we would look deeply into its mantras. That remains a viable option for us, if we would but look at the Rigveda through the vision of Yoga, meditation, and deep psychology, with a sensitivity to ancient myths, legends, and symbols.

The Centrality of the *Rigveda*

By the term *Veda* here, I mean primarily the *Rigveda*. The *Rigveda* is the oldest and longest of the Vedic texts, the one most frequently quoted in later teachings, and constitutes the core Vedic teaching. It is the pillar upon which all Vedic teachings are held. Of the other three *Vedas*, the *Samaveda* consists almost entirely of a selection of Rigvedic verses placed in a more musical chant. The *Atharvaveda* is formed like a supplement to the *Rigveda*.[1] The *Yajurveda* develops the ritualistic or action side of the *Rigveda* both at outer levels of fire offerings and at inner levels of mantra and meditation.[2] But none of the other *Vedas* carries the same extent, depth, and originality as the *Rigveda*, which is clearly the core Vedic text.

Without first deeply examining the *Rigveda*, it is not possible to speak of the *Veda* in an authoritative manner. There is a tendency today to use the term *Veda* loosely to refer to the Vedic tradition overall, to any of its many branches, or as a general term for Hinduism or Yoga. While such connections are important, to understand the *Veda*, one must go back to the original mantras of the *Rigveda*.

From the *Rigveda* and its powerful mantras, all other Vedic and Yogic branches have arisen, and perhaps surprisingly, maintained a continuity with Rigvedic insights, even when these connections have been forgotten. Yoga in all of its forms and branches of Knowledge, Devotion, and Action, as well as Yoga techniques, methods, and energy practices of all kinds are but the practical side of Vedic knowledge,[3] which refers to spiritual or yogic knowledge in the Rishi tradition. Without some sort of Yoga practice, *Veda* remains at best a theory, speculation, or belief, not the way of realization that is the real meaning of the term. *Veda* is the cosmic wisdom behind Yoga, without which Yoga lacks depth and profundity, and can easily become mechanical.

This "way of Vedic knowledge" has been transmitted through history mainly by the *Upanishads* of the late Vedic age, which were the scriptures behind all the Vedic philosophies, including Yoga in all of its forms. This Upanishadic knowledge in turn became developed and codified in the great philosophies of Vedanta that relied upon the practice of Yoga for their practical realization.

The way of Vedic knowledge forms the basis of modern Yoga-Vedanta movements, starting from that of Ramakrishna and Vivekananda at the start of the global diffusion of Yoga over a hundred years ago.[4] Yet Vedantic knowledge is not entirely new in the *Upanishads* as many scholars have thought it to be; Vedanta is but the philosophy hidden behind the symbolic Vedic mantras, which can be intuited in the earliest portions of the *Rigveda*. What is hidden in the Rigvedic mantras is made evident, clear, and rational in the *Upanishads* and *Bhagavad Gita*, which in turn formed the foundation for later Yoga and Vedantic teachings in all their diversity. The inner meaning of the mantras of the *Rigveda* is of the same nature as Vedantic philosophy, but expressed in a primal language of energy and light that is very different, and which requires a very different orientation of thought and language in order to appreciate.

The Importance of Vedic Sciences

Besides studying the *Rigveda*, I examined related Vedic sciences, particularly *Ayurveda* or "Vedic medicine," and *Jyotish* or "Vedic astrology." Yet I did not come to the *Veda* through these disciplines, but rather from an earlier study of the *Rigveda*. I studied the Vedic Agni, for example, before studying the Ayurvedic Agni or the digestive fire. This background in the *Rigveda* has caused me to look upon the Vedic sciences in light of the *Rigveda* as the prime interpretative model.

Ayurveda is perhaps the ideal system for introducing people to the principles of Vedic knowledge and the Vedic Yoga. Ayurveda takes prime Vedic deities like Agni and Vayu, or the cosmic Fire and Air powers, and explains how they function within our own bodies and minds. It turns these Vedic principles into practical realities for us to explore on a daily basis for our personal well-being.

Vedic astrology or *Jyotish*, the science of light, represents another aspect of the Vedic deities, which are powers of cosmic light, relative to the planets and stars. *Jyotish* provides the understanding of karma that is central to all Vedic mantras, as well as to our lives as a whole. Ayurveda is the healing branch of Vedic knowledge; Vedic astrology is its science of time.

Nature of My Vedic Research

My Vedic research began with a study of Vedic mantras, along with the cosmic forces reflected in them. From its inception, it required a giving up of the time and culture-bound intellect of my earlier education, letting go of the familiar self and society in order to understand the teachings of sages from a different *yuga* or world age. To understand the *Veda*, one needs to forget oneself along with the contemporary world and its turbulence.

This deeper study of the *Veda* is like a profound meditation, contemplation and inner dialogue with unseen forces – an encounter with the secret powers of light and energy beyond the ordinary life and mind. Only if the personal self is left at the surface and one turns within can the *Veda* come to life. That has been my continual experience. One cannot reach the secret of the *Veda* for the sake of any outer gain or recognition. It is not a question of the ordinary self but of discovering the *Veda* as one's true Self, with one's physical being as but a vehicle for the Vedic knowledge, which is the cosmic knowledge, to perpetuate itself in humanity.

In the beginning of the book I present the personal side of my Vedic experience—how the Vedic journey unfolded in my life and changed my awareness and my outer actions. This includes an inner experience of the Vedic deities, Rishis and energies. We have a deeper "Vedic Self" that is not bound by time, place, or culture, which has many births, and holds the knowledge of many forgotten times and places. There are Vedic connections that extend throughout human history and culture, with implications for future ages, and realms beyond the human.

I am sharing my "Vedic experience" with you, the reader, in order to make my encounter with the *Vedas* more understandable. Perhaps it can help create a pathway back to the *Vedas* that others can follow. But I do so with hesitation and discretion. We have too much of a tendency to relate the higher knowledge with personalities, when the true knowledge is impersonal. The Vedic knowledge is said to be *apaurusheya*, or non-personal, meaning not dependent upon or identified with any human personality. Yet it does need to be adapted on an individual level, and bring its own unique experiences for each disciple of the *Vedic Yoga*.

My Experience of the *Vedas*

What I have learned of the *Vedas* has been revealed not so much by effort as by an almost inexplicable flow of grace. Certain teachers, both living and from the past, have been crucial along this path. Perhaps strangely, I never had to work hard in order to appreciate and understand the mantras of the *Rigveda*. The meaning of the Vedic chants seemed clear from my initial encounters with them, as part of the symbolism of nature and consciousness – though unraveling their many dimensions has taken much additional time and effort.

The Rishis gradually became familiar to me as part of a greater spiritual family to which I in some way had always belonged. I came to know the different Vedic Rishis and the nuances of their thought, temperament, and frames of mind. What other people feel hearing the names of Jesus, Buddha, and Krishna, I can feel with the Vedic Rishis: Vasishtha, Vishvamitra, Vamadeva, Dirghatamas, Parashara, and Bharadvaja, among many others. The very sound of their names can evoke the Godhead within us.

I am not certain why this appreciation of the Vedic wisdom was seldom the case for others. But over time I learned to accept the Vedic view as integral to my life, and have developed various ways to introduce it to people from throughout the world. From a rare private study in the beginning, my examination of the *Vedas* has joined currents of global communication, where hopefully it can resonate and aid in the new Vedic unfoldment on the planet.

For me the *Rigveda* became full of light and clarity, with Yoga and Vedanta, and the mysticism of the entire world seeming more like its reflection or its shadow. The *Rigveda* became the most profound teaching for me, more so than the *Upanishads*, the *Bhagavad Gita*, or any other scripture or teaching, ancient or modern, East or West. If I had only one book in life, I would choose the *Rigveda*. The Vedic mantras, particularly to Agni and Soma, have a mantric power that seems unparalleled and reaches to the very core of the cosmic light.

There were many individuals in my generation of the late 1960s and 1970s in the United States who were interested in Yoga, and a few who carried that interest onto Vedanta. Yet those with any real knowledge of the *Rigveda* were but a handful. Even in India, individuals seriously looking into the original Vedic Yoga have been exceptional. Most Yoga students find it enough to follow recent teachers, for which the Vedic teachings are but a background influence from the distant past.

There have been a few scholars of the *Vedas* in the West, who did apply their minds to Vedic texts, but these were mainly individuals from the colonial era, and their Vedic works usually tell us more about their own opinions than anything significant about the Vedic Yoga. Most such colonial scholars had little appreciation for Yoga in any form or for any type of mysticism. Mainstream academia has rarely penetrated far beneath the surface of the ocean of the *Veda*, or come to suspect its profound yogic and cosmic knowledge. Of course, from a Vedic perspective, this is not surprising because such scholars have not been trained in the tools of insight and meditation necessary to uncover the mantric symbolism of Vedic texts.

There have been several important Vedic scholars from yogic backgrounds in India, but their work is little known and hard to find, particularly in English editions. Even spiritual scholars rooted in Yoga traditions have used the *Veda* mainly to support their own later yogic lines, in which the Vedic teachings can get lost or reduced.

Few people recognize how little of the *Rigveda* is actually known and used. This is not so much a criticism as a statement of understandable fact. No other spiritual teachings of such antiquity as the *Vedas* are still alive and practiced. Most of these like the *Egyptian Book of the Dead* have not been used for two thousand years. The *Veda* has survived in its branches and offshoots. Its root has been dormant, though showing new signs of awakening.

From the American Cow to the Vedic Cow

Those who know my background ask me this question: "How did an American born in the Midwest of the United States, with little in his background to stimulate such a search, discover the *Vedas* and find such a deep meaning in their arcane teachings – and this, starting around the age of twenty, before traveling to India or having any direct personal instruction?" The story makes a good justification for the validity of karma and rebirth, as there was nothing in my present life that could likely explain such an occurrence.

I was born in a small town in Wisconsin, the second of ten children, in a Catholic family in 1950. One of my favorite answers to *Why the Vedas?* is that it was the cows. My parents grew up on dairy farms and we frequently visited my grandparent's large dairy farm when I was a child.

This still does not seem to be a real answer to the question. There is no logical reason for my Vedic affinities, except that the boundaries between East and West, and the ancient and the modern are breaking down today. Examining the dissemination of eastern teachings worldwide, people born in the West now have access to and can progress on what were previously eastern spiritual paths, just as people born in the East now have access to and can progress on western scientific paths. The soul is not confined to a continent and can carry the knowledge of previous births to the lands of its new births.

I had a psychic sense when a child. I could pick up the thoughts of other people or sense events that had happened in a particular place that I was passing through, like what had transpired previously in a house that we just moved into. This inner sensitivity could be problematical. It made it difficult for me to be around crowds as I could easily sense the psychic energies of the people, including their agitation. Yet the same psychic sensitivity allowed me to tune into the ancient past, visualize life in the Vedic age, and gradually understand how the minds of the Vedic Rishis worked.

Later in life, in my travels to other countries, I could sense my own past life influences and those of the peoples of the area. Sometimes I have had to work hard to turn that psychic energy off, particularly when a surrounding psychic field was turbulent. Other times I learned to direct that sensitivity into particular areas of study and research. I had an inner life from an early age that dominated the outer life. I had a sense of another life, another time and place, which made modern America seem rather out of place, if not somehow alien.

Besides school when I was young, I developed my own line of special personal studies, starting with researching local libraries. These extended from history and geography to religion and philosophy, particularly to what was ancient. I took an ancient history class and memorized the complete line of the pharaohs of Egypt. For me ancient Egypt was more interesting than modern Europe or the United States.

I was exposed to eastern teachings as part of the counterculture movement of the times. I had a curious intellect and started to study European literature, art and philosophy. I added an examination of eastern spiritual teachings into my intellectual forays, first as a sidelight to European studies but soon as a dominant influence over them.

I gradually came into contact with a wide range of intellectual and mystical teachings, including Existentialism, Taoism and *I Ching*, Buddhism, Yoga, Vedanta, Sufism, Gurdjieff, and J. Krishnamurti. My curious mind looked into most everything available of this type. How this broad search would settle on the *Rigveda* was nothing that could be foreseen or predicted.

The teachings of Paramahansa Yogananda and his classic *Autobiography of a Yogi* were crucial in introducing me to the deeper practices of yoga, along with specific techniques of mantra, pranayama and meditation. Yogananda left an extensive set of lessons, which made his teaching particularly accessible. I studied these in 1970 and quickly learned the power of the methods that he taught, which helped me experience new levels of consciousness and prana.

Yet I had a philosophical mind that drew me into the study of Vedanta, the philosophy of Self-realization behind Yoga. For this, the teachings of Ramakrishna, the Indian avatar of world yoga, and Swami Vivekananda, his chief disciple who first brought Yoga to the West in the late nineteenth century, were very helpful. The many Vedantic texts translated by the Ramakrishna-Vedanta order introduced me to the classical teachings of the *Upanishads* and the Advaitic works of Shankara. I examined the main *Upanishads* along with Shankara's commentaries, and then moved on to Shankara's commentary on the *Brahma Sutras*, as well as his shorter works that were probably the most inspiring.[5] Shankara's influence came to dominate my mind and I could feel his presence and his guidance.

This study of Advaita (Non-dualistic) Vedanta led me to the teachings of Bhagavan Ramana Maharshi, probably modern India's most famous enlightened sage and the great exponent of a simple, direct path of Self-inquiry. I discovered Ramana's teachings later in 1970, and they have since been central to my practice. Ramana Maharshi is perhaps the most important spiritual figure in modern times, comparable to Buddha, Jesus, or any great teacher who has ever lived. He had his full realization after a short Self-inquiry of twenty minutes when a mere lad of sixteen, unlike the tribulations that most great teachers had to undergo in order to achieve their aims. I found related deep teachings of Advaita Vedanta like the *Ashtavakra Samhita* and *Avadhuta Gita* that like Ramana presented a direct approach to Vedanta, streamlining, and making Advaita accessible to all sincere students.

I was curious about the older Vedic teachings of India prior to the *Upanishads*. I felt that the *Vedas* must have had deeper teachings from which the *Upanishads* drew their inspiration and from which Advaita Vedanta arose. I had felt the presence of higher mystical teachings in the ancient *Egyptian Book of the Dead* and the Chinese *I Ching* already. I was aware of the myth of the Golden Age and traditions of ancient sages from throughout the world.

To my disappointment, however, I soon discovered that the *Vedas* were seldom afforded a high regard from a spiritual or philosophical angle. Even many Vedantic teachers looked upon the *Vedas* as mere ritualistic texts with little abstract thought or sense of any higher cosmic reality. This view occurred in spite of the great esteem afforded to the Vedic Rishis as sages of the highest order. Following my intuition of an ancient high global spirituality, I was not content with the opinion of the existing scholarship, which viewed the *Veda* as a primitive nature worship from which the *Upanishads* did not so much evolve as depart.

Fortunately, the studies I had been conducting helped me decode Vedic symbolism, particularly the work with poetry and symbolic language. I began writing poetry around the age of sixteen. I followed existential, surrealist, and symbolist approaches, particularly that of French poets like Rimbaud, Mallarme, and Yves Bonnefoy, as well as the German poet Rilke. I was aware of the symbolism in the novels of Herman Hesse like the *Glass Bead Game* (Magister Ludi) and *Journey to the East*. The images of the dawn and the night, fire, wind, and sun pervaded this early poetic inspiration along with the image of the muse or the Goddess.

I read the work of the renowned psychologist C.G. Jung, focusing on his esoteric volumes on psychology and alchemy from medieval Europe, in which he unraveled the spiritual meaning beyond the nature symbolism and the alchemical tradition with its inner processes of fire and water. I worked with the Chinese *I Ching* that presents an ancient symbolic language using the forces of nature, like its eight trigrams of Heaven, Earth, Fire, Water, Thunder, the Lake, the Mountain, and Wind. I wrote a few articles on that book in the succeeding years.

I took the symbolism of the *Vedas* in the same manner as other ancient mystical teachings, with the images of light and nature portraying cosmic and psychological forces, not simply outer concerns. I couldn't understand why so many scholars were unable to connect Vedic mantras with other forms of mystical symbolism, though the images were the same as those they honored as profoundly spiritual in other traditions!

Sri Aurobindo and the Secret of the *Vedas*

My poetic background set the stage for my entrance into the Vedic world, for which the doorway was the work of another great Indian Yogi and Seer, Sri Aurobindo. Sri Aurobindo was a unique Raja yogi of the highest order. He was able to experience the Supreme Absolute beyond all time and space, and yet understand the Divine Will in Creation, including potentials of higher evolution on earth beyond the human. Aurobindo's teachings affected my work in many areas, not only relative to the *Vedas* and Yoga, but also relative to ancient history, linguistics, modern social and political issues, and Vedic astrology, on which diverse subjects he had important and original teachings.

Sri Aurobindo was great philosopher and poet as well as a great Yogi who had explored all the planes of existence and put that knowledge into his teachings. His books were written originally in the English language of which he was a master. His epic poem *Savitri* is the longest blank verse work in English, a thousand pages in length, and is filled with yogic secrets of the highest order covering all aspects of the cosmos and every layer of consciousness.

Like Ramana Maharshi, Sri Aurobindo is an epochal figure. The legacy of his numerous writings is bound to remain crucial for guiding humanity for centuries to come. Mahatma Gandhi spoke of Aurobindo and Ramana as the two greatest gurus of his time, while the great poet Rabindranath Tagore touched Aurobindo's feet when he met him, though he was senior to him.

In the course of studying Aurobindo's writing, I became fascinated with the quotations from the *Rigveda* that he used to open the chapters of his monumental work, the *Life Divine*. These quotations presented the yogic and mystical meaning to Vedic symbolism that I had suspected was likely there. Aurobindo had also written two books on the *Vedas*, the *Secret of the Vedas*, which explained the background of the Vedic deities and Rishis, and *Hymns to the Mystic Fire*, which focused on the hymns to the sacred fire or Agni. These two books remain classics for any deeper study of the Vedic teachings and provided my entrance into the Vedic world. With my background in poetry and a love of symbolism, I could easily appreciate the spiritual explanation of Vedic symbolism that Aurobindo provided.

In February of 1971, as I first began reading his *Secret of the Vedas*, I was drawn into the Vedic mind in a state of heightened awareness. I experienced what I would call a "descent of the Vedic Dawn," a vision of a series of dawns representing not only my own spiritual aspiration as a soul, but also that of all humanity and all souls in the universe in a spiraling crescendo. I could feel the power of the Vedic Dawn, the original pristine light of creation, and the vista of ever unfolding planes of consciousness upward into the Infinite and Eternal. I felt like I had returned to the spiritual origins of humanity and entered into the heart of creation. This

Vedic experience was like crossing a great time barrier, learning to understand the humanity of a previous world-age long before our present materialistic civilization. From that point onward the focus of my studies remained the *Rigveda* and its teachings, as an experiential way of understanding the cosmic reality and its deeper spirit and Self. Yet I found myself in this vast new Vedic world almost alone, both as a new adventure and a great challenge!

While I had an intuition of the Vedic Yoga, there did not seem to be a practical way to go forward with it. Even Sri Aurobindo's Yoga used the Vedic teachings in a secondary manner. My main Yoga practices continued in the classical Yoga and Vedantic fields of pranayama, mantra and meditation, but now I knew something of their Vedic origins and continued to explore these.

I didn't know of anyone else in the United States that had a similar sense of the Vedic Yoga. My study of the *Rigveda* remained an intriguing sidelight to a more practical examination of Vedanta, Yoga, herbs, and astrology which, unknown to me at that time, would later become integral to my Vedic work.

Sri Anandamayi Ma – The Blissful Mother

I had felt a lack of a truly realized living teacher to guide and inspire me in my work. The great teachers of India that I resonated with, like Ramana and Aurobindo, were no more, though I did make important connections with their ashrams and their publications, including their current teachers and representatives. I did not seem to resonate with the gurus teaching in America at the time, though there were good teachers bringing out various yogic teachings, and I was able to meet several of them. I shied away from public gatherings and programs, given my independent and solitary bent of mind. I was looking for something more personal than any *en masse* instruction. Somehow my soul was seeking a different path— an approach of its own. Yet there was one great teacher in India who was still alive and who I was able to contact, though in the distance.

Starting in 1976 and up to her passing in 1982, I corresponded with the great Hindu saint, Sri Anandamayi Ma, the blissful mother of Bengal, through her disciples Nirvanananda and Atmananda.[6] Ma encouraged me in my studies and brought a great inner force into my work. I asked her to take the role of Ramana for me and draw me deeper into the Advaitic approach, which she encouraged me to follow wholeheartedly and with full faith.

I asked Ma for guidance in understanding the older Vedic teachings, and she encouraged me to pursue them. Her inspiration drew me into a study of the *Vedas* in the original Sanskrit and continued the trend that came earlier from my contact with Sri Aurobindo. I received my first Sanskrit copy of the *Rigveda* from India about that time (1977) and began to examine it regularly. As I had studied the Sanskrit of Vedantic texts, and that of Sri Aurobindo's Vedic translations, I was able to slowly make sense of this vast text and its archaic language. Just before Ma's letters would arrive, an electrical current of energy would move up my spine, signaling the arrival of her Shakti. She gave me the confidence to go forward with my esoteric studies that were far removed from the ordinary life around me.

Ma's inspiration brought me in contact with the teachings of Swami Rama Tirtha, another great Vedantin who came to the West for a short time (1902-1904), not long after Swami Vivekananda. Rama Tirtha brought the Himalayan inspiration and gave another view of Veda, Vedanta, and nature to me that was very helpful. He was a poet, an independent thinker, and a living manifestation of Vedantic knowledge.[7]

Unfortunately, I was not able to visit Ma in India while she was alive, though she sent me various gifts and was always gracious in her letters. Her spirit has remained with me and I continue to feel it behind all that I do. My work has always been based upon a devotion to the Mother, the Devi, or the Goddess, and Anandamayi Ma opened up that connection as a living reality. I see the *Vedas* as a manifestation of *Veda Mata*, the Mother of the *Vedas*, who is the great world wisdom Mother, as the ancient seers saw her. At first it was the Mother as dark Kali who guided me in my quest. Years later it would shift to the Mother as blissful Sundari. Anandamayi Ma holds the energy of both. Later I would stay at several properties in the Himalayas that Ma had frequented and would receive her grace from there as well.

The Early *Upanishads*

Shortly after I began to correspond with Anandamayi Ma, a curious event occurred. I regularly bought various books from India. Among these was a copy of the *Chandogya Upanishad*, one of the oldest and longest of the *Upanishads*. Whenever I looked at the book it literally began to sing to me, pouring forth mantric chants in a soft but definitive sound patterns. This occurred on numerous occasions. At first I just laughed and didn't take it seriously, but when it occurred repeatedly, I realized it was a message to begin a deeper study of the *Upanishads*, starting with this particular text. I was drawn not just to the philosophy of the *Upanishads* but also to the mantric and sound-based teachings, as the *Chandogya* was the main *Upanishad* of the *Samaveda*, the musical or song based Veda. This *Upanishad* would open many Vedic doors for me.

While most Upanishadic interpreters search out the roots of later Yoga and Vedanta in the early *Upanishads*, showing the forward development of these systems from the late point in the Vedic teaching that the *Upanishads* represent, I decided to take an opposite route. My goal was to use the *Upanishads* as a way back into the Vedic world. This required focusing on the Vedic terms and statements occurring in the *Upanishads*, and tracing them back to their origins in earlier Vedic texts and teachings. What I discovered was that most of Upanishadic thought – which was regarded by most scholars as a new invention – was based on older Vedic verses, quotations, and paraphrases, and was a reformulation of the Vedic mantric teaching in a later language. The main scholars of the *Upanishads*, East and West, had missed this Vedic connection, though I found it fairly obvious in the texts.

In the summer of 1978, I wrote my first book called the *Creative Vision of the Early Upanishads*, which traced Yoga and the Self-realization back from such Upanishadic texts to the Vedas.[8] The writing of the book followed inner experiences with the Upanishadic sages, notably Yajnavalkya, who derived his knowledge and his Yoga directly from the Sun.[9] It drew me to special Upanishadic quotations of the Vedic Rishi, Vamadeva.

My *Upanishad* book quickly expanded into a massive tome of over five hundred pages. Somehow the writings came easily. As I merged into a state of yogic concentration, the writing would flow for hours on end, done on a common typewriter some years before the computer age! I also wrote several shorter articles on Vedantic teachings that were published in the ashram journals of Anandamayi Ma and Ramana Maharshi. This had certain doorways open up to publishing in India. I had no idea, however, what to do with the information I had discovered and who might be interested in reading, much less publishing it, particularly in the western world.

M.P. Pandit and the Vedic Call

Although I had been familiar with Aurobindo's teaching and had visited a number of Aurobindo groups in the West, I had not yet met any of Aurobindo's major Indian disciples. About that time, a friend of mine had become a disciple of M.P. Pandit, the secretary of the Aurobindo Ashram, whose many books were well known to me. Pandit had written dozens of volumes, including several on the *Vedas* and *Upanishads*, which I found very helpful. If anyone might appreciate my Vedic work, I thought it would probably be Pandit. My friend informed me that Pandit was in the USA and was coming to San Francisco, not far away from where I was living at the time.

I arranged a meeting with M.P. Pandit in August of 1979. I explained the nature of my Vedic research to him, stating that it was not from an academic background but from my own inner quest. To my surprise, Pandit replied that because of my yogic approach, my Vedic studies were able to go deeper than existing academic works on the subject. He encouraged me to dedicate myself to this Vedic research and to share it with others.

I showed Pandit my manuscript on the early *Upanishads*. He examined it carefully and quickly said he would help publish it in India in book form. He asked me to write some additional articles about the *Rigveda* and said that he would get these published in the various Sri Aurobindo publications he was involved with.

Out of this meeting with Pandit, I was inspired to write an entire new book, which I called *Self-realization and the Supermind in the Rigveda*, following the approach of Sri Aurobindo's Yoga. In three months I managed to type over five hundred pages of translations and commentaries on a number of Rigvedic hymns, particularly those to Indra, the foremost of the Vedic deities. I sent a copy to Pandit by mail, who by then had returned to India. Pandit began serializing the book in various Sri Aurobindo Ashram publications starting in April of 1980 in the monthly, the *World Union*. Eventually, he had published several dozen excerpts of the book, up to the spring of 1984.

I was elated with Pandit's response and encouragement, which made me feel that the work I was doing privately had a greater value. The contact with M.P. Pandit brought about an additional flow of grace and helped increase my confidence in my obscure and difficult endeavor. Like Anandamayi Ma's contact before, it provided a sense of being part of a tradition, rather than just an isolated individual in the West, perhaps just reflecting his own imagination.

Pandit later wrote several favorable reviews of my Vedic books that were published in India, up to his passing in 1994. He encouraged me to continue with my 'Vedic mission' as he called it. Without his support, my Vedic work may never have gone far. Pandit himself was beyond any sectarianism or effort to manipulate others, and never tried to overtly influence me or direct my research. With the gentlest of manners, he knew how to bring out the deepest spiritual impulses in whomever he came into contact.

Along with Pandit came the grace of the Mother of the Sri Aurobindo Ashram, which became another great revelation and power in my life. Pandit was close to the Mother, a Frenchwoman called Mira Alfassa,[10] who passed away in 1973 in her nineties. The Mother or 'Mother Mira' as she was also called, was the spiritual counterpart of Sri Aurobindo and guided the Aurobindo Ashram after Aurobindo's passing. Pandit held the grace of the Mother with him, as he had worked with her for many years. I soon began experiencing the Mother's energy around me in the United States, even without seeking it, as powerful guiding force.

The Mother's grace has remained with me ever since, particularly in the form of the Goddess of the Flowers, as she deeply understood the spiritual power of flowers and wrote extensively on them – including in the form of Tripura Sundari, the blissful aspect of the Goddess in Hindu thought. Whenever I call upon her, she is quickly there. Mother Mira, though a western woman, became respected in India along with the great gurus of the country. She was the feminine counterpart of Sri Aurobindo and upheld his work until her death in 1973. Her energies can be of great value to us if we but call upon her sincerely.

M.P. Pandit directed me to the work of his own guru Kapali Shastry, who wrote extensively on the *Vedas* and *Upanishads* in both Sanskrit and English. Kapali was blessed to have both Ramana Maharshi and Sri Aurobindo as his gurus. Kapali was one of the main disciples of Kavyakantha Ganapati Muni, who was like a brother to Ramana Maharshi, and whose teachings had affinity with Sri Aurobindo as well.

Kapali left an extensive commentary on the first *ashtaka* (120 Suktas) of the *Rigveda* called *Siddhanjali*, along with several shorter works on the *Vedas* and *Upanishads*. Kapali's works elucidated Sri Aurobindo's view of the *Vedas* and went into greater detail with the Sanskrit texts and translations, taking Sri Aurobindo's method to a more precise level of examination. Strangely for me, a number of Kapali's comments on the *Upanishads* were very close, almost word for word, to what I had already written before knowing of him, a fact that Pandit was probably aware of.

About this time, a copy of the *Yajurveda* came to me by mail from India, and there I found another lost friend and guide. It was particularly surprising to me because Aurobindo did not include it among his Vedic studies. Within the *Shukla Yajurveda* I found a continuous flow of the same mantric knowledge as the *Rigveda*. I did a translation and commentary on several chapters of it,[11] as a short book that I called the *Heart of the Mystic Sacrifice*. These were also serialized in Aurobindo publications—mainly *the Advent*.

Continued Examination of the *Rigveda*

After examining Aurobindo's and Kapali Shastry's works, some mystery remained for me. The Vedic approach I took, though similar in many ways, was a little different. The Vedic hymns to Indra were most important for me as a symbol of the supreme Purusha. I did not regard Indra in the same way Aurobindo did as the force of the higher mind, though I can understand that perspective, as it is only through the higher mind that the Purusha can be perceived.

In my studies, I traced the way back from the early *Upanishads* to the Rigvedic hymns of Brihaduktha of the Vamadeva family, a seer of the tenth book of the *Rigveda*,[12] and to the hymns of Vamadeva himself, the main seer of the fourth book. Most important was Vamadeva's statement that "I was Manu and the Sun (*aham manur abhavam sūryaśca*),"[xiii] which is quoted in the *Brihadaranyaka Upanishad* relative to the great statement of *aham Brahmāsmi* or "I am Brahman." This is an obvious link between the Vedantic wisdom and Vedic mantras, and only one of many in the *Upanishads*. Other hymns of Vamadeva had similar statements, among his many hymns to Agni, Indra, and Varuna.

My Vedic approach reflected the two sides of my own Yoga practice. Though I had a strong affinity with Sri Aurobindo relative to my Vedic and poetic work (and later my social, historical and environmental work), I remained closer to Ramana Maharshi in my pursuit of Jnana Yoga (Yoga of Knowledge) and Advaita Vedanta. I was not as opposed to the Advaitic view of the universe as Maya, which Sri Aurobindo found misleading at times, though I could appreciate Aurobindo's own philosophy and his effort to bring the Divine presence into the earth consciousness. I also resonated with Shankara's Tantric works to the Goddess, notably his famous *Saundarya Lahiri* or "Ocean of Beauty" that outlined all the secrets of the universal manifestation, which I felt bridged the gap between Aurobindo and Shankara Advaita.

From my understanding, Ramana reflects more a Shiva energy of transcending the world at an individual level, while Aurobindo reflects more a Shakti energy of uplifting the world at a collective level, though some overlap between the two approaches always exists. Ramana reflects the immutable presence of the eternal and the absolute, while Aurobindo addresses the unfoldment of spiritual evolution through time and has a powerful futuristic vision. I feel a great validity in both their approaches that, however apparently different, can be viewed as complementary. One is reminded of the example of Shankara who not only promoted the Jnana Yoga of Advaita Vedanta, but also honored Shakti and worked selflessly for the renovation of India, its temples and its yogic traditions, mastering Bhakti Yoga, Karma Yoga, and Raja Yoga. Every great guru has a Shiva energy of higher realization and a Shakti energy of teaching, guiding, and uplifting humanity.

Yet Ramana had not addressed the *Vedas*, much less set forth any interpretation of Vedic texts as had Sri Aurobindo. Ramana's path was simpler and more direct, emphasizing silence and Self-inquiry, though not without a foundation in the traditional teachings of Advaita Vedanta. Ramana did allow regular Vedic chanting at his ashram when he was alive (which tradition continues today), but never appears to have given specific Vedic mantras or said much about the *Vedas*. He did honor the Sri Vidya, which I believe has strong Vedic roots, and reflects the power of Mantra Yoga. He identified the sacred mountain Arunachala where he resided as a form of the Sri Chakra. Ramana had the presence of Agni, but more through the power of silence.

I continued my research in the Vedic teachings and its deeper Yoga, looking for a connection with Ramana. My Upanishadic book came out in its Indian edition in 1984. My study of meditation, following more the teachings of Ramana, was the basis of my book *Beyond the Mind*, which appeared in an Indian edition of 1984. I continued with my sadhana of both the *Vedas* and Ramana's teaching but a dichotomy remained. I wondered how the *Vedas* would fit into Ramana's teachings.

I wrote another collection of Rigvedic hymns in a book originally called *Hymns from the Golden Age*, which was published first in India in 1986, in which I examined the yogic implications of the main Vedic deities.[14] The book's Indian publisher Motilal Banarsidass printed a number of my articles in its journal *Glory of India*, and would publish most of my other Vedic books in India in the years to come.

About this time, I began to visit India regularly, particularly the Ramanashram (Ramana Maharshi) in Tiruvannamalai and the Sri Aurobindo Ashram in nearby Pondicherry. I had notable inner experiences in Pondicherry at the Aurobindo Ashram. I remember meditating at Aurobindo and the Mother's (Mira Alfassa's) Samadhi, having their entire lives and teachings pour forth in front of my inner eye, with an experience of an inner solar force such as Sri Aurobindo had attributed to his Yoga. The Mother's presence in Pondicherry was particularly strong and sometimes overwhelming. One could feel her Shakti in many locations there as a palpable and pervasive force of light, which sometimes brought me to a state in which I had to sit quietly for hours in order to hold the energy. New directions in my Vedic quest would come from both these visits to the Ramanashram and the Aurobindo Ashram.

My Experience of the Vedic Yoga 2:

Kavyakantha Ganapati Muni and My Vedic Work

I had heard of Kavyakantha Ganapati Muni, the chief disciple of Ramana Maharshi, particularly relative to his Sanskrit translations of Ramana's teachings. I soon learned that he had written important works on the *Vedas*. The Muni was known as perhaps the greatest Sanskrit poet and composer of Sanskrit mantras in modern India. His Vedic insights would be most noteworthy, if I could track them down.

I asked M.P. Pandit about Ganapati Muni's Vedic works, as he himself was a disciple of Kapali Shastry, one of Ganapati Muni's main disciples. Unfortunately, Pandit did not have much information to pass on; as far as he knew, he told me, there was not much on the *Vedas* to be found in the scattered writings left of the Muni. It seems that little of Ganapati's Vedic work remained and it consisted mainly of shorter works or fragments.

Pandit did call Ganapati, "a luminary of the first order on the spiritual firmament of modern India. He was a versatile genius whose contribution in the many fields to which he turned his attention are yet to be fully assessed."[15] This suggested a monumental and independent stature for Ganapati, far more than his usual estimation as an important disciple of Ramana; I would learn to concur with that higher regard. I would come to see Ramana, Ganapati, and Aurobindo as three related great Rishis, with their unique messages, with Ganapati forming the link between the two.

Ganapati's monumental poem of a thousand verses *Uma Sahasram* was available in Sanskrit from the Aurobindo Ashram, along with Kapali Shastry's brilliant Sanskrit commentary, which I went over carefully.[16] This amazing massive yogic poem to the Goddess contains the main secrets of Vedanta, Tantra, mantra, Kundalini, prana, and meditation. It is one of the most beautiful, complex, and symphonic poems about Raja Yoga ever composed, and one of the greatest works in the art, literature, and philosophy of Yoga for all time. Studying and meditating on the text convinced me further of the greatness of the Muni not only as a poet, but also as a Rishi much like the Vedic seers. His *Uma Sahasram*, however, refers only to the *Vedas* peripherally, indicating that he possessed a deeper knowledge, outlining aspects of the Vedic Yoga but not explaining it in detail.

My continued visits to the Ramanashram suggested that there was something more about the *Vedas* for me to discover there. At the Ramanashram in January of 1988, I had an experience of Lord Skanda, the son of Shiva and the child of fire as

Ramana. The Agni-Skanda-Ramana connection came forth for me and I learned to surrender to its power, which was overwhelming, purifying, and inspiring. Later I would discover certain teachings of Ganapati Muni that explained this experience and provided special mantras to help it develop in a deeper way.

During this same visit to the ashram, I had a vision of the Divine Mother as Shiva's wife and Skanda's mother Uma. Uma appeared to my inner eye and passed on various weapons and ornaments to help me into my work, though at first I did not know their meaning. She connected me specifically to the Vedic Gods, the Maruts, indicating that the Maruts were her children. In the *Vedas*, the Maruts are the children of Rudra, the Vedic form of Shiva, and symbolize the ancient Shaivite Yogis, which I would discover more about later. Along with this experience of the Mother, certain verses of Ganapati Muni came to my mind, suggesting that I look more in his direction. Ganapati brought the blessings of Ma Uma into my Vedic work as a whole.

Mother Mira at Pondicherry, the New Tara: Towards a New Creation

In December of 1988 I took another trip to India, which took me to Pondicherry again. There I had an extraordinary vision during one of M.P. Pandit's programs. During the meditation phase that occurred after his public talk, I fell into a deep trance along with a natural form of Pranayama, as the breath suspended.

My mind was transported to a higher plane of consciousness, in which I saw Mother Mira of the Aurobindo ashram appeared as White Tara being worshipped by a group of Tibetan monks. She reflected to me the suffering of humanity, the need to change human nature, and the plea for a new creation and new humanity beyond the current divisions of the human mind that was an insufficient vehicle to bring the higher spiritual truth into the world. Her vision included a call for a new *Manu* and a new *Veda* to change the world. This would give a futuristic orientation to my Vedic vision as well.

After the meditation was over, when I was leaving his house, Pandit surprisingly handed me a white jasmine flower, the Mother's favorite, and said, "for a new creation," echoing the Mother's words from my trance. I would learn over time that this vision of Mother Mira, much like that of the Goddess Uma at the Ramanashram, passed on certain seed energies and insights for my later Vedic work. I would later experience her as Tripura Sundari, the great Goddess of bliss, though only after having undergone several fire ordeals of a strongly purifying nature. Sundari is represented by the white jasmine, which is the flower of the head or the crown chakra, and shows the descent of Soma or the immortal nectar.

Meeting with K. Natesan - Ganapati Muni's Vedic Works

I had inquired in the Ramanashram about Ganapati Muni's works, trying to find additional books of his, particularly anything on the *Vedas*. At first I did not have much success and was told that such works, if they did exist, were long out of print or never published. The Ramanashram had in print Ganapati Muni's Sanskrit renditions of Ramana's teachings like *Saddarshana* (Reality in Forty Verses) and *Upadeshasaram* (The Essence of Instruction), which the Muni had taken from the original Tamil and put into beautiful Sanskrit verses. There was the Muni's own *Ramana Gita*, which consists of answers from Ramana to questions posed by advanced disciples along with Ganapati himself, probably the best and most systematic book on Ramana's teachings. These all were very important works and I studied them carefully, but they did not provide the Muni's Vedic work that I was seeking.

Then, during another visit to the ashram in early 1991, I was directed to K. Natesan, among the oldest living disciples of Ramana, who was said to possibly have such teachings of Kavyakantha Ganapati Muni. Much to my happiness and inspiration, I finally received Ganapati's Vedic work that I had been looking for from Natesan. Natesan had been a disciple of both Ramana since the young age of twelve and of Ganapati from the age of sixteen. When I met him, Natesan was already nearly eighty years old. I would continue in regular contact with him until his passing at the ripe old age of 96 (K. Natesan 1912-2009). He carried the energy and the presence of his many decades with these two unparalleled great gurus. His ability to sustain the teachings of Ganapati Muni for many decades on his own, attests to his deep connection with the guru.

Meeting Natesan was a transformative experience, and provided a new understanding of the Vedic vision that had strongly motivated me. Natesan had carefully gathered Ganapati Muni's works from South India, where they were scattered as handwritten manuscripts or as out of print small privately published editions. He painstakingly transcribed by hand all of the Muni's writings in a series of notebooks of his own. Because Natesan was looking for someone to pass on the Muni's works to, he was happy to know of my interest. He told me that no one else from the West had sought him out seeking the Muni's works the way I had.

Natesan showed his notebooks of Ganapati's writings to me and gave me several of them of which he had duplicates, along with a few copies of Ganapati's rare published works that were no longer available. Natesan replied to my query about Ganapati's Vedic works that there were many writings of the Muni on the Vedas from various angles, and he began to direct me to these. In his notebooks and books of the Muni's writings could be found entire sections on the Vedic teachings.[17] Of most importance, as I studied these I happily discovered that my own Vedic interpretations followed an approach similar to that of Ganapati, though I had not read him up to that point. My interpretation of the Rigvedic hymns to Indra that dominated my earlier Vedic translations were mirrored in Ganapati's own many works on Indra.

To my greater surprise, the Muni had also written on Ayurveda, Vedic astrology, Vedic issues in ancient history, and contemporary challenges to Hindu Dharma, such as I had been working with in my other publications, studies and researches, although I had not known that these other interests of mine had any connection with Ramana or Ganapati. Natesan explained all these aspects of Ganapati's work to me, unraveling the many dimensions of the Muni's great personality. All my study, writing, and sadhana seemed reflected in Ganapati's writings in a way that was quite clear and detailed, like an encounter with one's higher Self or deeper soul.

I still did not entirely understand the full extent of my connection with Ganapati Muni. Because I shared a similar orientation, intuition, and state of mind as Ganapati long before I knew of him, this shaped the particular trend of my thought and motivation, almost as if reflecting a past life influence or an inner resemblance. This inner association with Ganapati further made me feel vindicated in my Vedic work and encouraged me in all other aspects of my endeavors.

K. Natesan was not just a scholar or mere intellectual compiler of Ganapati's written work. He had his own profound insights and yogic experiences, hidden behind his elderly frame and humble demeanor. He was a dedicated disciple of both Ramana and Ganapati with many years of devotion and sadhana, as well as contact with many of their important disciples. He often recited and explained various verses and mantras to me, from the Muni's numerous writings. He knew these quite well, including their deeper implications. In addition, Natesan had a great respect for Sri Aurobindo and told me of the Muni's encounter with Sri Aurobindo and the Mother, when Ganapati visited their Pondicherry ashram. Natesan's son lived in Pondicherry and was associated with the Aurobindo ashram.

Natesan used to call me 'Nayana,' a nickname for Ganapati Muni that meant father in Telegu, as I had some resemblance to Ganapati physically as well as sharing the same fields of interest and writing. The last time I saw Natesan, a few weeks before his passing in 2009, he held my hand and looked into my eyes and repeated "Nayana, Nayana, Nayana," perhaps aiming to draw in the spirit of Ganapati Muni to help me with my work. I do regard my work as carrying on the legacy of Kavyakantha Ganapati Muni – though I would certainly wish to have more of his power of tapas and his mastery of Sanskrit and Raja Yoga!

The Greatness of Kavyakantha Ganapati Muni

Kavyakantha Ganapati Muni (1878-1936) was probably the greatest Sanskrit writer of modern India, who we could only compare to Shankaracharya in his mastery of the language, mantra, philosophy, and the paths of Yoga. He composed many poems, sutras, essays, and a novel in the best classical Sanskrit. He invented a new language of his own as well. His *Uma Sahasram* or *Thousand Verses in Praise of the Goddess Uma* consists of forty chapters, each composed in a different classical Sanskrit meter, including the longest and most complicated among these. He composed many other hymns or stotras to Hindu Gods and Goddesses, particularly Shiva and Devi, displaying the full range of Sanskrit poetic devices that one does not see in any other Sanskrit writer.

As K. Natesan notes, "He (Ganapati Muni) gave the name Bhagavan Ramana Maharshi to Brahmana Swamy whose original name was Venkataraman."[18] The Muni took Ramana's Tamil teachings and rendered them into beautiful Sanskrit verses. He composed special verses in praise of Ramana (*Forty Verses in Praise of Ramana*).[19] He determined and directed the necessary mantras and performed the rituals to establish the Ramanashram and its temple that was the Samadhi of Ramana's Mother, Saundaryamba, who herself achieved liberation. Ganapati was close to her at an inner spiritual level that drew him deeper into the worship of the Goddess. Ganapati spent many years in sadhana and regular dialogue with Ramana, particularly before the ashram came into being. Later, when they resided in different locations, Ganapati wrote to Ramana regularly. These letters form another publication of the Ramanashram.[20] There are several important books about the relationship between the Muni and the sage.[21]

K. Natesan noted that Ramana took an active interest in his work transcribing the writings of Ganapati Muni. He states, "Bhagavan noticed it and kept track of my work. He would ask me if I had a specific writing. He would often ask for my notes, see them, and even make copies in different languages. I consider myself blessed, as there were occasions when Bhagavan Ramana himself would write some of the verses of the Muni (that I did not have in my collections) in my notebook in his own handwriting."[22]

Fortunately, K. Natesan fulfilled his youthful vow to Ramana and Ganapati, finishing only shortly before his passing at the age of 96. He was able to collect and publish Ganapati's Sanskrit works in eleven volumes, preserving the Muni's great writings for posterity. It remains for these volumes to be translated, commented on, and given the wider audience that they deserve.

Though a dedicated disciple of Ramana, Ganapati Muni was no mere imitation of the great sage, nor did he try to copy Ramana's approach. He retained his own personality, teachings, and insights, which honored Ramana's guidance but had his own original views and covered many topics in his writings, including the Vedic sciences, which Ramana did not address.

Ganapati was a great philosopher in his own right, with his own school of thought combining Advaita Vedanta, Shaivism, Shaktism, and the *Vedas*. He composed a number of original treatises in the field of Jnana Yoga, philosophy and cosmology, reflecting his deep yogic experiences. These writings not only articulated the teachings of Ramana Maharshi, but also brought in the Muni's own insights, with special explorations of the inner meaning of time and space as sound and light. He wrote a whole set of new sutras on many yogic, Vedic and Tantric topics, reviving this entire line of ancient literature, including his own Sutras on Yoga and a special *Raja Yoga Sutras*. They were somewhat different from Patanjali, but explained the place of Patanjali's teaching as well.[23] His views were close to that of Kashmiri Shaivism, the great sage Abhinavagupta. He did important work on the *Sri Vidya* and *Dasha Mahavidya (Ten Great Wisdom Forms of the Goddess)*,[24] which subjects I have brought into my books.

Yet more than a great poet and thinker, Ganapati Muni was a great Raja Yogi. All the secrets of Kundalini, mantra, and the chakras were well known to him and part of his own regular experience. He had a relationship with the Divine Mother and her Shaktis of the most direct type, with her revealing all her secrets to him, in both the manifest universe and the unmanifest Absolute.

Ganapati was in regular communion with the great deities of Vedic and Hindu religious practice, notably Devi, Shiva, and Krishna. He went to many temples in South India and performed powerful tapas or austerities for the *prana pratishta*, reinstalling the spirit in the temple icons, which had lost their spiritual aura from years of neglect. He revitalized many ancient temples, restoring their linkage to the higher lokas and Devatas.

Ganapati had a notable experience of "Kapala Bheda" or the opening up of the skull, a rare yogic experience that one finds mentioned in the *Upanishads*,[25] in which the Yogi's actual skull bones parted, allowing an easier access to higher states of consciousness. Unfortunately, this opening of the skull makes life in the physical world very difficult and was a cause of his short of life of only fifty-eight years. His Shakti was so powerful that it was hard to keep it in a physical body. Yet Ganapati vowed to continue his presence in the world at a subtle level in order to guide aspirants and help spiritually awaken India. Ganapati's spirit remains with us, as one of the inner guides of this era. He had no concern for his own liberation and realization, but was dedicated to working out the will of the Goddess or Shakti for helping the world and her children.

Ganapati was a master of Ayurvedic medicine and Vedic astrology,[26] and sought to revive India and its culture through restoring the ancient Vedic teachings and reviving the Vedic sciences. He lived during the Indian independence movement but not long enough to see India free from British rule. His devotion to Bharat Mata or Mother India, such as many great Yogis of that time felt, was extraordinary and is found in many of his verses.

Relative to the *Vedas*, Ganapati composed several notable works including the *Thousand Names of Indra* (Indra Sahasranāma),[27] in which I found a similar approach to Indra as I had taken in my Vedic translations. He wrote shorter poems or *Gitas* and special works on Indra, Agni, and Vayu that explained the yogic meaning of these deities with depth and profundity. He composed wonderful hymns in praise of the Goddess Indrani, Indra's consort, who he also identified with the Tantric deity Chinnamasta and Renuka of the *Puranas*.

Ganapati wrote a longer work on ancient history through the *Vedas*, in which he connects the *Mahabharata* to the *Rigveda*.[28] In addition, throughout all of his works are references to Vedic teachings and their Vedantic, yogic, and Tantric connections, which he saw as a single stream of knowledge. For example, he found special verses in the *Rigveda* for all the Ten Wisdom Forms of the Goddess (Dasha Mahavidya).[29] While Ganapati's Vedic teachings only contain direct commentaries on a small number of *Rigveda* hymns, he provided a complete system of Vedic interpretation in his explanation of the Vedic deities.

Ganapati and Ramana: Ganesha and Skanda

Ramana and Ganapati were very close, as were their teachings, as the following story illustrates. Ganapati Muni decided to finish his *Uma Sahasram*, his *Thousand Verses in Praise of the Goddess Uma*, within a certain period of time. He found himself more than two hundred verses short with only one day left. He took a vow to finish the work that very night. He then came and sat at the feet of Ramana and a stream of inspiration arose, in which he quickly finished the work, reciting the new verses while Ramana sat silently nearby. When he had completed the work, Ramana opened his eyes and, surprisingly to all present, said to Ganapati, "Have you finished what I have dictated?"[30] This means that Ramana's grace is an integral part of Ganapati's work, of which *Uma Sahasram* was his greatest composition. When Ganapati passed away in 1936 Ramana wept and said that such a person as Ganapati could not be found. Ramana often spoke highly of the Muni's humility, his great personality, and his profound knowledge.

Kavyakantha Ganapati Muni perceived Ramana Maharshi as the Agni of the *Vedas*,[31] particularly Agni's Vaishvanara form as the liberated soul (Mukta Purusha). Ganapati identified this aspect of Agni with Lord Skanda, the son of Shiva, called

Murugan in Tamil, mentioned in the *Chandogya Upanishad*.[32] Ganapati composed special Vedic and Tantric mantras for invoking Skanda-Ramana as the supreme guru. He associated the *Dahara Vidya* (Secret Knowledge of the Cave of the Heart) and *Hridaya Vidya* (Heart Knowledge) of the Upanishads[33] – Upanishadic teachings about Self-inquiry and the spiritual heart that Ramana emphasized – to Agni hymns of the *Rigveda*, particularly those of the Rishi Parashara.[34] Through the Vedic teachings of Ganapati Muni, I learned the Vedic basis of Ramana's teaching and better understood the Agni energy that Ramana reflected and why I had first experienced Lord Skanda when I initially visited the ashram.

Ramana as Skanda and Ganapati Muni as Ganesha were like two brothers, and the two sons of Shiva and Parvati. Ramana, like Skanda, held the highest direct knowledge of what could be called *Jnana*, that of the Supreme Self, which he would not scale down or compromise. Ganapati Muni, like Ganesha, held the comprehensive knowledge of what could be called *Vijnana*, which includes all the Yogic, Tantric and Vedic sciences. Ramana taught mainly through silence, while Ganapati had the power of the Divine Word in all of its expressions. Yet Ramana and Ganapati performed tapas together for long periods of time, in which their influences crossed over in many ways. One could say that Kavyakantha Ganapati Muni was the poetic voice of Bhagavan Ramana Maharshi and brought out the Vijnana that corresponded to the Maharshi's Jnana.

A true understanding of the Vedic teachings requires both *Jnana* and *Vijnana* as I would define them: both the direct knowledge of the Self-absolute (Jnana), and the integral knowledge of the Self in its cosmic manifestation, which is cosmic intelligence (Vijnana). Through the Jnana or direct knowledge, we can perceive our true nature as the Self Absolute, such as in Advaita Vedanta. Through the Vijnana we can grasp all the Vedic sciences, through the Mahat Tattva or cosmic intelligence that underlies the manifest worlds.

The *Vedas* deal with both Jnana and Vijnana, with both the direct and comprehensive forms of knowledge. Ramana and Ganapati reflect these two aspects in their teaching. Ramana reflects more the pure Jnana, while Ganapati explained the Vijnana. Generally Jnanis develop more the pure transcendent knowledge, while Yogis explore the dimensions of cosmic knowledge (Vijnana) as well, which can serve as steps to reach the transcendent knowledge that, like a high mountain, is hard to realize directly.

Yet while the Jnana or direct knowledge of the Self is simple, the Vijnana, that comprehends the entire universe, is necessarily complex and covers a variety of disciplines. For this reason, the *Vedas* reflect more of the Vijnana, which extends to all the Vedic sciences. These are not simply intellectual fields but arise from intuitive perception and the higher logic, the logos of cosmic intelligence. Understanding the Vedic mantras allows the Vijnana to unfold in all of its vastness. The Jnana or direct knowledge of the Self in the *Vedas* is hidden in the Vedic mantras and approached by degrees through the Vijnana, including all the Vedic sciences. It is approached more simply and clearly through Advaita Vedanta.

In Vedic thought any Vijnana or Vedic science, including Ayurveda and Vedic astrology, can be used as a way of Jnana, Self-knowledge, or Self-realization. Similarly, the attainment of Jnana or Self-realization affords the soul access to the Vijnana or cosmic knowledge. While Ramana did not overtly teach the details of Yoga practice or any of the Vedic sciences, when questioned on the subtleties of these teachings, he always knew the answers, no doubt because through his Jnana he could access the Vijnana as needed.

Jnana, or direct knowledge of the Self, has the ability to transcend or even nullify the Vijnana or comprehensive cosmic knowledge. In the Self Absolute there is no world and the entire universe disappears into the unborn or uncreated. From the standpoint of the Supreme Self there is no need for any Vijnana or cosmic knowledge as there is no cosmos existing from its perspective. That is why some Jnanis may not show personal interest in any form of Vijnana, including the Vedic sciences, though they may appreciate their value in the spiritual quest. Sometimes they may discourage their disciples from studying the Vijnana and orient them to the Jnana by itself. This was often the case for Ramana, who would first offer the Jnana or direct knowledge of the Supreme Self to all who visited him.

For this reason, some followers of Ramana have not looked into Ganapati's teachings relative to other Vedic disciplines or looked to him for guidance. Ramana himself, however, honored Ganapati's knowledge. He took careful note of the verses that Ganapati wrote in praise of him, and was quite aware of Ganapati's commentaries on his teachings and other subjects.

Sometimes, the Vijnanis or Yogis of the cosmic mind find that the Jnana or direct knowledge, particularly if taken by itself, can be impractical or narrow in its application, not affording adequate scope for cosmic knowledge and cosmic evolution. This seems to have been the view of Sri Aurobindo, who found Shankara's Advaita Vedanta to be excessive in its negation of the importance of the external world manifestation.[35] Both perspectives of the Jnana and the Vijnana have their validity. Jnana is more simple and direct but has its full expression with the Vijnana, which can serve as a means to access it.[36] If students are given the direct knowledge before their minds and bodies are prepared to handle it through preliminary teachings, they can get caught in their own imagination and speculation.

Ganapati, Ramana and Sri Aurobindo

Relative to the *Vedas* and to Yoga, Ganapati had some similar teachings to Sri Aurobindo, though he only knew Aurobindo late in his life. Sri Aurobindo, like Ganapati, reflected more the Vijnana or 'integral Self-knowledge' as he called it. Ganapati, like Aurobindo, had a special concern with uplifting humanity and the earth consciousness as a whole through bringing down the Divine Shakti to counter the forces of ignorance in the world. Similar to Aurobindo, Ganapati had a strong vision of India and its future through Bharat Mother or the Shakti of Mother India, particularly the need to reawaken the country to its spiritual mission as the guru of all nations. He directed much of his energy for the benefit of the nation.

Like Sri Aurobindo, Ganapati Muni had a strong connection with Tantra and the worship of the Goddess as Shakti. Yet Ganapati was a master of Vedic and Tantric practices and Yoga techniques, while Aurobindo sought more to work with a direct flow of grace not dependent upon specific techniques. In this regard, once Ganapati used his yogic power to draw the subtle body of Ramana from the Tiruvannamalai Ashram to near Madras where he was staying. From this, Ramana noted Ganapati's yogic powers that drew his awareness that distance without any effort on his own part.

For me, Ganapati bridged the gap between Ramana and Aurobindo. I came to see the three as a great trinity of spiritual Rishis of the highest order in modern India, with Ganapati not merely a disciple of Ramana but a teacher of his own line of yogic and Vedic teachings that preserved Ramana's core insights as well.

Ganapati Muni identified Ganapati as a deity first with Brihaspati of the *Rigveda*.[37] Brihaspati is the Vedic lord of speech from whom all mantric powers arise. Brihaspati is also the original and foremost of the Vedic Rishis, the head of the important Angirasa line, identified with the planet Jupiter, the guru among the planets. Ganapati was much like a new Brihaspati of a new Vedic line of Vedic Rishis, and possibly of a new line of Vedic mantras. At a broader level of interpretation, Ganapati Muni related Brihaspati with Indra, the foremost of the Vedic deities, with whom he was also personally identified.

In Ganapati Muni was contained the prototype of the work that I had unknowingly followed of my own accord. Now I understood where the main Vedic insights that had come to me were probably based. Ganapati's spirit came to me and continues to be with me, guiding and motivating me in accord with a deeper connection to Ramana, and reflecting the insights of Aurobindo.

Ramana is like Agni; Ganapati is like Indra; and Aurobindo is like Surya, the prime trinity of Vedic deities. Ramana reflects the Self-inquiry line of Agni or Fire, Ganapati reflects the lightning perception of Indra, and Aurobindo reflects the comprehensive and integral knowledge of Surya or the Sun. Yet each is unique. We need not compare them, debating who is better, or try to combine their teachings together, but rather to appreciate their differences and unique orientations. Such monumental figures stand on their own and must be approached according to their own teachings.

Brahmarshi Daivarata is revealed to me

In January 1994 a reception was organized for me with the staff of the Bharatiya Vidya Bhavan in Mumbai (Bombay), an important spiritual and cultural center in India. My Vedic work was discussed and honored. As a special gift for my Vedic research I was given a book on the *Vedas* that the Bhavan had published in 1968, which had been long out of print. To my surprise and delight, it was the *Chhandodarshana* of Daivarata, an important disciple of Ganapati Muni and Ramana Maharshi. I had not previously known of Daivarata's contribution, and the people at the Bhavan did not know of my connection with Ganapati. Such a fortuitous event could only have occurred by Divine Grace.

Later returning to Ramanashram, a friend and colleague there presented me a copy of an additional book of Daivarata, *Vak Sudha*, and another monumental work on the *Vedas*. Daivarata's two works on the *Vedas* were profound and inspired. They were more systematic and detailed than Ganapati's writings and followed a similar line. Daivarata, unlike Kapali Shastry who joined Aurobindo later, remained with Ramana's teachings for the rest of his long life. Along with K. Natesan, Daivarata, and Kapali were perhaps the three main disciples of Kavyakantha Ganapati Muni.

Daivarata's work completed Ganapati's for me, filling in some details that the Muni had only alluded to. Daivarata was said to have created his own new and authentic Vedic mantras, something that Ganapati himself confirmed. *Chhandodarshana* consists of Daivarata's new Vedic mantras, mainly to Brihaspati and Sarasvati, but covering the full range of Vedic deities and formulations, with a language like that of the *Yajurveda*, complete with an extensive commentary by Ganapati Muni.

His *Vak Sudha* or "the Nectar of the Word," is a study of the Vedic speech, both as a Goddess and a cosmic power, written in beautiful classical Sanskrit meters, explaining the Vedic language in depth. *Vak Sudha*, continuing the approach of Ganapati, further connected Vedic mantras to Tantric deities, especially forms of the Goddess and manifestations of the Divine Word, notably Tara, reminding me of my vision of the Mother at the Aurobindo Ashram as the White Tara.

Brahmarshi Daivarata and Maharishi Mahesh Yogi

In recent decades, most of the people in the West who have come to appreciate the *Vedas* and the Vedic sciences like Ayurveda and Vedic astrology discovered the *Vedas* through the teachings of Maharishi Mahesh Yogi and his TM (Transcendental Meditation) movement. That was not the case for me, but I learned to recognize the importance of Maharishi's work in making people more receptive to Vedic ideas of all approaches. Eventually I discovered an important bridge between my Vedic Yoga gurus and Maharishi.

Around 2000, I learned that 'Brahmarshi Devrat', as they called him, was one of the main inspirations for the Vedic approach of Maharishi Mahesh Yogi of the TM movement. Maharishi had brought Devarat to the West several times as an important traditional representative of the Vedic teachings and modern Rishi.[38] Perhaps our thought waves crossed as Daivarata crossed the US! In any case, the Vedic side of the TM movement connects through Daivarata to Ganapati Muni and Ramana Maharshi – a fact that few people in the TM movement know.

Daivarata was like the new Vishvamitra Rishi, the seer of the Gayatri mantra, whose Rishi line he was part of. Like Ganapati Muni, his works need to be collected and published in the original Sanskrit, translated and better distributed. We hope that there are scholars and devotees who will take up this work. From what I know, there are many unpublished works of Daivarata, like those of Ganapati Muni, including much on the Vedic Dhi Yoga or Yoga of meditation. I am hoping to find some of these.

Ganapati and Daivarata show that the Rishi power can come again and is likely to descend more often as humanity ascends in consciousness in the coming ages of light. Yet besides the Aurobindo and Kavyakantha Ganapati Muni lines of modern Vedic research, I discovered several other important modern Vedic movements that would become part of my Vedic vision.

B.G. Tilak

B.G. Tilak (1856-1920) was a monumental figure in modern India, socially, politically, and religiously. He was the head of India's independence movement in the late nineteenth and early twentieth century before Mahatma Gandhi. In fact it was largely owing to Tilak's labor that the movement was developed. He spent many years in some of the worst jails in the British Empire for his efforts to liberate India but never lost his inner vision. Of utmost importance to our current discussion, Tilak wrote on the *Vedas*, extensively exploring the astronomical references in early Vedic texts.

Sri Aurobindo was one of Tilak's closest associates and his likely heir apparent before Aurobindo renounced politics to devote himself to Yoga in 1905. Later, Mahatma Gandhi succeeded Tilak as head of the Indian independence movement and continued Tilak's focus on the *Bhagavad Gita* as a book of Karma Yoga.

Tilak's work helped me examine the historical side of the *Vedas* further, though I eventually took a different angle. His *Orion or the Arctic Home in the Vedas* is an important work on Vedic astronomy and shows that the Vedic texts mirror ancient astronomical eras. His idea of an arctic home for the *Vedas*, however, is not of the same order of accuracy. This idea occurred before the Sarasvati River was known and reflects mistaken views of his time, that the Polar Regions were warm and inhabitable fewer than ten thousand years ago.

Swami Dayananda - Arya Samaj

One cannot look into the *Vedas* without coming into contact with the Arya Samaj, one of the largest movements in modern Hinduism. The Arya Samaj line is probably the largest contemporary Vedic line of teachings, has the most teachers, the most books, and has done the most research, and produced the best new editions of Sanskrit Vedic texts.

The founder of the Arya Samaj, Swami Dayananda Sarasvati (1824-1883) electrified and awakened India in the late nineteenth century by his call for a return to the *Vedas*. His approach to the *Vedas* was simple yet profound. He taught that the various Vedic deities were not separate Gods but simply different names, qualities, and functions of the same Supreme Being, which is perhaps the main factor that we need to understand in order to understand the *Vedas*. He explained the spiritual relevance of the Vedic deities and connected the *Vedas* to the *Bhagavad Gita, Upanishads*, and *Yoga Sutras*.

The Arya Samaj Vedic revival in India was strongly involved in the independence movement in the country. Tilak and Aurobindo owed much of their Vedic emphasis to the pioneering work of Swami Dayananda. Swami Vivekananda followed Swami Dayananda's lead as a fiery monk promoting the Vedic knowledge. Swami Dayananda and his Arya Samaj was not only a return to the *Vedas*, but also a great social movement in modern India, initiating many important social reforms.

I studied Swami Dayananda's *Satyartha Prakash*, which is a commentary on the Vedic teachings in Sanskrit. I have worked with several Arya Samaj and related groups in India and the West, giving talks at their various centers and conferences. They strongly promote Vedic rituals, particularly Agnihotra, or daily fire offerings and regularly study and chant Vedic mantras.

Ram Swarup

Ram Swarup was called by the magazine *Hinduism Today* as "the foremost modern teacher of Hinduism." When he passed away in 1998, Atal Behari Vajpayee, the Prime Minister of India, called him a 'modern Rishi'. Among his many publications, Ram Swarup did an important work on mantra, the *Word as Revelation: Names of God*, discussing the *Vedas* among various spiritual traditions of the world. Swarup followed Aurobindo's approach to Yoga and the *Vedas*. He was connected with Sri Anirvan and brought me more into contact with the Vedic side of Anirvan's work.

Ram Swarup like Sri Aurobindo was involved with the social and cultural issues of the *Vedas* and Hinduism, as well as the spiritual side and yogic dimension. He was a strong defender of Hinduism from the attacks of leftist scholars and Christian missionaries. Swarup was perhaps the leading Indian intellectual to oppose communism in the country in the post World War II era, when it was fashionable to be communist and when the communists came to dominate Indian academia.

I had a number of important discussions with Ram Swarup in Delhi when I met him in 1992, to his passing in 1998. He said that the entire Hindu tradition, and most of Buddhism, is rooted in the *Vedas*. He encouraged me to emphasize the nature of Sanatana Dharma, the eternal and universal tradition of yogic knowledge behind Hinduism and Vedic knowledge. Ram Swarup wrote forewords for two of my books *Hinduism, the Eternal Tradition* and *Awaken Bharata*. Later I wrote the forewords to four volumes of his works that were released after his passing.[39]

I came to write a number of books for Voice of India (Bharata Bharati), the company founded by Ram Swarup and his colleague Sitaram Goel, and its affiliates like Aditya Prakashan. This included titles on ancient India like *Myth of the Aryan Invasion* and *Rigveda and the History of India* as well as titles on Hinduism and Sanatana Dharma. Voice of India expanded the influence of my Vedic work, particularly in India and relative to Hindu youth worldwide.

Sri Anirvan

Sri Anirvan was a great Bengali Yogi who wrote original works on the *Vedas* and on Samkhya philosophy, as well as translating Sri Aurobindo's works into Bengali. Notable was his *Buddhi Yoga of the Bhagavad Gita*. He wrote on the poetry of the Bauls, the mystic singers of Bengal. Some years later (2002) when I was visiting Shilong in the northeast of India (Meghalaya), I happened to visit a Sri Aurobindo Center there. I asked them if they knew of Sri Anirvan who had spent time in the northeast. They replied that the cottage next door was his place of residence for many years. It seems that Anirvan had welcomed me. I communed with him in his cottage for some time through meditation. His three volume study of the *Rigveda*, called *Veda Mimamsa* is unfortunately only available in Bengali and Hindi; it should hold many secrets.

Vedic Astrology and Interpreting the *Vedas*

I began studying astrology with western astrology, with an inspiration from C.G. Jung's writings in 1968, and added Vedic astrology in 1970, from the books of Dr. B.V. Raman, and have continued to work with it since then. After 1984 I began teaching Vedic astrology through various books and courses. I was also an amateur astronomer and at a young age learned the positions of the stars, which became particularly helpful because Vedic astrology is star based, not equinox based like western tropical astrology. Because of my knowledge of astrology and astronomy, I was able to appreciate astronomical references in the *Vedas*, including planetary positions of great antiquity relative to solstices and equinoxes, which became another important part of my Vedic studies.

Over time I met with many noted Vedic astrologers in India like Dr. B.V. Raman, Gayatri Devi, Niranjan Bapu, K.S. Charak, and K.N. Rao.[40] I contacted special Bhrigu and Samhita readers that related to me secrets of my past lives and important future indications. India's great astrologers had similar ideas about the history of India and the antiquity of the Vedic astronomical references involved as I did, providing them great antiquity.[41] They provided important keys on areas of archaeo-astronomy.

Dr. B.V. Raman (1912-1998) was more than a great astrologer but an important spiritual, cultural, and intellectual leader of India to whom many national dignitaries went for guidance, including several Prime Ministers. He became my main astrological teacher and I had a number of important visits with him in India. I became close to the Raman family and Dr. Raman would organize public talks for me in Bangalore during my visits, often relative to historical issues of the *Vedas*. He read my astrological chart according to a special text the *Dhruva Nadi* that he had, which divided the zodiac into fifteen hundred parts. He encouraged me in my Vedic work and asked me to continue promoting Vedic astrology.[42]

The *Vedas* have an astrological side to their interpretation, primarily through the 27 Nakshatras or lunar mansions, which are ruled and defined by Vedic deities. Vedic deities are also star Gods and sky deities. Late Vedic texts, particularly the *Brahmanas*, highlight the vernal equinox in the Pleiades (Krittika) or Taurus, a date of around 2000 BCE, while much earlier references are found in the Rigveda, going back perhaps ten thousand years.

The mathematical symbolism of the *Rigveda* – with numbers like 720, 432, 360, 180, 120, 60, 12, and 7 common in the hymns and their meters – reflects astrological factors and, particularly with 360, a zodiacal division of the heavens. The *Rigveda* speaks of the "four times ninety (360) names of Vishnu that revolve like a wheel or chakra,"[43] suggesting a special Vedic name for each degree of the zodiac. The *Vedas* gave the world the decimal system, which aids in all manner of astronomical calculations that are otherwise difficult to compute.

I brought this astronomical and astrological dimension into my interpretations of the Vedic hymns.[44] Vedic deities are related to the stars, to movements of the Sun, phases of the Moon, seasons of the year, and times of the day. They are part of a profound understanding of natural time cycles. This Vedic view of time enabled me to establish a new relationship with nature and the stars. We live according to cosmic rhythms and if we can attune ourselves through them through ritual, mantra and meditation, they can help us move into the eternal and universal.

Ayurveda: The Vedic Key to Right Living

Along with my study of Yoga, I had a special interest in herbs and plants, extending to a mystical sense of their spiritual energies. My study of herbs gradually took me into nutrition, natural healing, western herbology, Chinese herbal medicine, and Vedic medicine or Ayurveda.

My study of Yoga, the *Vedas*, and herbal healing formed my initial approach to Ayurveda. In Ayurveda, I found my familiar Vedic friends like Agni and Vayu but in a biological terminology. In fact, before I had learned Ayurveda in detail, I had already written extensively on the Vedic deities of Agni, Soma, and Vayu that are the basis for Ayurveda. Ayurveda was one of the later portions of the Vedic teaching that came into play for me, though it would become central for my writings and for my work, particularly in the West.

In 1983 I moved to Santa Fe, New Mexico, which had perhaps the only extensive Ayurvedic training program in the country under the guidance of Dr. Vasant Lad, one of the greatest Ayurvedic teachers to come to the West. Through Ayurveda, I was able to see how the Vedic knowledge that I had already studied in depth, as well as my work with herbs, nutrition, and Yoga, was relevant as a natural healing approach that could be appreciated by a larger audience.[45] I began to bring Ayurveda into my Vedic work in a primary way.

Dr. B.L. Vashta in Mumbai, India, became my main teacher of Ayurveda and provided me with the guidance and inspiration to teach Ayurveda throughout the world. I visited Vashta in India regularly for ten years up to his passing in 1998. In another coincidence, Vashta was a noted journalist in Maharashtra, India, and opened up a greater audience for my writings in India, including my books on the *Vedas*, which he appreciated and promoted.

I discovered that there is considerable Ayurvedic knowledge present in the *Rigveda*, and that the Vedic deities are easier to understand from an Ayurvedic background, following the same threefold understanding of nature's forces. Ayurveda has remained alive through the centuries as a Vedic discipline, reflecting Vedic terminology like Agni and Vayu, while other aspects of the Vedic Yoga have faded with time. Ayurveda remains perhaps our simplest and most practical doorway to the Vedic world and to a Vedic lifestyle, one that is in harmony with the great triune forces of nature. If we can understand the Vedic energies through Ayurveda, we can approach them in the *Rigveda*, not simply as biological forces but as cosmic principles. My understanding of the Vedic Yoga is rooted in the energetics of Ayurveda. We can call the Vedic Yoga an "inner Yoga of Ayurveda," or an "inner Dosha-balancing." The Vedic teaching shows us how to understand these three forces and work with them for the transformation of mind and consciousness.

Archaeology and Ancient History

Along with my translations and interpretations of Vedic hymns from a spiritual standpoint, I gradually put together a new view of ancient India based upon the type of culture that I found existing within the Vedic texts. I could not accept the prevalent textbook Aryan Invasion/Migration Theory (AIT, AMT), for which I found no basis in the Vedic mantras that laud the Sarasvati River region as their ancient homeland. My study convinced me that the Vedic civilization was largely a maritime culture rooted in India going back many thousands of years.

By 1980 I had written a short manuscript on ancient India. I did an expanded work in 1987, which eventually became the book *Gods, Sages and Kings: Vedic Secrets of Ancient Civilization* in 1991, my first published book on ancient history. In the book I traced over one hundred and fifty references to the ocean (samudra) in the *Rigveda* alone, along with many references to ships and ocean travel.[46] Manu and the seven Vedic Rishis appeared as part of a massive flood myth that reflected the end of the Ice Age. In addition, from my appreciation of the sophisticated nature of the Vedic language and philosophy, I was convinced that the Vedic mantras reflected an advanced spiritual and poetic culture, not a group of primitive nomads as was the Aryan Invasion theory!

The publication of *Gods, Sages and Kings* in India and the West opened a new historical dimension to my work. It brought prominence as well as criticism to me as an historian. I discovered that many scholars are sensitive to those who may criticize the Western world as the origin of civilization, and who would connect the origins of civilization to the yogic culture of India. Though I was largely repeating what the great Yogis of India had previously said – including modern figures like Sri Aurobindo and Paramahansa Yogananda – I found little willingness in the academic world to examine the yogic dimension of the Rigveda, or to recognize the need for a great ancient culture in order to produce it. I wrote a short book for India publication called *Myth of the Aryan Invasion of India* (1994) that summarized these views; it was widely circulated in India and on the Internet.

Help from Other Scholars

While finishing *Gods, Sages and Kings*, I came into contact with noted Vedic scholar and scientist Subhash Kak. Kak has discovered much significant new information in the *Vedas* on astronomy and mathematics, particularly relative to the building of Vedic fire altars. His work on the astronomical code of the *Rigveda* is most significant, and shows the deep scientific knowledge that the Vedic Rishis had.[47] Kak has written several important books and many articles that have been published in major scientific journals. In addition to his Vedic research, he has many new insights on the role of consciousness in the physical universe, and like the Vedic Rishis, is an excellent poet as well.

Georg Feuerstein was one of the foremost western scholars of Yoga, detailing its different branches, philosophies and history. After *Gods, Sages and Kings* came out challenging the Aryan Invasion Theory, I called him and related my views to him. To my surprise, though he had presented the Aryan Invasion Theory in his earlier writings, he responded favorably and remarked that he had doubts about the Aryan Invasion anyway, and was acquainted with Sri Aurobindo's views on the subject. Feuerstein, Kak, and I soon collaborated on a book on ancient India, *In Search of the Cradle of Civilization* (1995), highlighting these new views and discoveries.

N.S. Rajaram, an India-born scientist who worked at NASA for many years, had similar views and contacted me a little later after he had returned to live in India. I provided him with information on the Vedic literature for another book *Vedic Aryans and the Origins of Civilization*.

Surprisingly for me, these historical issues came to dominate over the yogic side in the response to my Vedic work. I encountered more interest in the *Vedas* from the standpoint of world history than from the yogic meaning of the hymns. My work as a Vedic historian seemed to take precedence over my work on the Vedic Yoga. My Vedic views became part of a larger debate on ancient India and the Indo-European or Aryan question, which has long been part of European political and social thinking, and has many strong opinions on various sides.

This same phenomenon occurred relative to all the writers in the field that questioned the scenario of an outside-of-India origin for the Vedic people. Anyone who challenged the Aryan invasion/migration idea was likely to become the target of personal attacks. I began to realize the powerful cultural issues behind such theories and how they have been used to discredit the yogic depths of Vedic thought.

Help from Religious and Spiritual Organizations

Yet I had many allies in this new view of ancient India. Most notable among supportive publications has been *Hinduism Today*, which has helped my work in many other ways as well. Sivaya Subramuniyya Swami, the magazine's founder, whom I visited on several occasions, worked tirelessly to connect the Vedic and Shaivite visions. I owe a great deal to his inspiration, which supported my efforts to align the two traditions.

Self-Realization Fellowship (SRF), the Sri Aurobindo Ashram, the Ramanashram (Ramana Maharshi), many members of the TM (Transcendental Meditation) movement, and many followers of the Krishna or ISKCON movement have similarly been supportive, as their gurus also have not accepted the Aryan Invasion/ Migration theory. In addition, most of the great gurus of India firmly hold to the idea of the Indian origins of the Vedic teachings, though it is not usually taught in the Indian educational system, which tends to follow western educational views.

Most important for my work has been Swaminarayan (BAPS), one of the largest modern Hindu movements and the builder of the largest Hindu temples in both India and the West.[48] I eventually wrote a book with them along with N.S. Rajaram called *Hidden Horizons: Unearthing 10,000 Years of Indian Culture*,[49] designed for their monumental Delhi temple, the largest in modern India. For the book they gained the endorsement of important spiritual, religious, and cultural leaders of India today. They have distributed this book to more than twenty thousand people, gifting it to many dignitaries and several heads of state. A number of times in the past more than twenty years I have received the personal blessings of Pramukh Swami, the head of the order. His young Swamis have been enthusiastic supporters of such Vedic work.

In India there has been much confirmation from leading Indian archaeologists, notably Professor B.B. Lal, the former director of the archaeological survey of India, and S.R. Rao, the famous excavator of Dwaraka.[50] My historical work received the recognition of noted author Graham Hancock, who included references to my writings in his book *Underworld: Flooded Kingdoms of the Ice Ages*.[51] Clearly there are many mysteries of ancient history that we can no longer ignore.

Sri Sivananda Murty

Sivananda Murty is one of India's greatest gurus, yogis and Jnanis today. He is well known in Andhra Pradesh, the region of India where he lives. His ashram is located along the coast by Vishakhapatnam (Bheemli), though he frequently visits Hyderabad and other parts of India. He has visited the West several times, both the United States and Canada. Sivananda Murty has a special knowledge of the *Upanishads* and their Vedic roots, which is quite profound. He was strongly influenced by Ramana Maharshi and carries the blessings of Trailanga Swami, a great Raja Yogi of the nineteenth century.

Sri Sivananda Murty is the head of the Shaiva Mahapeetham order of Shaivism and has over ten thousand families who follow him. I joined that order under his blessings. It is a Vedic Shaivite order that reflects the same Vedic and Yogic approach that I follow, and the same philosophy. It follows the *Vedas*, a philosophy of non-duality or Advaita, an honoring of Shiva, and of Shakti as the Supreme cosmic Power. It is based on daily worship of the Shiva linga, which is a symbol of the supreme consciousness. Sivananda Murty's inspiration has helped me understand the nature of Vedic Shaivism and the connection of Shiva with the *Vedas*.

Sivananda Murty has a great knowledge of Vedic astrology. He has organized a number of events, notably the World Conference on Mundane Astrology in October 2010, which I attended, which discussed the issues of 2012 and the change of world ages. I have had many profound discussions with him over the years since 1994 when we first met, and these discussions have helped me in many ways. I edited and wrote the introduction to his *Katha Yoga*,[52] his interpretation of the famous *Katha Upanishad*, which reveals many yogic and Vedic secrets. He wrote a forward to my book *Universal Hinduism: Towards a New Vision of Sanatana Dharma*. He shows that Vedic knowledge and the line of great Vedic Yogis is alive and flourishing.

Swami Veda Bharati

The most recent revelation of a modern Vedic Rishi has come from someone surprisingly close by, whose work I had known of for many years before becoming aware of the specifics of his Vedic writings. This is Swami Veda Bharati of the Swami Rama Sadhaka Gram India, formerly known as Pandit Usharbud Arya. While visiting his ashram in Rishikesh several years ago, Swami Veda gifted me with several small Sanskrit works of his own, including *Chhandasi*, his own meditative vision of Vedic mantras.[53] I found the book to be one of the most important and original works available on the *Vedas* in modern times, reflecting the deeper meaning of the Vedic mantras in terms of Raja Yoga and mirroring the ancient Vedic language in a very faithful manner. The book suggests an entire new school of Vedic interpretation, which I would call the "Swami Veda Bharati school of Vedic interpretation," after the great Swami, having the same depth and insight as the Aurobindo line or the Ganapati Muni/Daivarata line of Vedic interpretation that we have been discussing.

Veda Bharati in Sanskrit means the 'voice of the *Vedas*'. Swami Veda was a Vedic prodigy in India as a child, coming out of a staunch Arya Samaj family background. He later joined Swami Rama of the Himalayan Institute in the United States and took up the Raja Yoga/Advaita Vedanta path through Rama's influence. Swami Veda has the ability to compose original Sanskrit and Vedic verses of several types, to which his contribution is noteworthy. His work *Chhandasi* is not a commentary on specific Vedic verses but a re-creation of Vedic teachings, reflecting the main Vedic deities and their yogic implications, in an inspired Rishi language. It resembles Daivarata's *Chhandodarshana*, a samadhi-based creation of Vedic-like verses.

Swami Veda's Sanskrit verses seem closer to the Vedic language than the others I have seen, having a certain richness and compactness of the Vedic style. Like Daivarata, his verses reflect more the cadence of the *Yajurveda* than the *Rigveda*, but add many yogic implications. Notably, Swami Veda reveals what was likely the ancient original Yoga of Hiranyagarbha, the reputed founder of the Yoga Darshana system, which the *Mahabharata* connects to Vedic verses. We will discuss this later in an upcoming chapter.

Swami Veda is also probably the greatest living scholar of the *Yoga Sutras*. His study of each of the four *padas* or section of the text comes to about a thousand pages each. He examines all sides of the *Yoga Sutra* teachings and their many implications in Yoga practice and Indian philosophy. His Vedic mantras show how the yogic tradition is rooted in the *Rigveda* itself, and is not simply the product of later currents and developments. His teachings can connect us not only with the essence of the *Yoga Sutras*, but the earlier Hiranyagarbha Vedic Yoga on which it is based. We could call Swami Veda's work the restoration of the original Hiranyagarbha Yoga Darshana.

Swami Veda's personal blessing has been important for the continuation of my Vedic research. He once told me, whom he calls his Vedic brother, that he would try to take care of Yoga and I should aim at taking care of the *Veda* – certainly a tall task but an inspiring encouragement to proceed. In any case, he has shown the way to accomplish both.

My View of the *Vedas*

The great Vedic teachers that I have mentioned have all encouraged a deeper research into the Vedas. They emphasize the application of the Vedic teachings in our own sadhana or Yoga practice, not simply as an intellectual endeavor. It is important that we recognize their deeper Vedic approaches and apply these in order to arrive at a broad understanding of the Vedic Yoga. The Vedic Yoga contains many options for different temperaments of individuals. It holds a great synthesis of yogic teachings of all types. Though it has enduring principles, it does not reflect merely a single philosophy or approach.

One may find apparently disparate inspirations in the *Vedas*, covering yogic approaches of mantra, ritual, devotion, meditation, and the application of energetic techniques. One can find the origins of later systems of philosophy and metaphysics, dualist or non-dualist. This need not be a problem. The One Truth is always infinite. Its unbounded Shakti is always seeking new forms of expression and creating new paths to draw people in. It is not concerned with mere outer agreement but with inner transformation. The *Vedas* are meant as a resource guide for all temperaments, not as a specialized teaching or Shastra for one line of approach only.

The entry into the Vedic world cannot be achieved by the mind alone, though a good intuition is essential in the process. It requires Yoga in the sense of holding the mind in a calm, concentrated, and silent space so that the eternal *Veda* can be mirrored within it. Vedic mantras reverberate in nature and are not simply a human production. They reside in the Sun and other cosmic light forms, and pervade all space. The true *Veda* is not a particular text or one of the many compilations of the *Vedas*. The *Vedas* are in fact said to be endless.[54] The Vedic mantras arise in the silence of the heart as the vibration of space. Only when we discover the cosmic *Vedas* can we claim to have access to the true *Vedas*.

We should remember that the Vedic teaching is the root of later Yoga and Vedanta teachings and requires an understanding of these in order to appreciate it. Over the years I have continued my study of Yoga and Vedanta as well, and have worked with a number of other important teachers and teachings in these fields. This has helped me deepen my approach to the *Vedas*, which I see as a mantric expression of Yoga/Vedanta.[55]

Part II

Background of the Vedic Yoga

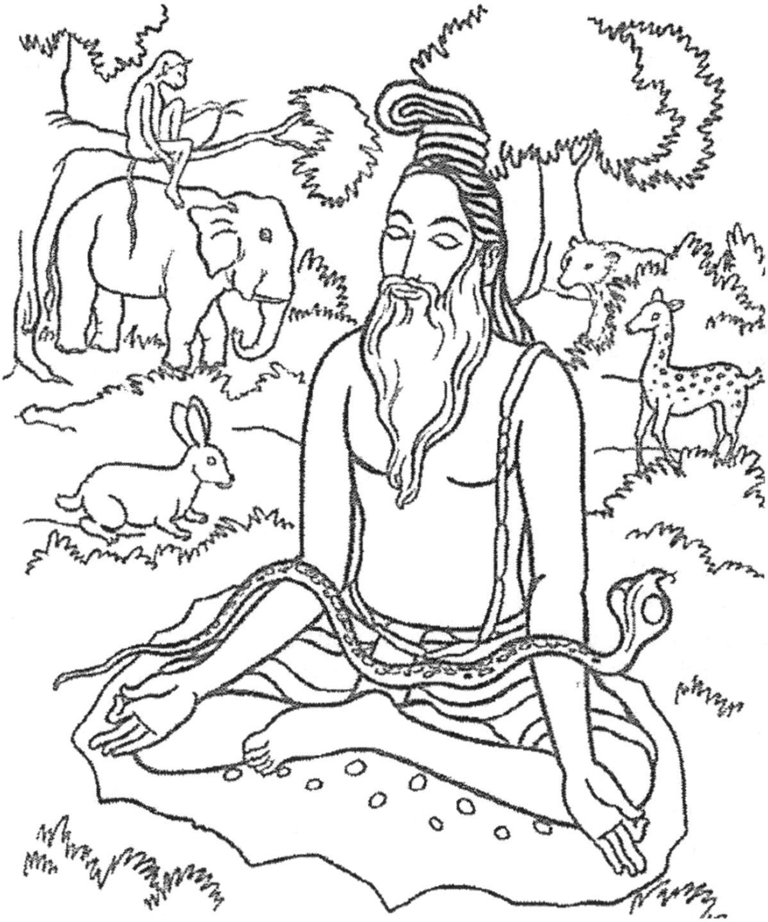

Yoga and the *Vedas*

Sanatana Dharma: The Eternal and Universal Tradition

The Yoga tradition, originally called *Yoga Dharma*, presents a remarkable system of spiritual and healing knowledge that can help us reach our highest potential in all aspects of our being. Whether it is practices of bodily postures, breath, mantra, or meditation – or a deep knowledge of the cosmos of energy, mind, or consciousness – the scope of Yoga is as vast, detailed, and profound as the universe itself. Yet with all the different Yoga teachings that have become available over the recent decades of its global spread, only a small portion of the greater Yoga tradition is truly understood or practiced today. Above all, we still do not know the basis of this great tradition or its place in the ancient world.

What is the origin of this profound system of yogic wisdom? From where did its inspiration arise? There are a number of different opinions on the issue, but the Yoga tradition itself from the *Yoga Sutras* to the *Bhagavad Gita* firmly places its foundation in the *Vedas*, the oldest scriptures of India.

Yoga rests upon the extraordinary cosmological and psychological understanding that we find in the Vedic mantras. These arcane mantras represent the meditational insights of the Vedic seers called *Rishis*, who are said to have looked over our planet since its beginning as world creators and culture makers. Yoga is the gift of the Vedic Rishis to humanity to help guide us in our inner quest toward Self-realization that is the real purpose of our existence. The Vedic Rishis were no mere ordinary human beings with mundane ambitions, but great yogis who could manifest the power of cosmic intelligence in our human realm. Yoga arose from the mantras of the Rishis that reflects the metalanguage of the Gods, the Divine forces that rule the universe externally as forces of nature, and inwardly as powers of consciousness.

The greater tradition of Yoga is not limited to what we see in Yoga books or in public Yoga classes today. Yoga in its true essence remains hidden deep within our minds and hearts as part of the older spiritual heritage of humanity. Yoga forms a great human potential, a major continent in the human psyche that is as old as our species and carries our highest aspirations for the future.

As we begin to explore this greater universe of Yoga, we will discover that the entire universe dwells within us. We can break through the barriers of time and space, and conquer death, suffering, fear, and doubt. We can understand all cultures and civilizations, all history and human development as part of our own evolution to a higher awareness.

Sanatana Dharma: the Universal and Eternal Teaching

Yoga places itself in a universal approach to spiritual knowledge called *Sanatana Dharma* or the 'Eternal Tradition'. The term *Dharma* stands for the laws of truth and consciousness that uphold the universe, including the great law of karma. *Sanatana* refers to the eternal, perpetual, universal, and holistic aspect of Dharma. *Sanatana Dharma* is the traditional name for the Vedic tradition or Vedic Dharma starting with the oldest Vedic texts. It is the name for the Hindu tradition in the broadest sense beyond any local limitations.

All Dharma is, in a sense, Sanatana because only a truth that is enduring and eternal is real. This Eternal Dharma dwells in the cosmic mind and is the foundation of all manifestation. It is impersonal, transcending all personal and cultural biases. It is beyond all names and forms, organizations and institutions, available to all those who are receptive to it within their own minds and hearts. As the great Vedic Rishi Vishvamitra states in the *Rigveda*:

> *For the universal soul, whose power is vast, the seers ordain the insights and the treasures that we may travel to the foundations of the world. The immortal sacred Fire gives power to the Gods so that the Eternal Dharmas cannot be violated.*[56]
>
> *Gathina Vishvamitra, Rigveda III.3.1.*

The Yoga tradition or *Yoga Dharma* rests upon this greater *Sanatana Dharma* tradition of living in harmony with the conscious universe, all living creatures and all the forces of nature in matter, energy, and mind. The highest human dharma, which is the highest dharma of all creatures, is the pursuit of Self-realization, or direct awareness of the cosmic Being. We exist to further the unfoldment of the supreme consciousness that is the true Self of all beings. Yoga is the means of fulfilling our highest dharma or duty of inner spiritual growth, called Moksha or liberation in Sanskrit. Yoga Dharma teaches us the necessary principles and practices to help us grow in consciousness and bring the Divine into manifestation within and around us.

This *Sanatana Dharma* or Yoga Dharma is called *Satya Dharma*, the natural law of truth. It is not the creed of one community or another.

> *Two guardians of truth, you ascend your chariot, the Satya Dharma in the supreme ether. Whom Mitra and Varuna you protect, for him the honey like rain pours from heaven.*[57]
>
> *Mitravaruna, wise in consciousness, by the power of Dharma, you guard the laws by the magic wisdom power of the Almighty. By the truth you rule over the entire universe. You have placed the Sun in heaven as a lustrous chariot.*[58]
>
> *Archanana Atreya, Rigveda V.63.1,7*

The *Vedas*

The *Vedas* in all their branches represent our best preserved corpus of spiritual and religious knowledge from the ancient world, consisting of several thousand pages of teachings. The *Vedas* form the largest set of texts that have survived from the early ancient world, the world's oldest library as it were, dating back long before the time of the Buddha, Krishna, or Rama. This means that the *Vedas* are probably our most authentic voice from our ancient ancestors, which we can still access in their original language. The Vedas constitute a living link with the ancients that remains accessible today – a great doorway through time and history. We can use the *Vedas* to speak directly to our ancient spiritual progenitors.

The *Vedas* constitute a living connection with the early spiritual era of humanity, such as many ancient traditions indicate, long before our civilization had fallen into the materialistic striving and religious dogmatism that has characterized the last two thousand years. The *Vedas* consist not merely of fragments of ancient writings haphazardly reconstructed by the modern mind, but of complete texts from the ancients themselves, along with extensive commentaries and detailed applications in daily life.

The massive Vedic compilation contains several layers and suggests a long period of development, extending over many centuries. The *Rigveda* alone contains a thousand hymns by dozens of great sages. In addition, there are later portions of the Vedic corpus down to the *Upanishads*. In addition, many other branches and recensions of Vedic teachings are mentioned traditionally that have been lost over time.

Various dates have been proposed for the compilation of the *Vedas* from 1500BCE to 3100 BCE or even to ten thousand years ago. The *Rigveda*, at least in its older portions, appears to reflect the conditions at the end of the last Ice Age, when a great geographical transformation occurred throughout the planet, with ocean levels rising more than three hundred feet, triggering great migrations and cultural changes.

The *Vedas* contain the oldest form of the great Sanskrit language, which became the prime medium of India and South Asian culture throughout the centuries. Many thinkers regard Sanskrit as the most perfect language in the world, the most scientifically formed and mantrically powerful. It reflects the deeper knowledge behind the Vedic understanding of sound and vibration. Sanskrit as a Rishi language requires such a great Rishi culture to produce and sustain it.

Historical Implications

Archaeologically speaking, the *Vedas* can be linked to the monumental "Indus-Sarasvati culture" or "Harappan culture" that flourished on the banks of the great Sarasvati River in Northwest India up to its drying up around four thousand years ago. The antecedents of this culture go back to the beginning of agriculture in the region some ten thousand years ago.

The Sarasvati River, which flowed east of the Indus and parallel to it, was a large river in North India in early ancient times, fed by the end of the Ice Age glacial melting and stronger regional monsoons. It began to decline by 3000 BCE,[59] near the beginning of the main urban Harappan era. By 1900 BCE or the end of the Harappan era, it had diminished into a seasonal stream. For those interested in a detailed account of the *Vedas* relative to ancient history, there are several books that can be consulted for more information.[60] For archaeological information, note the books of Professor B.B. Lal.[61] I will provide a short summary of this information here.

Many readers may be familiar with the Aryan Invasion Theory (AIT) that has been used to explain the history of ancient India, and which still occurs in history textbooks worldwide. This theory proposes that a group of people it calls Aryans, generally regarded as a Caucasian ethnic group and identified with the Vedic people, entered Northwest India around 1500 BCE as intruders from Central Asia, and overthrew the existing culture (often regarded as Dravidian in nature).

To put the case briefly, however, no solid evidence to prove this theory has ever been found. Whatever evidence of this type has been proposed has not stood the test of time. To date there is no evidence of any Aryan skeletons, Aryan horses, Aryan chariots, encampments, or native cities destroyed by the invading Aryans. There is so far nothing in the archaeological record that can be identified with any incoming Aryan peoples apart from the existing populations of India. Such proposed evidence like Wheeler's massacre at Mohenjodaro was found to have been only a graveyard, not a massacre. There is also no conclusive genetic evidence of such an influx from Central Asia. In fact, genetic evidence shows the continuity of the same peoples in India going back tens of thousands of years, with a greater gene flow out of India than into it.

Given this lack of solid data, some scholars have proposed instead of an Aryan Invasion, some sort of migration of small groups of so-called Aryans, an "Aryan Migration Theory." Such incoming Aryans were said to be able to change the language and culture of India, but came in such small numbers that no evidence of their arrival is likely to be found, either archaeologically or in terms of genetics. Their entry is usually placed after the end of the Harappan era, as there is no sign that this great civilization came to an end by external interference.

This Aryan migration theory, however, seems to be an attempt to avoid the need to produce any positive evidence, and cannot stand on its own without some hard data to support it. A small, largely pastoral group such as the Aryans are proposed to be, cannot change a subcontinent that has already been highly civilized and populated, without more solid evidence of their movements.

The decline of civilization in India in the period from 2200-1500 BCE at the end of the Harappan age is now attributed to ecological changes and the drying up of rivers, notably a large river in the northwest of India that is described in Vedic texts as the Sarasvati homeland of the Vedic people. No intruding Aryans are necessary for this. The *Rigveda* reflects the geography of India when the Sarasvati was a great river "pure in its course from the mountains to the sea,"[62] which was probably before 3000 BCE, with later Vedic texts, noting the progressive drying up of the river. The *Mahabharata* speaks of the Sarasvati as *vinaśanam* or disappearing, no longer reaching the sea, but broken in its middle course, much as it was in the later Harappan era.[63] *Manu Smriti* speaks of the Vedic sacred land as between the Sarasvati and Drishadvati rivers, but has the Sarasvati disappearing in the desert and not reaching the sea.[64] The Vedic people not only knew of this great Sarasvati River, but also were aware of the phases of its drying up over long periods of time.

The Indus-Sarasvati or *Harappan* culture, the culture of north India from around 3500- 1500 BCE, was the largest urban civilization of the world at the time, greater in extent than contemporary civilizations such as Egypt and Mesopotamia, and it hosted a larger population. It was more uniform in its building standards and designs. We should note that Harappan seals and artifacts abound with fire altars, water tanks, swastikas, pippal tree motifs, sacred bulls, Shiva lingas, deities in sitting meditation postures, and other Vedic symbols and artifacts, showing a continuity of art and spirituality into later times.[65]

It must be remembered that the Vedic tradition is a massive, pluralistic tradition carried on over thousands of years, and cannot be identified with a single culture or one particular historical era only. Similar to later Hindu culture that looks back to it, the *Vedas* contain a great abundance of deities, great teachers, and teachings. We cannot simply identify the *Vedas* only with the Harappan era. Harappan culture likely reflects later phases of the Vedic age, not its full extent or its origins. There were probably other civilizational trends in ancient India as well as the Vedic, as India as a vast subcontinent has always had a variety of cultures. In the late Vedic age, other influences arose, including trends that we see in non-Vedic schools like the Buddhist and Jain.

The existing compilation of the *Vedas*, which is attributed to Vyasa Krishna Dvaipayana, is said to be the twenty-eighth, reflecting a much larger teaching and greater antiquity. Earlier Vedic compilations are attributed to great sages and

Rishis going back to the time of Manu.[66] Similarly, ancient lists of kings in India, such as occur in the *Puranas*, are extensive and suggest a very ancient culture. Megasthenes, in the fragments of his *Indika* quoted by classical sources, records that the Hindus then had a record of 153 kings going back 6451 years and three months before the time of Alexander the Great to Dionysus, the reputed first Indian king.[67] This takes us back to a time before 6700 BCE.

The *Rigveda* as we have it does not represent the beginning of the Vedic teaching, but demonstrates a complex, integrated, and diverse teaching of many sages and seers that must have taken considerable time to evolve. This means that existing Vedic texts, notably the *Rigveda*, are a window into a vaster ancient culture, not simply the first such teachings to come into existence.

The Vedic corpus as a whole is the most extensive literary work out of India until the time of the *Mahabharata*. The Vedic corpus requires a great civilization to produce, support and sustain it. This would be a great kingdom or empire and long dynasties, not simply haphazard productions of wandering nomads. The *Vedas* are like spiritual pyramids of the mind and require a great and enduring culture like that of ancient Egypt in order to explain their existence and perpetuation.

Universality of Vedic Dharma

If one examines Vedic literature, one does not find the idea of religions in the modern sense of the term, as competing belief systems or theologies of salvation, seeking to convert all peoples. The Vedic approach is that of *Sanatana Dharma*, an eternal dharma, a universal order of enlightenment that is relevant to all creatures. The Vedic sacred fire or Agni, the foundation of both outer Vedic rituals and inner Vedic Yoga practices of mantra and meditation, is first of all a power of Dharma, a Dharmic striving to truth.

> *Enkindled according to the original Dharmas, he who carries all blessings is anointed with light, whose hair is radiant, who is anointed with ghee, the purifier, the good sacrifice, Agni to worship the Divine powers.*[68]
>
> *Kata Vaishvamitra, Rigveda III.17.1*

The *Vedas* emphasize *Manava Dharma*, the "Dharma of humanity," which is inwardly to seek the Divine and outwardly to care for all life as sacred.[69] The *Vedas* speak to all humanity and to all nature, through the Divine power that pervades the universe. The Vedic hymns are mainly directed to the deity in order to help it manifest within us, which their mantras seek to invoke. The *Vedas* constitute a "dialogue with Divinity," offering everyone who is sincere and receptive the opportunity to participate in that dialogue. The deity though One in essence is accessible through many names, forms, and practices. It is not an abstract principle but a living reality within each person, reflected in all the rhythms of life.

The *Vedas* constitute a mantric *Dharma Shastra*, or guidebook to right action in life. There are many levels of dharma in the universe, reflecting our right relationship with all of existence. There is a dharmic way to use the human body, which is as a tool of conscious evolution, such as Ayurveda teaches us. There is a dharmic way to structure society. This means a society that aims at the development of consciousness as its prime value and allows each individual to unfold this according to her or his nature. Of most importance, our highest dharma is to seek the eternal truth and bring it into our lives. The Vedic tradition emphasizes liberation or *Moksha Dharma* as the ultimate goal of all our strivings. Yoga dharma is key portion of *Moksha Dharma*, its practical side, and is the highest dharma (principle and duty).

The *Vedas* and the Goals of Life

The *Vedas* are concerned not only with the spiritual quest, but also contain teachings on culture, art, science, and society, including guidelines to right living for all types of individuals. The *Vedas* teach Moksha or liberation through Yoga practice, but also honor the ordinary goals of life as *Dharma*, *Artha* and *Kama*.

There are Vedic hymns that extol wealth accumulated dharmically, with a sense of sacrifice and charity, as a worthy goal, the 'Way of the Merchant' or *Vaishya Dharma*. There are Vedic hymns that extol victory in a righteous battle, the 'Way of the Warrior' or the *Kshatriya Dharma*. This is more evident in the *Brahmana* texts that outline specific rituals for the ordinary goals of life of wealth, progeny, and marriage. Such Vedic rituals for all the goals of life are still commonly performed in India today.

Unfortunately, some scholars fail to see that in honoring the lower goals of life in the *Vedas* that the higher goal of liberation is not excluded. They would reduce the *Veda* only to a seeking of wealth, victory, or outer success in life. It should be noted that the *Vedas* can teach different goals in the same mantras, relative to how we understand the symbolism. The same Vedic hymns that at an outer level may appear to be extolling wealth or victory can have an inner meaning relative to the wealth of spiritual knowledge or victory over the forces of ignorance.

This multileveled teaching is not unique or surprising in the *Vedas*, which themselves refer to different levels of interpretation. In later Hindu thought, extending to the *Puranas* and *Tantras*, a deity like the Goddess Lakshmi can be pursued for the outer wealth of gold or the inner wealth of devotion. The same classical Sanskrit hymns to the deities can be used to gain Dharma, Artha, Kama, or Moksha. The same is true of the *Vedas*.

While the *Vedas* can be used for the ordinary goals of life, that constitutes their secondary or outward application. The Vedic teachings derive from the samadhi of the Rishis, from the flow of Soma through the Sushumna or central channel of the subtle body into the mind and heart. Vedic mantras reflect a yogic language for which a yogic meaning can be found in verses that seem to be of outer value only. While it is wrong to deny the value of the *Vedas* for the outer goals of life, it is a greater mistake to think that this outer pursuit is the true import of the *Vedas*. The *Vedas* use the veil of the outer human life, just as an outer nature, to conceal the inner search for a higher realization, which was the prime focus of the Vedic Rishis.

The *Vedas* and Later Teachings in India

The *Vedas* form the core teaching of many later ways of knowledge in India and many branches of spiritual literature. The *Vedas* are the foundation for the other branches of Vedic knowledge, the *Brahmanas, Aranyakas*, and *Upanishads*. They are accepted as authoritative by Ayurveda and Vedic astrology, which count among the various *Upavedas* (secondary Vedic teachings) and *Vedangas* (limbs of the *Vedas*). The *Vedas* are accepted as authoritative for the *Six Darshanas*, or "six schools of Vedic philosophy," including Samkhya, Yoga, and the many schools of Vedanta, which constitute *Smriti* (remembered) literature that follows the Vedic revelation or *Shruti*.[70]

The *Vedas* contain the seeds from which the *Upanishads* developed their direct approaches to Self-realization, along with the core insights from which the different types of traditional Yoga arose. The *Rigveda*, understood at an inner level, is the first *Upanishad* and the first *Yoga Shastra* or guidebook of Yoga. Yet the *Rigveda* relates to other branches of sacred literature as well. The *Rigveda* is the original or seed form of the *Puranas*, the massive encyclopedic texts of Hindu knowledge and culture. In the Vedic hymns one can find the origins of classical Sanskrit poetry and Hindu devotional chanting. The *Vedas* do not reflect an intrusive culture imposed upon India from the outside, but an organic development of spiritual knowledge and culture inside of India.

The Vedic Yoga in the Modern World

Many people in the world today have studied Yoga in one form or another, and know something about it. Many have heard of the *Vedas* and their spiritual value. Yet few of these understand the Vedic roots of the Yoga tradition or the Vedic Yoga that exists behind the earliest Yoga teachings. Most Yoga students and teachers today focus on contemporary asana approaches, and emphasize recent Yoga movements.

A few fragments of the Vedic Yoga are known to modern Yoga students, such as the Gayatri Mantra and the chanting of Oṁ. Even in India, the full extent of the older

Vedic Yoga has been largely forgotten after several thousand years of derivative teachings. The original Vedic root has been obscured by the very luxuriance of its leaves, flowers, and fruit. Though a number of Vedic mantras continue to be recited by many groups in India, particularly for ritualistic purposes, the deeper Yoga behind these mantras is rarely examined.

A few notable efforts to present Vedic teachings to the world at large, however, have occurred in recent years. Most popular and influential has been the 'TM' or 'Transcendental Meditation' system of Maharshi Mahesh Yogi that emphasizes the importance of the *Vedas* along with Vedic sciences of Ayurveda, Vedic astrology, and Vastu. These have become known worldwide largely because of his efforts. Maharishi's global work has brought the eminence of Vedic knowledge to the global mind, bringing a recognition of humanity's global Vedic heritage.

Many other Yoga and Vedanta groups throughout the world have brought attention and respect to the *Vedas*, even if they have not overtly taught Vedic mantras or offered interpretations of Vedic deities. Great Yogis from India like Paramahansa Yogananda, the first great Indian guru to live in America, and his guru Sri Yukteswar, have indicated the Vedic Yoga as the basis of their own teachings.[71] Yukteswar dates Manu of the *Rigveda* well before 6700 BCE[72] and has similar ideas about the antiquity of the *Vedas*. Yogananda's famous Kriya Yoga pranayama technique represents an inner Vedic fire sacrifice that is yogic in nature.

This global Vedic movement arises from a "Return to the *Vedas* movement," which began in earnest in nineteenth century India. The first major impetus for a Vedic revival in modern India came from the 'Arya Samaj', founded by Swami Dayananda Sarasvati in the nineteenth century. The Arya Samaj remains one of the largest movements in modern Hinduism and is based on a study and practice of Vedic teachings going back to the *Rigveda*. Sri Aurobindo – one of the dominant figures of modern India and its renaissance – based his new Supramental evolutionary Yoga on a Vedic model.[73] Sri Aurobindo brought out new translations and interpretations of many Vedic mantras, a trend that his disciples continue to follow.

The call to "Return to the *Vedas*" had a strong impact on the Indian independence movement from its inception. Sri Aurobindo himself was originally an important political figure who could have become the leader of the Indian independence movement, but chose to retire from politics to pursue his integral Yoga. Aurobindo's approach to the *Vedas* was aimed at a global audience as well as for reviving the soul of India. B.G. Tilak, the main figure in the independence movement before Mahatma Gandhi and a mentor of Aurobindo, wrote on the *Vedas*.

The value of the *Vedas* was taken up by several western spiritual groups in the nineteenth century, notably the Theosophical Movement, which was active at that time throughout the world. Its founder, H.P. Blavatsky, speaks highly of the Vedic Rishis and states that the *Vedas* were composed largely at Manasarovar, by Mount Kailas in Tibet.[74] She connected the Vedic Rishis with a group of ascended masters, several of whom had Vedic names. A good example of this Vedic influence is the importance of Agni, the prime Vedic deity, in the writings of Alice Bailey from whom much of western New Age thought arose. The New Age movement in the West reflects a Vedic influence, embracing the ideas of karma, rebirth, the higher Self, and oneness, though it does have other trends and associations.

Meanwhile, the colonial era in India brought about a new western Vedic scholarship, with European and American Vedic scholars arising, often working under government patronage. However, this western study of the *Vedas*, we should note, was not born of Yoga, mantra, or meditation. It followed new approaches derived from new western disciplines of linguistics, anthropology, comparative religion, and comparative mythology for which the *Vedas* were museum pieces, not living sources of inspiration. Such western scholars largely dismissed the Indian and Yogic scholarship on the *Vedas* and took their own angle of approach. They opposed or ignored the Vedic views born of the new Vedic renaissance in India.

This colonial Vedic scholarship was followed by several western educated scholars in India, especially the Indian Marxists, who remain a strong force in India's educational system to the present day. It formed the background for modern psychological interpretations of the *Vedas* following Freudian approaches. Curiously a Jungian approach to the *Vedas* was not developed, though it would likely have had a deeper sensitivity to the spiritual meaning of Vedic symbols. I would not say that such academic work has no validity, but it does not provide an adequate vehicle for uncovering the yogic secrets of the Vedic mantras.

This means that most of the available scholarship on the *Vedas*, particularly in the West, reflects an intellectual and cultural orientation that cannot likely appreciate the depths of Yoga, or reveal its ancient roots. Such scholars placed the *Vedas* within the same group of primitive religious teachings that they did the Native American, ancient Egyptian, Gnostic, and other ancient and native traditions (which they similarly failed to appreciate as possessing any deeper mysticism).

The result is that the Yoga community in the West and in India rarely understands the Vedic Yoga or the Vedic roots of the Yoga tradition. This is in spite of the fact that many of the same individuals recognize that ancient cultures East and West had deeper spiritual teachings, that have much in common. Just as there has recently been a positive reevaluation of many native traditions, the time is ripe for a new look at the *Vedas*.

The Rishis and the Ancient Seer Orders

Throughout the ancient world we can discover stories of extraordinary sages, seers, and Yogis possessing great wisdom and magical powers, who gave early humanity its first religion, culture, language, and medicine. Whether it is China, Egypt, Babylonia, Mexico, Peru, Hawaii, or India, the names of these figures vary but their essential teachings and practices remain similar, connecting humanity with the sacred universe and the powers of light and consciousness behind it.

These early ancient sages founded priestly orders and sacred families to carry on their legacy and transmit their knowledge to future generations. They developed secret teachings and mystical traditions, mainly oral in nature, even when writing was known. Such esoteric teachings were deliberately veiled to protect the sacred lore from the worldly-minded. The teachings required special initiations and the following of strict disciplines in order to receive and understand their real import. Such early ancient teachings set in motion our collective spiritual aspiration at the dawn of history. The great religions and philosophies of the later ancient world – such as those of classical Greece, Israel, or India two to three thousand years ago – appear to be but sparks or embers of these greater traditions from their closing period.

The Rishi Tradition: The Legacy of the Ancient Seers

The *Vedas* reflect the teachings of the Rishis and represent the Rishi tradition. *Rishi*, which literally means a seer, stands not only for the ancient sages at the beginning of this world-age, but also for the very principles or dharmas of conscious evolution.[75] The Rishis are not merely human sages but spiritual powers of the cosmic mind. This Rishi tradition is far more extensive than the Vedic texts that have been preserved. The Rishi tradition is a continual tradition of spiritual and cultural knowledge that comprehends the very fabric of creation as well as the Absolute beyond time and space. The Himalayan Yogis have maintained this core Rishi knowledge across the millennia, dispensing it in many forms through Yoga, Vedanta, Ayurveda, and Tantra. The Rishis remain as a continual light of truth for the world, some in human bodies, and some guiding us from higher planes of consciousness.

The Rishis represent the seed-consciousness behind our world. It is said in the *Vedas* that the Rishis created these worlds and we are their progeny. The Rishis reflect the core creative intelligence behind all that exists. In this sense the Rishis are co-creators with the Gods. We could say that the Rishis represent the DNA or archetypal powers of consciousness that are necessary for any world to come into existence. The Rishis remain inside of us as our deepest essence of spiritual knowledge and aspiration.

Towards a Reassessment of the Ancient World

Current science now estimates that our human species dates around two hundred thousand years, based on the "Out of Africa" theory. Alternative theories of multiple locations for the human species may put the time of our species back to two million years. Up to the twentieth century, scholars were working on a largely five thousand year time line for human civilization. Now scholars are willing to place the origins of agriculture back more than ten thousand years or prior to the end of the last Ice Age.

A glaring time gap remains, however. What did human beings do for the previous 190,000 years or more? Was there no language, culture, civilization, art, or spirituality during that long period? All ancient traditions – whether of China, India, Egypt, Mesopotamia, or the Americas – speak of earlier humanities, civilizations, and world ages (yugas). What we regard as the first civilizations had a memory of advanced humanities and great sages long before them, often prior to a great flood or deluge that can easily be identified with the end of the last Ice Age some ten thousand years ago. There are now many tens of thousands of years for humanity in which such prior cultures can be possibly placed, and probably all over the world.

Was the beginning of civilization that we see starting after the end of the last Ice Age the beginning of civilization overall, or just the beginning of a new era in civilization? The ending of the Ice Age was a cataclysmic event much greater than anything that we could imagine today through current Global Warming and Climate Change scenarios. At that ancient time, ocean levels rose more than three hundred feet, flooding extensive areas of the world. Global temperature and rainfall patterns changed radically, with massive melting of glaciers and warming up of northern regions. Such powerful climate changes could easily disrupt or destroy any existing civilizations, particularly if these were centered in coastal regions as most urban areas have been historically. It would have caused people to move to new regions inland and new cultures to arise in these areas.

I have always aligned my examination of the *Vedas* with an examination of the ancient world as a whole. I would not view Vedic India as a completely unique or isolated phenomenon. The same type of yogic spirituality that we find in the *Vedas* has its counterparts throughout the ancient world. Other Indo-European traditions, like the Persian, Celtic, and Greek, have Vedic affinities that include traditions of great sages, druids, or spiritual masters. A similar great tradition existed in ancient Egypt that had a profound occult and spiritual knowledge. Ancient Egypt shares many symbols with the Vedic including the falcon, the Sun, the sacred bull, and the cobra. India and Mesopotamia were in extensive trade contact well before 2000 BCE, giving the opportunity for many cultural interchanges.

Looking to East Asia, we find that the Taoist tradition of China has much in common with the Vedic. It has a similar tradition of seven sages and great Yogis in the Himalayas, along with special Yoga practices. Shinto in Japan is similar with its worship of the Sun. All native traditions even today have much in common with ancient spirituality like that of the *Vedas*, honoring all nature as sacred. The native traditions of Africa, the Americas, Asia, and the Pacific Islands resemble the ancient nature religions of Europe, India, the Near East, China, and Japan.

The Rishi, the Yogi and the Shaman

The Vedic Rishi is a Raja Yogi, one who knows and has mastered the inner Yoga of mantra, meditation, pranayama, ritual, and service. Yet the Rishi is also a bit of a Shaman, in the sense of one who is able to work with the forces of nature, fire and water, Sun, Moon, stars, and lightning.

It is likely that the Rishi, Yogi, and Shamanic traditions of humanity are linked together and are all very ancient. Beyond what may appear to us as primitive Shamanistic cults contained deeper traditions of Yogis and Rishis, though perhaps limited in numbers and secretive in nature. There were likely Rishis and Yogis present in many Shamanic traditions going back tens of thousands of years.

We should note that the pursuit of higher consciousness has never been limited to technological cultures, much less to literate cultures. It is as old as humanity. It is hard to imagine that over the last two hundred thousand years there were no great sages in humanity, even if outwardly there was not much by way of technology. The great Rishi did not need technology but could control his own body and mind as well as access occult forces in order to understand the cosmic mind directly.

The *Vedas* likely preserve the ancient Shamanic traditions of humanity, showing their spiritual dimensions. The cult of the sacred fire, the sacred plant, sacred baths and waters, sacred mountains and rivers, sacred music, dance and drumming are not only Vedic, but also part of the natural religion of all humanity. They have an inner reality, not just an outer form, with the sacred fires and waters that exist within our own psyches.

This Shamanistic side we find not only in Vedic deities, but also in Lord Shiva. Shiva, the supreme Vedic deity, is very much the great deity of Shamanic traditions. Shiva as the sky God, whose forms are the Fire (Agni), Moon (Soma), Sun (Surya), and Lightning (Indra), resembles the Shamanic sky God as well. The search for any original Shamanic tradition of humanity should be aligned with the idea of older yogic and Rishi traditions, noting their similarities.

The *Vedas* and the Search for a New Evolutionary Transformation

In the Vedic view we live in a "conscious universe," not merely a matter, energy, or mind based cosmos. Consciousness is the underlying substance, force, and reality that creates, sustains, and dissolves all things in the world, constituting their inner essence. Consciousness, we could say, is God, not in a mere theological or faith-based sense, but as the supreme principle of life and existence. We are all aspects of this supreme consciousness reflecting itself in various forms and manifestations, like sparks from a single fire.

This underlying universal consciousness the *Vedas* call the *Purusha*, meaning the cosmic person, the Supreme Being for whom the entire universe is its expression, which is lauded starting in the *Rigveda*.

> *The Purusha is everything, what has been and what will be. And he is the lord of immortality.*[76]
> *Rishi Narayana, Rigveda X.97.2*

The *Vedas* use the term *Atman* as a synonym for *Purusha*, meaning the true Self behind every creature or object in the world. The entire universe consists of a single being, and the world of nature is but the body of the greater cosmic spirit. The universe is a single organism energized by a single consciousness that resides at the core of all creatures and behind the inanimate world as well.

What we call Nature is primarily a force of consciousness in manifestation. Nature reflects the unfoldment of an organic intelligence, through which the One Being expresses itself through innumerable forms of becoming. We can observe this natural intelligence in the wonderful order of the universe that transcends the rational mind and its limiting concepts. Who has not confronted the magic, mystery and awe of existence? It is obvious in the mountains, the clouds, the stars, and the ocean. It is also there in the marvelous workings of our own bodies and minds, in the wonderful intricacy of our organs, tissues, and brain.

Nature operates according to a natural law or Dharma, which has both a material and a spiritual basis, as a law of consciousness. The conscious universe has not only physical laws like gravity that link various material bodies together, it has spiritual laws like *karma* that link various minds together as well. The *Vedas* mirror this natural intelligence and teach us the true laws of nature, the universal *dharmas*, which are also the laws of consciousness.

Consciousness is our true nature, our higher Self beyond body and mind. Consciousness is also the natural state or original condition of all beings. It is the basis of our sense of self internally and constitutes the ground of all existence externally. The forms that we observe in the outer world do not represent the true essence of reality, but are only intimations of a greater spirit and awareness lighting them up from within. Consciousness is the inner space that informs all aspects of space within and around all things.

At the core of nature as its underlying energy and secret intelligence is this universal consciousness. When we look at the world, we are looking only at the shapes and colors created by the light of consciousness. It is the light of consciousness that we see reflected in objects, filtered through the limited lens of the mind. It is also the light of consciousness that constitutes the true seer or observer within us, and allows us to see.

True spirituality works with the entire conscious universe and seeks grace and guidance everywhere. It is not time-bound, human-bound, or culture bound. This is the basis of the Vedic and yogic heritage that belongs to all beings. The Purusha, which literally means person, does not refer simply to the human person, but to the principle of light and awareness that endows all beings with their sense of self, the conscious being overall. In the Vedic view, the universe is light and light is consciousness. This is the 'Purusha principle'. The goal of classical Yoga as stated by the sage Patanjali, as well as the goal of all other Vedic philosophies, is to return to the state of the Purusha, pure consciousness or the seer, which is to return to the highest light.[77] This echoes the Upanishadic view, "The Purusha in the Sun beyond, He am I."[78] This inner vision takes us beyond the outer forms and laws of the universe to the awareness, freedom, and creativity behind it.

The *Vedas* teach us that consciousness is the ultimate essence hidden in all things and evolving through them by the vehicle of the mind. The *Vedas* teach a Yoga of light for extracting the light of consciousness within ourselves and from the world around us. They show us how to move from our lower nature to our higher nature, which is the natural development of our being and its inner light. Matter is crystallized light. Life is light in motion. Mind is light that perceives. Yet consciousness is the supreme light beyond and behind all.

Vedic philosophy discriminates between the Purusha, the cosmic person, and Prakriti, the organic mechanism of nature. Prakriti is the natural force governing the body and mind, and the forces of the universe. It constitutes the body and mind of the Purusha at a cosmic level as the different worlds or lokas. Our true nature, which is the true nature of the entire universe, is the Purusha or pure consciousness. There is a Purusha in every natural phenomenon. The *Vedas* speak of the Purusha in the Sun, Moon, Fire, Lightning, and Water, or the Purusha in all the forms of light. The Purusha is not only within us, but also within all that we see.

The *Vedas* work to lift our awareness from the outer movement of nature or Prakriti to its higher yogic realization in the Purusha. To this end the Vedic Yoga helps us let go of the habits, addictions, and inertia that weigh down body and mind, which are but the shadow of Prakriti, and develops our higher nature in consciousness that is not mechanical. It teaches us to look within, and to recognize the inner dimension in all that we observe externally.

Yoga as the Natural Unfoldment of Consciousness

Yoga is a science of Self-realization, a methodology of returning to our true nature that is neither body nor mind but pure consciousness. Consciousness is our internal real nature as opposed to the body and mind that constitute our external apparent nature. Consciousness is our eternal nature as opposed to body and mind that are our transient nature. We could say that we are the ocean of consciousness and the body and mind are but waves at its surface that come and go without affecting our true essence. It is our basic ignorance that we confuse who we really are with our changing instruments of outer expression.

The true practice of Yoga consists of moving from nature to nature, going from our outer nature as a physical being to our inner nature as conscious awareness. Yoga is not about the denial of nature or the suppression of natural tendencies. It is about reaching the higher levels of our nature, in which the lower levels are transcended. Each aspect of our nature exists like a step for us to rise in consciousness, towards the eventual goal that is beyond time and space. While each step has its purpose, merely to stay on that step and not continue to climb becomes regressive. Each step is a means of ascent, not an end in itself. At the highest step we move beyond all stages altogether!

This means that Yoga, though using nature, does not accept following our natural tendencies blindly, as we ordinarily experience them to be through our ordinary desires, habits, and beliefs. Nature contains many potentials, of which our actual current given nature is only one possibility – and generally not the highest. Hidden in nature is an evolutionary power that compels creatures to go beyond their evolutionary programming and strive for new and higher levels of action, expression, and self-realization. Yoga requires harnessing nature's evolutionary power and secret intelligence, which means going beyond our past to the higher future hidden within us.

Yoga works with the forces of nature for their higher possibilities within us, not merely for what these may appear to be at the present moment. Everything in the universe is not what it appears to be. We ourselves are not what we appear to be. Appearance is as much a veil as it is a manifestation, as much a covering as a revelation. Just as fire is hidden in wood, so behind all appearances are inner powers and higher possibilities. Each one of us can be much more than what we currently are. We contain in our inner consciousness the power of all things, the omnipotential of which the current time-space universe is only one manifestation.

Yoga teaches us to use nature to transform nature. It employs the forces of the body, breath, speech, and mind in order to develop a higher consciousness beyond them. Yoga works with the capacities that we have, seeking to develop them in an organic manner. It does not reduce us to our current state of development or status quo, but takes the seeds of the higher light within us in order to draw us to our highest potential. We could compare our ordinary nature to the condition of milk. Yoga is about churning out the butter inherent in the milk. It is not about accepting milk as it is. Nor is it trying to turn milk into something that it is not, like wine or water.

The world of nature is filled with many different capacities for transformation, hidden substances and energies that can manifest under the right circumstances. Another example is that of metal, like gold hidden in an ore. Yoga is about extracting the gold from the ore. It is not about accepting the ore as it is as gold. Nor is it about trying to get something from the ore that is not there, like trying to extract wood out of it.

Nature is never in a static condition. We are always evolving, which is the dimension of Shakti or creative power. Yoga propels us in our conscious evolution toward Self-realization. Yoga enables us to develop our higher qualities and faculties, which requires an application of heat, the "fire of Yoga" or *Yogagni*, to use Vedic terms. That is why Agni is the first deity of the *Vedas*. It is the fire that quickens, ripens, and develops all other potentials. The *Vedas* are a means of developing our own higher nature, not merely some foreign or ancient religion.

Vedic View of Evolution: The Return to the Absolute

The Vedic view of the universe, like that of modern science, is evolutionary in orientation, recognizing a progressive development of subtler powers and beings throughout the universe. But the Vedic view differs from materialistic science in its understanding of who and what is evolving. In the Vedic view, evolution is primarily an evolution of consciousness or spirit through the instrumentality of the mind. Any evolution of matter or form is a by-product of a deeper inner evolution, not the main movement, as it usually has been in the view of modern science since Darwin.

Ultimately in the Vedic view, we are inherently one with the supreme consciousness that transcends the mind, that exists in its own nature beyond all time and space, and all outer experiences, energies, and phenomena. Our true awareness is one with the Absolute and Supreme Brahman. It is the mind that is evolving in its ability to recognize and reflect that immutable truth.

Evolution is but a changing outer appearance of an inner reality that is beyond all change and limitation. The evolution of consciousness is but a return to one's true Self and awareness beyond time and space. It is not the production of anything new, but a recognition of who we really are. This means that though the Vedic view of the universe is evolutionary, its view of reality and of the Self transcends all evolution – an important distinction to remember. Evolution is a play of Maya or illusion through which the Divine consciousness hides itself in the manifest world and then rediscovers itself through the human being.

Devas and Souls

For the ancient Vedic seers, the great forces and formations of nature are houses of the Gods or cosmic powers. The indwelling deity is the main factor, not the outer temporary structure in which it may reside for a time. These invisible Godheads or powers of consciousness are the real factors behind the world development, shaping it from within by their will and concentration. The Vedic teaching aims to further the evolution of consciousness by aligning the human being with the cosmic energies that are hidden behind all that natures does.

The Devas or Divine powers work to unfold the potentials of consciousness and intelligence in nature, through a progressive layer-by-layer development. They provide the background support for the evolution of living creatures, shaping their bodies, senses, and minds. The Devas sustain the worlds in which the individual soul takes birth and gains experience, governing the elemental processes behind them. The Devas are the great lords of light, life, mind, and consciousness.

Yet just as the Devas sustain the evolutionary process from behind, the individual soul (Jiva) takes birth in the worlds in order to carry the evolutionary process forward from within. The evolving soul holds the power of the Devas in an embodied form, just as the Devas oversee the process in non-embodied forces. There is a hidden divinity in all creatures, particularly in the human being that has the power of self-determination. We are incarnated in this world not for personal enjoyment but for the unfoldment of the cosmic spirit, of which the individual soul should be the power working at the forefront.

Evolution is brought about by the descent of the soul (Jiva) or consciousness principle into matter, which enters like a spark or flame that carries the seed of all that is to be evolved over the long course of time. That seed gradually ripens and grows in power and subtlety, unfolding new levels of manifestation hidden deep within itself. The soul gradually evolves and ascends through the kingdoms of nature, like moving up various steps, layers, or strata, which it also deposits along the way, just as fire creates ash as it burns. For each vertical ascent, the soul deposits a horizontal layer, which like a step becomes the means of its ascent to the next level. This constitutes the homeward journey of the soul to the Godhead from which it has arisen, but carrying all the powers of nature that it has developed along the way.

These layers that the soul creates are, on a general level, the different kingdoms of nature of the mineral, plant, animal, and human. On a specific level, they are the different bodies that the soul takes birth in and fashions further, the physical, pranic, emotional, mental, and spiritual forms that the soul works through. The process of the rebirth of the soul is the driving power in nature and provides continuity to the evolution of life and consciousness.

The Devas, like the soul, can descend into creation, but as governing spirits within the forces of nature in order to support the soul's ascent. The soul can call the Devas into manifestation out of knowledge and devotion, for their grace, guidance, and assistance. The Devas enter into matter in a general sense as pervasive powers, and presences. They do not take birth within the worlds as embodied creatures, but rather wear the forces of nature as their subtle vestures. Divine powers create and sustain the worlds that are the fields of evolution for the souls born into them.

This movement of the Devas is what we could call "celestial evolution." Its goal is the formation of various worlds like the planets and stars, along with the energy currents that link them together. The movement of the soul is what we could call the "creaturely evolution." Its goal is the formation of various bodies, until the soul has a sophisticated enough instrument to manifest its underlying cosmic consciousness and divinity that is rooted in the Supreme.

Yet these two movements of the Gods and the souls (Devas and Jivas) are interrelated. We could say that the soul is the instrument of the Gods for evolution inside the worlds, while the Gods are the powers of the soul for shaping the evolution of the worlds on the outside. Souls prior to their descent into matter can play the role of various Gods or cosmic powers. In their higher evolution through Yoga, they can experience the powers of the Gods once again inside themselves. In deep meditation, the soul can commune with any of the Devas up to the supreme Divinity.

There are innumerable souls latent in the kingdoms of nature, starting with the mineral kingdom that is spread throughout space and the stars. These souls are individualized powers, forms of embodied or creaturely existence. In addition, there are innumerable deities in nature, which are portions or manifestations of the cosmic Divine, not individualized and creaturely in nature.

Cosmic evolution sustains both a vertical and horizontal movement, spreading out the worlds and ascending through them. The vertical movement consists of developing new and more sophisticated species. The horizontal movement consists of expressing the full range of possibilities for each species within its field. We can examine this process in human beings. The force of vertical evolution drives us to the development of a higher consciousness beyond our current body and mind development, such as occurs in Yoga and the spiritual path in general. The force of horizontal evolution drives us to fully explore our bodily and mental faculties, such as in science and technology. Evolution continues on both horizontal and vertical planes. For example, some human beings will seek to develop a higher consciousness, while others seek to expand their physical, emotional, or intellectual powers further. Both levels can overlap, but the horizontal force usually predominates as it is hard to ascend without a base to rise from.

Nature seeks to develop all possibilities on both horizontal and vertical levels. The two processes can be complimentary, though the ascending evolutionary leaps in consciousness are the most significant in furthering nature's growth. The vertical ascent, like a new adventure, involving a radical change, a vertical leap beyond the human, will naturally be for only the few. The masses of human beings will naturally gravitate towards a horizontal expansion of ordinary human possibilities, which mainly consists of external forms of enjoyment. The few who take up the daunting and daring vertical ascent are aiming at the creation of a new consciousness, or perhaps a new more intelligent species. The *Veda* addresses both vertical and horizontal movements, while making the vertical movement central and the essence of the Vedic aspiration.

There is a complexity and intricacy of life-forms and species on all levels both horizontal and vertical. Lower life forms continue to evolve as higher life forms develop, though the lower life forms tend to diminish in prominence as higher life forms come to predominate. For example, flowers have evolved only with mammals. The plant kingdom has continued to develop though the animal kingdom has long surpassed it in the complexity of life expression.

Of most importance in this movement of cosmic evolution of life, the human being is a transitional species designed at its highest expression to facilitate the vertical ascent from matter to spirit, from nature to super-nature. This we can observe in the fact that only very rare human beings can attain Self-realization and God realization. In its normal condition, the human being is the ultimate form of the material manifestation, seeking its greatest expansion in the outer world, only sensing inner spiritual realities in the distance, if at all, preferring its own worldly pleasure, power, and possessions. The human species overall has more a horizontally expanding energy than a vertical ascending force, and can become inimical to the spiritual ascent which appears destabilizing to its worldly urges. That is why the masses of human beings have often opposed or oppressed the few spiritual masters that have been able to take birth in the human world.

Devas and Asuras

Natural evolution proceeds from the lower to the higher, from the gross to the subtle, from the unrefined to the refined. It strives to develop divine energies out of what are at a lower level materialistic, elemental, and animal forces.

Besides the "evolutionary force," however, both complementary to it and serving as a restraint upon it, is an "anti-evolutionary force." This anti-evolutionary force works to sustain existent forms and forces in the universe and resist their change, sublimation, and evolution. While the evolutionary force tends to move upwards, ascending to a higher level, the anti-evolutionary force tends to move outwards, expanding potentials on the same level of manifestation. At times, the anti-evolutionary force can even move downwards, trying to reverse the course of higher evolution, particularly resisting new developments that can challenge the existing evolutionary order. The anti-evolutionary force can work to bring out egoistic and undivine energies, extending into what we can call "evil." It can have a negative affect, seeking to suspend the development of consciousness and make the minds of creatures more ignorant and destructive.

While the evolutionary force in Vedic thought is that of the *Devas* or Divine powers, the force that resists evolution is that of the *Asuras* or "anti-Gods."[79] The Devas are the powers of light and truth, whereas the Asuras are the powers of darkness and falsehood. The Devas represent our Godward aspiration, whereas the Asuras represent our worldly ambitions. The Devas reflect the virtue and receptivity of *sattva guna*, the quality of purity. The Asuras reflect the turbulence of *rajo-guna*, the quality of aggression, leading to tamas, darkness, and inertia. The Devas bring about an evolution of higher capacities, while the Asuras bring about expansion on the plane on which they exist. For example, the urge to transcend the world is largely of the Devas, while the impulse to conquer the world is largely Asuric.

The Devas relate to those souls who believe that consciousness is the Self, who are connected to the Deva forces within and around them. The Asuras are those souls who identify the Self with the body, who are connected to the Asura forces within and around them.[80] The Devas are the powers of Yoga and Self-realization, whereas the Asuras are the powers of Bhoga or enjoyment, and ego assertion. The Asuras strive to develop negative thoughts and emotions, expanding egoistic urges, rather than calming them, as do the Devas. The Devas relate to our higher intuitions and feelings; the Asuras relate to our baser instincts, desires, and aggression. The Devas represent our spiritual urges and sense of self in pure consciousness; the

Asuras represent our bodily identity. The Deva force is more present in the mind and sense organs and their perceptual capacities. The Asuric force is more present in the motor organs and pranas and their active tendencies.

Yet the Asuric force can serve a positive role in the evolution of consciousness. It can prevent the evolutionary force from moving too quickly. It assures the full development of horizontal evolutionary potentials, so that the movement of nature does not just simply jump from species to species but allows each species its development. However, on the spiritual path, the Asuric force is a primarily an obstacle that progressively grows as one ascends higher on the ladder of the worlds. Its power and danger should not be underestimated.

The Ongoing War Between the Devas and Asuras

Vedic thought reflects the clash or battle between the Devas and Asuras, though the term "Dasyu" is more common for the Asura in early Vedic literature.[81] The Vedic Yoga works with the Devas in order to further the ascent of the soul. For this reason, the Vedic Yoga gains the wrath of the Asuras or undivine forces that work to keep the soul from developing its higher potentials. Asuric energies frequently attack the Yogi and seek to weaken his practice, creating various obstacles, doubts, and contrary desires. This battle between the Devas and Asuras on the subtle planes is reflected on the earth, where the two powers struggle within the human soul and within human civilization, as the forces of dharma and adharma, truth and falsehood.

The human being in its soul is ultimately a Deva, a portion of the supreme Divine that can manifest its entirety. The more we move into our deeper being and core consciousness, the more the Deva force arises within us and the Asura energy is correspondingly weakened. Yet the more we get caught in the outer world through our identification with the physical body, the senses, and the motor organs, the more the Asura force rules us and draws us into greater Asuric currents of aggression and conflict.

Unfortunately, our present humanity by way of its culture and civilization, is predominantly an Asura species and has been so for thousands of years – at least since 3000 BCE when the greater materialistic era began. Our society is dominated by ego identity, conflict, violence, self-assertion, and self-aggrandizement. We have bred within our species, both in our karma and our physical DNA, violence against our own and other species: eating of meat, extensive use of drugs and intoxicants, gambling, sexual excesses and perversions, mind control, and black magic – indications of the Asura force. Even in Vedic times, the Asura force was strong and the Deva force could only defeat it with great effort and through a continual battle.

Yet there are Deva elements in all human beings and Deva aspects to humanity as a whole, extending to individuals, cultures, and communities. Each human being, however possibly Asura in behavior, contains the seed of the Deva on the inside that must eventually develop outwardly as well. In addition, there is always a special Deva humanity of mystics, yogis, artists, and free thinkers, regardless of the time or culture, including during what are considered to be dark ages. This Deva or yogic group, however, usually remains in the minority, in the background, and is commonly oppressed. It rarely exercises ruling power in the outer world.

Asuric powers usually dominate humanity at outer political, military, and economic levels, with few notable exceptions. The worldly power-seeking aspect of the Asura is quite comfortable with and easily becomes skillful in realms of political, military, and commercial influence and control. The Deva person is rarely a match for the Asura in worldly wiles or in the tenacity to promote himself.

The mass media today – with its powerful combination of illusion and technology – easily lends itself to the Asura force, which is comfortable with sensational outer displays. Our modern cult of media personalities – whether athletes, actors, politicians, or religious leaders – easily becomes a fertile ground for the Asura. The Asura, we should note, often has more charisma, or at least is a subject of more fascination than the Deva, whose mild and gentle manners are not as dramatic or stimulating! This we see in our culture fascination with bad boys, bad girls, graphic violence, and horror stories. In this regard, we should remember that the Asura has a strong relationship with the planet Venus for a power of seduction, hypnosis, glamour, and personality. The Asura is not simply a demon or an ogre but a powerful ego and mind, with a strong vital force that can lure and hypnotize.

Given the strong Asuric tendencies within the human race, even religion and spirituality can be taken over by Asuric forces and turned into instruments of conquest, war, and genocide. This is what we have seen throughout history, particularly in organized religion, with blind faith and dogma, crusades, and holy wars. The Asura force, with its outward orientation, is better at organization and developing material structures, resources, and institutions than is the Deva force that is introspective in nature. The *Vedas* tell us that whatever the Gods create, the Asuras make a counterfeit form of and then go on propagating it for their own benefit. Such Asuras in the guise of Devas are perhaps the greatest problem for humanity.

The Asura force does have its own mysticism. The Asura, being militant in nature, can take to strong ascetic and Yoga practices, mantra, and pranayama in order to achieve worldly power and prestige. At the extreme form, Asuric mysticism can degenerate into black magic, or the dark Tantra that seeks to harm, dominate, and hypnotize. Such militant and manipulative forms of mysticism can have their triumphs, which aim not to enlighten the individual but to control the masses. Yet at times an Asura can shift his passion to a Divine energy and become able to transcend his limitations and surrender to the Divine. While this is rare, the Vedic literature has examples as in the case of Prahlada.

The battle between the Devas and Asuras occurs at intellectual and cultural levels of humanity. The Devas promote yogic arts and sciences and a deeper seeking of truth, looking for a spiritual meaning to life and the universe. The Asuras promote the dominance and power of the body, senses, and outer mind, looking for a materialistic or political meaning to life and culture. Most of our current views of humanity, history, and civilization reflect an Asuric mindset that values outer technology over inner spirituality as the main movement of human history, which can end up glorifying the machine over the spirit.

It is clear to those whose inner eye is open: a new war between the Devas and Asuras is occurring today, with science and technology so far holding more an Asuric force, though Deva energies are struggling to emerge within them. We can expect this spiritual conflict to intensify in the decades to come, as global forces collide. The Deva force is aided by the fact that the earth itself is a Deva planet, and its planetary energies can arise to keep the Asuric forces in check, which the coming century is likely to experience. But the Asura force will remain difficult to defeat and seems always to find new ways of coming back and reinventing itself. We should carefully note that we cannot simply identify the Asuric force with any one group in humanity. It is a potential within all of us and can arise whenever we fail to honor a higher truth and compassion.

Our current largely Asuric humanity is hopefully coming to the phase in which more people will take to the Deva force and help it exert a greater influence in society. The Deva force must eventually triumph, though this is more a matter of long term human evolution, than the battles of a single generation. Though the current situation can seem dire and the Asuric force is well entrenched, the Deva force cannot be extinguished, and will always remain accessible to those who are sincere in their search for truth. What we need today is not pessimism facing the difficult challenges of our times, which will only make us weaker, but a new idealism to provide the positive energies to face all obstacles and promote a positive future for humanity, even if it may take some time to fully manifest.

The Power of the Vedic Mantras for a New Humanity

It is said that Vedic mantras have the power to destroy the Asuras, meaning to dispel the Asuric force of ignorance, aggression, and division. Certain Vedic verses form *astra mantras* or "weapon mantras" to eliminate these negative Asuric powers at a subtle level. Kavyakantha Ganapati Muni spoke of having rediscovered these astra mantras and knowing how to use them.

To overcome the Asuric force, we must first purify ourselves. The Asuric force dwells within each one of us. We cannot simply look upon it as the power of other people that we may not approve of. The weapons of the Gods work first of all for our own self-purification, not for attacking other people, though they can be used to promote the Divine force over the undivine for purification of the society. First the astra or weapon mantra must burn up one's own impurities and dissolve the ego. It awakens the purifying power of the inner Fire or Kundalini Shakti. Anyone who attempts to use astra mantras must accept this self-purification first or the mantras may be disturbing. These astras are the weapons of the Rishis and the Devas, not of us as individuals for our personal benefit. The ultimate astra is the 'Brahmastra', or the weapon of the Supreme Brahman, which eradicates all ignorance and Maya, revealing the sole reality of the Godhead.[82]

Vedic mantras, applied as part of a deep Vedic sadhana, have the power to create a new world age or *yuga* and a new humanity. They hold the keys to cosmic creation. Our higher evolutionary potential as a species can be unlocked through the right understanding and application of Vedic mantras. For this purpose, however, a mechanical repetition of the mantras is not enough. One must repeat the mantras along with the consciousness of the Rishis, which means that one needs to create an inner link to the Rishi consciousness and higher awareness in one's own heart.

The *Vedas* can take us back to the "consciousness of Manu," the primal human being or root state of human consciousness, in which a new Manu or new humanity can arise – implying a new mind and consciousness. This is perhaps the greatest gift of the *Vedas*, to seed a new *Veda* for the future. To bring about this inner revolution in humanity, we need a new group of Vedic Yogis, who have mastered deep sadhanas on all levels, as well as possessing a deep knowledge of Vedic mantras.

Sri Aurobindo alluded to this impending global change in his call for a Supramental humanity, a new type of human being reflecting divine energies rather than the powers of ignorance and karma that presently dominate us. Many yogic and spiritual traditions have looked to create such higher human beings. Clearly our current species needs to undergo a radical transformation at a very deep level, so that we can truly fulfill the ultimate human destiny of divinity. This is not a matter of one generation, but is a millennial concern.

The Rishis themselves are said to be manifestations of Manu and each Rishi carries special energies of human culture and spirituality. The Rishis are called world-makers, meaning that they can help create new species and new cultures. The Rishi does this through the power of consciousness within, not through genetic manipulation on the outside. The Rishi has the power to change karma, not simply to alter physical DNA.

Avatars, like Rama and Krishna, are also manifestations of Manu, and connect to the Rishi vision, helping to develop new human potentials. We need to open up to their flow of grace. Today we do need a new avatar, not as a new hero figure or savior, but as a new creative consciousness to enlighten the planet present within everyone. Such an avatar mind and avatar consciousness is required, not just a single sage to guide us.

Manu is the earthly manifestation of the cosmic intelligence that comes through the Sun. Manu brings us the evolutionary power inherent in the Sun, which is responsible for the unfoldment of the solar system. The Sun is the source not only of light and life, but also of intelligence, consciousness, and spirituality. The Sun is the abode of the Vijnana, Buddhi, Dhi, Supermind, and cosmic mind, all of whom are connected in Vedic thought. The Kundalini is but a portion of the solar energy latent within our deeper consciousness.

The Vedic seers drew in this solar transformative force through Vedic chants and mantras, notably the Gayatri Mantra to the Supreme Light. The Gayatri Mantra is directed to the aspect of the Solar Deity called *Savita*, which is the most important manifestation of solar intelligence. Savita governs all transformations, daily and seasonally, outer and inner, including all higher evolutionary potentials through the process of Yoga.

A new Manu and a new Rishi order can help us create a new humanity that can better reflect the cosmic intelligence and its enlightened dharma, and help us move beyond the vagaries and violence of the ego-mind. Developing that vision of Manu and creating such a new humanity is the need of the times, however one may look at the details. This new humanity is a species that reflects and develops a new planetary consciousness, based upon an inner Self-knowledge as linked with an outer cosmic knowledge.

A new Rishi order implies not only a new Manu, but also a new Brihaspati, who is the leader and primal guide of the Rishis. A new human consciousness needs a new seer-order, a new Rishi consciousness and Rishi community. We need a new Brihaspati or new founder of such a new Rishi order for a new *Vedas*. The works of Ganapati Muni and Brahmarshi Daivarata on Brihaspati can aid us in this direction.[83]

The Theosophists from the nineteenth century like H.P. Blavatsky were influenced by this Vedic inspiration towards a new humanity. A number of New Age groups have taken this in various directions. While one may argue that their work is mixed with wishful thinking, it is still pointing in a positive direction and can be developed further.

Such a new humanity would have a connection to the old priestly families and monastic orders of the past, but consist of their renovation and transformation for a new era, no longer bound by local or regional boundaries and limitations. It would create new spiritual communities, such as Sri Aurobindo and Swami Yogananda foresaw. These new spiritual communities would have a semi-monastic orientation, in that they would aim at the primacy of the inner life, but also be creative and innovative in the outer realms of art, science, healing, and culture building. They would be forces not simply for renouncing the world but for a new spiritual and intellectual renaissance for the planet. They would consist of families, but like the ancient Vedic Rishi lines, of a more spiritual than emotional nature, with ties of the soul, not simply of the body or blood.

Such new Vedic communities would aim at restoring and enlivening the ancient *Vedas*, but also bringing into consciousness a new Vedic vision, with a vision of future *Vedas* as well. These groups would not rest upon emotional fervor or expectations of an external savior, but on the ability of serious individuals to dive deeply into their inmost consciousness and reality, looking not only to elevate the human, but also to create a path beyond the human to the Divine.

A Yogic Humanity

How can we change our nature, one might ask, from the Asura to the Deva, and bring about a higher yogic humanity as the natural state of human beings? Is our nature not something fixed? Can't we be only what we are? The complication is that we as human beings have two natures, an outer material nature caught up in the inertia of physical existence, and an inner spiritual nature that transcends time and space. We contain both the Deva and the Asura within us.

We can align ourselves either with our outer nature or with our inner nature. And our outer nature can be oriented toward the world of nature or toward various human social orders. The *Vedas* show us how to link our biological nature with our spiritual nature. Most of modern civilization, with its commercial orientation, on the other hand, strives to link our biological nature to conditioned social imperatives, including many that are not natural, such as the commercial world cleverly promotes. The *Vedas* do not try to change our nature artificially, but rather show us how we can link our outer nature with our inner nature as spiritual beings, which affords a higher evolution in consciousness.

Our biological nature is always changing with the movement of life. The nature of a child is different from the nature of an adult. Our biological nature mirrors all of nature with its seasons, layers, births, and deaths. Our outer nature is always changing, not only gradually, but sometimes radically, particularly at key transformational moments like birth and death. The Vedic Yoga shows us how to use the natural changes of our biological nature to achieve higher evolutionary transformations and a greater connection with our inner being. It shows us how to use transitional forces like sunrise and sunset, inhalation and exhalation, falling asleep and waking, birth and death, in order to carry us to a new level, not simply to keep us on the level at which we currently are.

This Vedic change of nature is a shift from our outer bodily nature to our inner spiritual nature. It requires understanding what our true nature is apart from our outer nature conditioned by the external world. This shift or change of nature is portrayed in organic metaphors, such as bringing fire out of wood, gold out of gold ore, or butter out of milk. This Deva potential can be brought out naturally through the process of Yoga, but that must be done on a daily basis and with all aspects of our being. Vedic Yoga can help us bring about the radical change not only of the individual, but also of the entire human species that the world needs today. It remains evolutionarily speaking relevant and futuristic, not a mere cult of the past. We must learn to visualize our Vedic future, which is aided by the memory of the ancient Vedic vision.

The call to return to the *Vedas* should not be a mere nostalgia for the past, but should become a foundation for building a greater future, a new golden age — an age of enlightenment to come. This hope of humanity must be fulfilled, though it may be a matter of centuries and may not be understood by the events of a few recent decades. It requires much more than information technology, computers, or new chemicals for the brain. It requires a living link to the cosmic intelligence that pervades us on every side.

Yoga as the Inner Sacrifice

Nature is always practicing Yoga in her processes. In nature there is an ongoing movement toward greater integration of the individual and the universe, a seeking of greater forms of wholeness. We can see this in the evolution of life itself, with each new species being a new expression of the totality. The ultimate form of wholeness is consciousness itself, in which we can see our self in all beings and all beings within ourselves. In all the processes of nature there is a greater unfoldment of light, through life, mind, and consciousness. As human beings we can embody the whole, the Purusha, or the cosmic Being. We can reflect the universe itself, through its core awareness that is already hidden within us.

Yoga works with the intelligence of nature that is impersonal and universal, not simply with our human intellect or creaturely cunning. Our current human intelligence cannot take us out of our creaturely limitations; rather, it is their product and must reflect their compulsions. For the universalization of our being, which is the true process of Yoga, we must connect to the higher intelligence within and around us that transcends words and thoughts as we know them to be. This entails a different learning process than going to a school, examining the outer world with the tools of the senses, or the skill of the intellect. It requires opening up to the language of nature as the expression of a greater awareness of the All.

A true Yoga of nature must employ the language of nature, which resides far from our ordinary forms of human discourse. What is the language of nature? It is not our language of abstract concepts, personal discourse, or dictionary-defined words. It is not the language of science or art, though these may touch upon aspects of what nature may be. The language of nature is first of all the language of light. Light is the presence of cosmic intelligence and carries the visible world on its hidden screen. The pattern of light is a pattern of intelligence working for the unfoldment of all life. Light in its subjective action is consciousness or the seer. In its objective action, light creates the forms of the outer world or the seen.

The *Vedas* are based on the prime images of light as Fire, Dawn, Sun, Moon, and Lightning. These are not simply the ordinary forces that we ascribe such names to. They are analogical tools for understanding all the powers of the universe. The Sun (Surya) indicates the all-revealing light of consciousness. The Moon (Soma) is the reflective light of bliss. Lightning (Vidyut) is the energy of consciousness, which is the power of perception. Fire (Agni) is the consciousness or soul hidden in all manifest objects like fire in wood. The Dawn (Ushas) indicates the awakening of our soul to its deeper spiritual aspiration, including its past-life strivings.

Besides a language of cosmic light, the language of nature is a language of cosmic sound. Sound is the vibration of the cosmic mind, which pervades the infinite space of awareness. When primal sound and transcendent light come together in universal meaning, the deepest level of mantra is created. Mantra is the light-sound pattern of the cosmic mind that creates, sustains, and transforms the universe, impelling all creatures towards the Divine. The Vedic language of light is a language of mantra or spiritually empowered speech. In mantra the sound and meanings of words reflect one another and mirror all the forces of cosmos and psyche.

The Vedic Yoga as a Yoga of nature is built upon the language of nature, which at an inner level is the language of mantra. The *Vedas* speak in terms of deities or Devatas, who are regarded superficially as nature Gods and Goddesses. While this idea of many Gods provides a sense of their outer qualities, it creates confusion and misunderstanding. The term Deva means, first of all, a being of light, which to the Vedic mind implies consciousness and intelligence, a manifestation of the supreme light of awareness. Deva is related to the term Dyaus, meaning heaven, and refers to the heavenly or celestial lights. Vedic deities represent the main forms of light that can be found everywhere in the universe and underlie the workings of all natural processes that involve light and energy. Our cognitive powers of the mind and senses are Devas at an individual level. The stars in the sky are Devas at a cosmic level. All such Devas are linked together in the supreme deity that is the highest Light, which ultimately transcends all manifestation and all duality.

Analogical Language and Symbolic Thinking[84]

The *Vedas* are composed in a cryptic mantric language – a secret code as it were – which cannot be understood without the proper background and orientation. The teaching is not only hidden, but at times is deliberately veiled to protect it from those who are unawake or uninitiated and could possibly misuse it.

Vedic texts are not written in a philosophical style, much less a scientific or psychological manner. They cannot be looked upon according to the strict logic or abstract terminology of later Indian philosophy as in Vedanta and Buddhism, with their sophisticated philosophical dialectics. The *Vedas* are not practical books like Yoga Shastras, outlining specific techniques and methods. The Vedic language is mantric, symbolic and unique, reflecting its own profound vision of reality that must be understood in its own right.

Without first recognizing the background worldview and spiritual vision of the Vedic seers, little can be gained by literally translating Vedic mantras. Yet today we expect the *Vedas* to yield their secrets to us by a causal reading or through translations done by scholars who have little affinity with or appreciation for the Rishi mind. We assume that the *Vedas* should reflect a language or a mentality that is easy for us to access by our current high tech cultural standards. A little thinking shows that, given the difference of time, civilization, and mentality, the

Vedas cannot easily make sense to us, without first some fundamental shift in how we see the world. Without deep meditation and questioning the limitations of our current civilization, it is very difficult to gain access to the Vedic world.

The key to the language of the *Vedas* is the world of nature, not according to the views of a naturalist but that of a poet, yogi, and mystic. The *Vedas* take simple images of nature like Fire, Wind, and Sun, but use them as part of a vast cosmological and spiritual symbolism. Fire is not just the earthly fire, but also that of the atmosphere and heaven. In the human being, it is the digestive fire, the fire of prana, the eye, and the fire of the mind. In Yoga practices, fire is mantra and Kundalini. To lump all of this diversity together under primitive fire worship does not at all reflect the multileveled vision of the Vedic mind.

Every object in nature is in some way a mirror of the entire universe. In this universe of consciousness, the whole is present in every part. It is not that each object is just a part of the whole. Each individual object can express and reveal the whole. Each object can awaken us to the meaning of the whole and reflect the comprehensive Divine reality to us that imparts wholeness to all aspects of life.

The Vedic Fire is inherently the cosmic Fire. The Vedic tree is the cosmic tree. The Vedic waters are the cosmic waters of space. The *Vedas* work with archetypal energies, not simply particular manifestations in our transient human world. For the Vedic mind, everything is indicative of the cosmic whole and its development on all levels. Each thing is a gateway to the great mystery beyond all manifestation. The Vedic seer notes the universal essence in each thing, not merely the practical reality of the object. Once we perceive the cosmic wholeness in the object, we will regard it as sacred. Each phenomenon in nature is a message from the Divine to reveal its reality to us. The Rishi understands the message and does not stop short by judging the envelope.

The *Vedas* rest upon a principle of what could be called "cosmic analogy"; "as above, so below"; "as without, so within," as many mystical traditions reflect. For example, the Vedic fire represents the Sun on earth. The outer fire reflects the inner fire, which is primarily speech and the Divine Word. Each Vedic deity is mirrored in every other, and is never a separate God or Goddess. The *Vedas* abound in associations and contain several formulas for how the universe works as a single organism. Often inner connections are implied rather than overtly stated. If we do not first draw the analogy in our own minds, we are likely to miss its presence in Vedic texts.

The *Vedas* reflect a series of connections between the individual human being and the greater universe. We could say that each thing that we see is a "cosmic analogue." It is not an object in itself but a way of knowledge, a doorway of perception, allowing us to understand not only what the object itself may represent, but also how it serves to unlock all the processes in the universe. Central to these cosmic connections is the broader idea of the Purusha, or cosmic person, that the universe forms a single organism like the human being. The process governing this interrelated universe is *Yajna*, which means not only worship, ritual, and sacrifice but also mutuality, one in all, and all in one, an interrelated sacred presence.

Images of the Vital Plane

Vedic hymns reflect the common life images of the people of that ancient historical era. These images include a seeking for wealth in terms of cattle, horses, servants, food, gold, land, and victory in battle – which is what the Vedic ritual seems to be mainly about if we look at it only superficially. Sometimes these vital plane images seem quite unspiritual to us, a glorification of manly power, weapons, chariots, and conflict. This is particularly true in the case of Indra, the most important Vedic deity, who is portrayed as a powerful warrior. Add to these martial images the Vedic glorification of the intoxicating powers of Soma, like some Shamanistic drug, and it is easy to find the *Veda* to be primitive.

Many translators are content in presenting this mundane dimension of the Vedic language. However, to the inner view, each of these outer life images has a higher symbolic value, like the cow as a symbol of light and the horse as a symbol of energy. These life images in the *Vedas* always have cosmic dimensions. The Vedic cow can mean the earth, a ray of light, perception, the sense organs, or the soul. Such a vast tapestry of associations does not arise in our minds when we read the word cow in Vedic hymns!

We can compare these earlier Vedic life images with those of later Hinduism, like Lord Shiva who appears only as a deity of male energy, a bit like a primitive shaman, with his matted hair, drums, dancing, and ecstasy. Yet if we examine the deeper associations in Hindu texts, we find that Lord Shiva represents the Supreme Self beyond all time and space, the Absolute and the Unborn, and the great lord of Yoga. Another example of this type of symbolism occurs in hymns to the Goddess that glorify her physical female features much like ordinary poets do, yet connect her with the power of pure consciousness as a manifestation of the formless Supreme Brahman.[85]

It is clear that even in Vedic times, the majority of people lived at an outer level of vital plane fulfillment in terms of family, wealth, property, and social recognition. Yet there was a smaller group, the yogic humanity of the Rishis that had much prominence and power in Vedic society. The outer meaning of the Vedic ritual was for the ordinary person who was content with happiness of the body and senses during life, and a heavenly world beyond after death. The inner meaning was for the children of the Rishis who saw the outer world as a symbol of the inner light, and pursued a path of Self-realization. To understand the *Vedas*, we need a Rishi vision to take us beyond these outer forms to the inner essence of Divine light. We need to take the Vedic images in all their complexity and depth.

Karma and Ritual: Nature in Action

All life is ritual, by which we mean a repeated rhythmic movement expressing harmony, interrelationship, and transformation. We are all linked together in the cosmic chain of interaction and evolution that is a kind of ritual or sacred unfoldment. Ritual is not merely a special set of ceremonies that people may do by way of duty or routine, but a way of understanding the greater universe along with its sacred and interrelated energy patterns.

The Vedic term for ritual is *karma*, which is better known as referring to the effects of our actions through our various incarnations, the cycle of rebirth. According to the Vedic view, all actions constitute a kind of ritual because they produce an occult force that creates long-term karmic results for the soul. Our actions have enduring effects, both outwardly and inwardly, so it is important that we perform them with awareness and a sacred intent.

Action tends to follow a pattern of repetition, rhythm, or season in alliance with the forces of nature that affords it a ritualistic quality and effect. Vedic rituals begin with simple biological rituals like eating and breathing, as well as simple natural rituals like fire offerings performed at sunrise and sunset, new and full Moons, equinoxes and solstices. Ritual is the very rhythm of life extending to the stars. Ancient rituals included a journey into the inner worlds or world of the Gods in search of guidance for our life and actions.

The term *karma* originally meant action of a ritualistic nature, particularly offerings to the sacred fire, but as symbolic for all actions of life that consist of various mutually related processes. Vedic rituals are powerful orchestrated actions designed to produce specific and lasting effects upon the world as well as upon one's own person and soul. One could say that ritual is a conscious or empowered form of karma. The more empowered our action, the stronger are its positive karmic affects. Vedic rituals achieve this empowerment of action by bringing the forces of nature into all that we do.

Action tends to be a repeated phenomenon that builds up a certain mode of behavior or learned response. Doing something once establishes the impulse to do it again, until a regular pattern of action is set in motion that becomes our very way of life. Action leads to involvement in the world, because in performing actions we enter into the world and become part of its movements and powers.

Action is essentially interaction in which we both put out energies and receive them back into ourselves. As our greater field of action is the sacred universe itself, all action must ultimately be sacred or ritualistic in nature, connecting us with all existence. Action that is not sacred is action performed in ignorance of these cosmic connections, and it thereby becomes egoistic, divisive, separative, and destructive in its effects.

All actions in nature are kinds of rituals, just as human rituals largely arise from an imitation of the rites and rhythms of nature. All natural actions are interactive sacred dramas moving with the rhythm of life. Such natural rituals are eating, breathing, sleeping, and reproducing. They include daily, monthly, seasonal, and yearly changes reflected in the skies. They include the passages from conception to birth, from childhood to maturity, from maturity to old age, from old age to death. That is why, for indigenous people who live in nature, all actions are rituals and all actions are sacred.

Karma is the very movement of nature, the rhythm of life, which follows a cyclical pattern of return like the rising of the sun after the night, the phases of the moon, the fluctuations of the seasons, and the births and deaths of creatures. All these rituals involve some sort of fire, heat, light, or transformation as the determinative force. Ritual action is the very natural expression of the movements and cycles of light, whether in the outer world or in our own bodies and minds.

Our karma reflects our interaction with the universe in either a supportive or resistive manner. Our karma either moves along with the rhythm of nature, which is towards the unfoldment of life and consciousness, or against it, in the direction of destruction and ignorance. Our karma, though having its individual consequences, is connected to the karma of all living beings and to the fate of the universe itself. Vedic rituals are a special means of working with karma in a transformative way on both individual and collective levels. They are a means of embodying the sacred in our daily existence, raising our awareness into sacred time and sacred space, in which we become an integral part of all that is.

All ancient cultures were highly ritualistic in nature, as are traditional people today, reflecting their recognition of the sacred presence in the universe. We moderns, on the other hand, tend to dislike ritual, which we associate with something artificial or contrived, a mere social ceremony or show. If we are attracted to spirituality or yoga, it often goes along with a dislike of ritual that we associate with institutionalized religion and its dogmas. We have forgotten the deeper dimension behind the practice of rituals. At the same time we create new modern rituals unknowingly through forming gangs, fan clubs, political parties, or in the adulation of the beautiful, talented, rich, famous, and powerful as our new Gods and Goddesses.

Traditional Yoga usually begins with Karma Yoga, which implies ritual or action done out of worship. Traditional Karma Yoga involves Seva or service, but as part of ritual, which is often regarded as the main action that we can do for the upliftment of the world because it brings the Divine into our endeavors. Yet ritual has an important place in traditional Yoga. Asana originally had a ritualistic connection, employing a series of gestures, movements, and poses also used in various rituals. Mantra Yoga is the basis of all rituals that usually consist of mantras, prayers or recitations of Divine names. Devotion or Bhakti Yoga naturally inclines us towards ritual worship of the Deity, using chants, movements and gestures. Tantric Yoga is highly ritualistic as part of its orientation, honoring the cosmic masculine and feminine powers.

Yoga as a whole arose as an internal ritual or sacrifice, in which we use our own speech, mind, and prana as instruments of worship for the Divine within us. Classical Yoga is not opposed to ritual, which is traditionally part of Karma Yoga, but includes an internalization of ritual through the mind. If we do not have an appreciation of ritual for making our outer actions sacred, our Yoga practice may lack the proper foundation. Ritual in the true sense is symbolic or analogical action, which is the embodiment of the mantra in our outer life and expression.

Karma and Rebirth

Some scholars hold that karma and rebirth are not known in the *Vedas* but that karma only reflects ritual in Vedic texts, particularly primitive fire worship. They fail to see how ritual or return in nature can lead us to an understanding of rebirth or the return of the light of the soul. There are, however, many Vedic verses that do suggest rebirth, as well as the weight of the Vedic symbolism of the return of the light.

> *For the eternal Gods, O Solar Creator (Savita), you first created immortality, and then as a bondage for mortals a succession of lives (anūcīnā jīvitā mānuṣebhyaḥ).*
>
> *Vamadeva Gautama, Rigveda IV.54.2* [86]

The Vedic ritual's emphasis on cyclical return of the day, month, and seasons of the year provides a good basis for understanding the process of karma and rebirth for the soul – the phases of return of the soul's journey from life to life. The ancient seers observed nature at a deep level and learned the secrets of its many cycles of birth, death, and rebirth.

Agni, the sacred fire, which is the root of the Vedic ritual, is symbolic of the individual soul, which is hidden in the body like fire in wood. Each life of the soul is like one day of the fire in which it is enkindled anew. One of Agni's prime forms is *Jatavedas*, which means "one who has knowledge (veda) of birth (jata)." Vishvamitra states that Agni is hidden in every birth.

> *Agni as the Knower of birth is hidden in every birth (janmañjanman nihito jātavedāḥ).*[87]
> *Gathina Vishvamitra, Rigveda III.1.20*

Jatavedas is Agni's form in the middle world of the atmosphere, connected with the forces of life and prana. The very name *Jatavedas* implies one who has the knowledge of rebirth. Agni is the inextinguishable Divine Fire that comes into this world at birth and leaves at death.

The Vedic ritual of the daily relighting of the sacred fire reflects the many lives of our souls and the deeper spiritual aspiration that constitutes our inner immortal flame. The real Vedic ritual requires an awakened soul in order to perform it. Its practice is Yoga or seeking of union with the whole of light. This inner fire of the soul gradually awakens by the power of the dawn of spiritual aspiration to eventually expand into the Sun, the solar Self of pure awareness. This is symbolic of transcending rebirth and returning to the inner light of the Self. According to the *Rigveda*, mortals can become immortal, which occurs by manifesting the Divine light inherent within us, especially as uniting with the inner spiritual Sun, a process symbolized by the resurrection of the Sun out of darkness.

Yajna, the Way of Sacrifice and Transformation

The *Veda* speaks of *Yajna*, usually translated as 'sacrifice', as the underlying principle of life, which views the universe as following a sacrificial order. The ancients perceived a sacred order behind all the movements of life, with each creature serving as an offering to the entire universe, and the entire universe providing a support in turn for every creature. We can see this process in our own lives that are part of a greater social and natural order, in which the rocks, plants, animals, and other human beings as well as the water, air, Sun, and Moon contribute to our own well-being.

The English term "sacrifice" is derived from the word "sacred." It does not mean to destroy or to eliminate, but to worship, pray, and sanctify. It implies offering something up in which it is transformed, losing its lower or impure nature but gaining a higher or pure nature. Sacrifice means offering to the Divine in order to spiritualize, not simply bringing something to an end. Self-sacrifice is considered one of the greatest virtues that both helps others and ennobles ourselves.

Yet the term "sacrifice" can be misleading for Yajna. It implies violence, as in animal sacrifices, and does not reflect all the different aspects of the Vedic Yajna.

Yajna refers to all aspects of worship, not just to literal animal sacrifices that were meant for the less evolved levels of society (or were symbolical with the animal offered being our own lower nature). Vedic Yajnas include not only outer fire offerings, but also internal offerings of prayer, mantra, pranayama, and meditation. Along with outer sacrifices like giving wealth for charitable purposes are inner sacrifices, offering our own minds and hearts to the Divine. The Vedic Yoga is such an internal offering or sacrifice. Any Yoga approach should begin as an internal sacrifice of the ego or it cannot awaken and manifest the soul.

In the Vedic language, "Yajna" means the "Divine" or "the Deva." Yajna is *Vishnu*, the Divine force that preserves and protects the universe, as the *Vedas* say. Yajna is *Brahma* or *Prajapati*, the Divine force that creates all beings and provides them with their means of sustenance.

> *The Lord of Creation, generating these creatures together with the Sacrifice, said "By this you will expand, this will be your wish-fulfilling cow."*[88]
> *Bhagavad Gita III.10*

Yajna is also Shiva or Rudra, the Divine force that transforms all things. Death is the highest sacrifice in which we can offer our entire lives for a greater universal transformation. All Vedic deities are personifications of various aspects of the sacred movement of the universe, which is not a mere human ritual, but represents the cosmic order of Oneness. Each deity reflects an aspect of the Yajna, a power or principle behind it, or some energy or quality gained through performing it.

As embodied souls, we are all sacrifices to the Divine, with our short life being but a ritual offering to the whole. We exist to contribute to the sacred order of the universe, which is to support the well-being and light in all that is. Our first duty in life is to give, which is to serve. By giving we receive, and we enter into the sacred order of life that is ever full and never dies. Naturally, this is a very different life value than our current commercial and ego-based society whose prime rule appears to be to take what we can. Yet even in our non-sacred social order today, sacrifice, particularly as service to others, is where we find the greatest meaning and happiness in life, and is often regarded as the highest societal goal.

Yajna and Evolution

Yajna is an offering of one thing to another for the purpose of transformation. The rule in nature is simple. In order to achieve a higher level of evolution, we must be willing to give up and step beyond the lower. To reach our higher nature, we must be willing to offer up, purify, or renounce our lower nature.

The inner power of this Yajna transformation process is Agni, which outwardly is the fire element. The fire element purifies and transforms, just as the power of heat is able to bring gold out of crude ore. Whatever is offered into the inner fire must be transformed to a higher and subtler level of substance. Developing a transforming heat, light, pressure, friction, or vibration is the key to the Vedic process. The Vedic Yajna is called *tapas* or the purifying power, another synonym for Yoga or an important aspect of it.[89]

Yoga develops this process of the sacred fire. It shows us how to move beyond our ordinary states and conditions of being to something higher. This is not a matter of denial or repression but of honoring our ability to grow and to move beyond. It is like learning how to churn butter out of milk. It does not require denying the nature of milk, nor does it involve accepting milk as it is.

The Five Great Vedic Yajnas and Yoga

There are five traditional daily Great or Mahayajnas that should be practiced to remove our karmic debt to all existence:

1. *Brahma Yajna*
   Study and teaching the *Vedas* or sacred teachings.

2. *Deva Yajna*
   Worshipping the Divine and cosmic powers.

3. *Manushya Yajna*
   Helping fellow human beings, particularly taking care of guests.

4. *Pitri Yajna*
   Honoring one's ancestors, culture and societal traditions.

5. *Bhuta Yajna*
   Serving living beings, making offerings to animals, plants, and the mineral kingdom, as well as protecting the earth, her lands and waters.

Proper performance of these five types of Yajnas frees us from our karmic debts in life, enabling our soul to move beyond them. We can see here that the Vedic concept of Yajna is one of worship and includes outer rituals, prayers, and inner rituals (meditations). It encompasses all aspects of caring for nature, other creatures, other human beings, and charity. The Vedic Yajna is hardly a matter of slaughtering animals. None of the main Vedic Yajnas are sacrifices in the ordinary sense. Some like study and teaching the *Vedas*, which is the highest of these five Yajnas, are very different from anything that we would call a sacrifice.

We can call these *Maha Yajnas* or Great Sacrifices as *Maha Yogas* or "Great Yogas," as each implies Yoga practices of Knowledge, Devotion, and Service (Jnana, Bhakti, and Karma) that constitute Yoga in the broadest sense of the term. Brahma Yajna is mainly the Yoga of Knowledge. Deva Yajna is mainly the Yoga of Devotion. To study the *Veda* we must purify ourselves and develop the powers of higher perception and awareness. For the Deva Yajna, we must develop devotion and offer our own minds and hearts to the deity, not simply external offerings. The other three, the Yajnas for human beings, ancestors and other creatures are mainly forms of Karma Yoga or the Yoga of Action and Service. Though they have an outer activity associated with them, these Yajnas rest upon an inner attitude and orientation to the Divine.

Yoga first arose from the inner sacrifice of the *Vedas*. The inner Yajna (*Antaryaga*) consists of internal worship through Yoga and meditation. Inner Yajnas involve offerings of speech, breath and mind, through mantra, pranayama, and meditation to the Deity within. Yet the outer sacrifice properly performed is a type of Karma Yoga. Krishna in the *Bhagavad Gita* comments on these inner Yajnas that consist of meditation, control of the senses (pratyahara), pranayama, and Yoga specifically as a Yajna.[90]

The Vedic Ritual Order of the Cosmos

The priests of the Vedic Yajna reflect the sacred order of the universe and its Divine powers, and how these forces work within the individual human being. This begins with a primary threefold order.

Earth	Agni, Fire	Vak, Speech	Hota, Invoker
Atmosphere	Vayu, Wind/ Lightning	Prana, Breath	Adhvaryu, Master of Action
Heaven	Surya, Sun	Manas, Mind	Udgata, Master of the Chant

Our outer world is threefold as earth, atmosphere, and heaven, which are ruled by their three light forms of fire, wind, and Sun. These are the three aspects of God or the cosmic Being, the supreme Light. The outer ritual honors the three worlds and their guiding lights and links human activity with the sacred world order. This is done mainly through various fire offerings because fire can convey our messages to the higher worlds and powers of light. As human beings we live on earth and can contribute to the earthly fire and its unfoldment. That is our point of origin and initiation into the cosmic process.

Our inner world or psychological nature is similarly threefold as body, prana, and mind, which are ruled by their three light forms of speech, prana, and intelligence. These constitute the three aspects of the Soul or the individual Divine. The inner ritual honors the internal Divine through mantra or sacred speech, pranayama or sacred breath, and meditation or sacred thought. It is not the ordinary faculties of speech, prana, and mind that are indicated here but their spiritual counterparts that arise from self-control and silence.

We can observe this threefold order in our own human body, which has three spheres or levels. The sphere of the earth is centered in the belly. Its ruling power is fire that is based in the navel as the digestive fire. The sphere of the atmosphere is centered in the chest. Its ruling power is prana or the bioelectrical force that runs the body from its position in the heart. The sphere of heaven in the head, which is round like the Sun and is dominated by the eyes that project the solar force above.

The same pattern is reflected in the human head itself. The lower part of the head, the jaw is the realm of earth governed by fire which is the tongue or speech. The middle part of the head, the nose, is the realm of the atmosphere governed by wind or the breath. The higher part of the head is the realm of heaven governed by the Sun through the eyes.

In some Vedic correlations, prana is associated with the Sun and the mind is associated with Vayu or wind, a reversing of these two principles. This is because the mind is like the wind or Vayu and serves to make connections between all aspects of our experience. The Sun is not just the source of light and perception, but also of life and vitality or prana.

The Fivefold Sacred Order

Besides the basic threefold scheme of the worlds and deities, there is also a fivefold order:

1. Agni – Fire	Speech – Vak	Hota – Invoker
2. Vayu – Wind	Breath - Prana	Udgata – Singer
3. Surya - Sun	Eye - Chakshu	Adhvaryu – Performer
4. Chandra – Moon	Mind - Manas	Brahma – Guide
5. Dig - Directions of Space	Ears - Shrotra	Agnidh – Fire starter

In this fivefold order, the Sun stands for the eye and the perceptive part of the mind, not just for the eye as a sense organ. The Moon stands for the reflective part of the mind, which relates to the emotions. The directions of space relate to the receptive part of the mind and our ability to listen. All five are integral parts of the same cosmic being that is the basis of our own psychic being.

These five faculties refer not only to their physical counterparts but are the main factors of the subtle body that continues after the death of the physical body. It is not just the physical aspects of these faculties that the *Veda* is developing. The Vedic ritual and mantra purify the subtle body both for spiritual practice in this life and for attaining a higher plane of existence after death. We discover higher powers of speech, prana, mind, hearing, and seeing.

The *Mahabharata* presents other Vedic sacrificial orders, connecting the Vedic ritual and its priests with various internal processes in its *Yoga Yajna* or "Yoga Sacrifice."[91] We should remember that such cosmic connections cannot be reduced to a single fixed formula, any more than a gem with many facets can be reduced to a single view. What may appear to us as inconsistencies in different Vedic formulas are variations on the same truths, designed to help us develop a many-sided perception, so that we can understand the One in all and the all in One. Vedic unity is not an abstract principle or an emotional assertion, but an integral oneness that holds all diversity as complementary expressions of itself. Vedic unitary thought teaches us to draw connections, not simply to look at one set of correspondences as the final or the ultimate.

Vedic Yoga and Classical Yoga

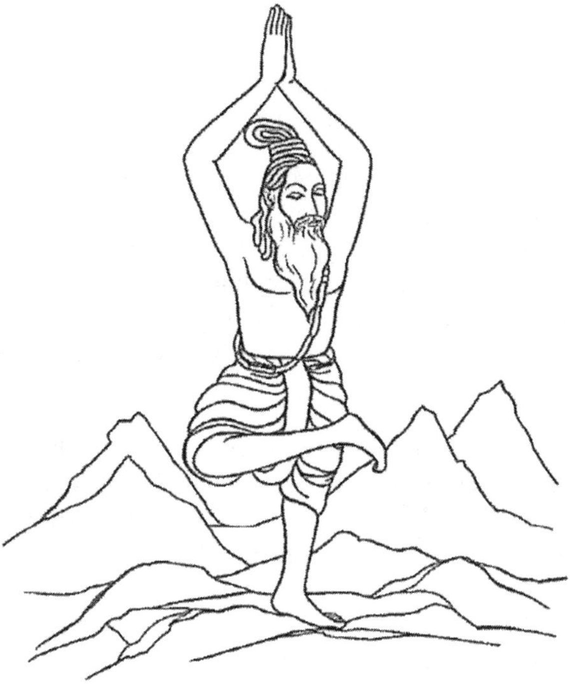

In this chapter we will introduce the Vedic Yoga relative to classical Yoga, as a foundation for a more detailed examination of these topics later in the book. Yoga is a term with several levels of meaning that we should consider carefully when we look into the Vedic Yoga. In classical Indian thought, Yoga in the general sense refers to a particular integrative way of spiritual practices. The term Yoga suggests asana, mantra, pranayama, and meditation, as well as principles like ahimsa or non-violence, aligned with philosophies of Self-realization and communion with the Divine.

Yoga in this broader sense as spiritual practice has five basic types, to which many secondary types can be added.

1. Jnana Yoga – the Yoga of Knowledge, using meditation and Self-inquiry for Self-realization

2. Bhakti Yoga – the Yoga of Devotion, seeking union or communion with God as the Divine Father or Divine Mother

3. Karma Yoga – the Yoga of Action, emphasizing ritual worship of the Divine and selfless service to living beings

4. Raja Yoga – the Royal Yoga of higher techniques and methods, mainly mantra and meditation.

5. Hatha Yoga – the Yoga of Effort of outer techniques and methods, mainly asana and pranayama.

All schools of Indian spiritual thought, Vedic or non-Vedic, employ one or more of these approaches of Yoga, which they may define relative to different philosophical backgrounds. Many employ an integral approach using aspects of all five. The integrative approach of Yoga pervades the culture of India along with its literature, drama, music, dance, science, medicine, and even grammar. We find this broader meaning of Yoga in Vedic teachings going back to the *Rigveda*, not simply Yoga as asana in modern parlance.

However, besides this general meaning for Yoga and not to be confused with it, Yoga in a specific sense refers to Yoga as one of the six classical schools of Vedic thought, those philosophies that accept the authority of the *Vedas*. This is the Yoga school or *Yoga Darshana*, also called 'Samkhya-Yoga' owing to its connection with the Samkhya school of Vedic thought. In addition there are Shaivite, Vaishnava, and other Yoga approaches, which have their own Yoga texts and teachings, and do not always emphasize the *Yoga Sutras*.

Yoga and the *Vedas*

It is difficult to think of the *Vedas* without thinking about Yoga. The *Vedas* promote spiritual knowledge born of meditation, the way to achieve which is the practice of Yoga. Yoga is a term that is first found in the *Vedas*. Some scholars – generally not trained in the inner meaning of the *Vedas* - have tried to separate Yoga from the *Vedas* because Yoga as a specific term is not common in the *Rigveda*. While the term Yoga as a noun, though it does occur is not common in the *Rigveda*, the root for Yoga, "yuj," meaning "to unite, yoke or harness" is very common, not only relative to horses and chariots, but also relative to the mind and senses, taking it in the direction of Yoga practice. The yoking of the Vedic chariot can be symbolic of Yoga practices of controlling the mind or energizing the subtle body and its chakra centers.

Besides the many Vedic words deriving from the root for yoga as "yuj," the *Vedas* contain many terms for Yoga practice, including karma, yajna, mantra, tapas, svadhyaya, and dhyana, as well as Purusha, Ishvara, and Atman. Vedic deities like Agni, Soma, and Vayu commonly relate to the inner energies of Yoga practices in later yogic and Tantric texts. The Vedic Rishi is also a Yogi who has higher powers of consciousness, can commune with the deities, and becomes a deity himself.

Sometimes people fail to see the yogic nature of the *Rigveda* because they are defining Yoga according to a modern idea of Yoga as asana or physical postures. Asanas do not have a dominant role either in the *Vedas* or in classical yogic texts like the *Yoga Sutras*, which only devotes two of two hundred sutras to them.

The *Vedas* do address Yoga in an obvious but different manner. *The Vedas as chants can be defined first of all as Mantra Yoga*. The practice of mantra is important for Yoga as a whole and its different approaches. The *Yoga Sutras* similarly emphasizes *Pranava* or the Divine Word (Oṁ) as a prime principle of Yoga practice, implying the importance of Mantra Yoga.[92] The *Vedas* are mantras and reciting them is a path of Mantra Yoga. Mantra Yoga in India continues to use Vedic mantras like Gayatri Mantra as well as resting upon the Sanskrit language, the origin of which is in the *Vedas*.

Mantra is one of the inner sacrifices that constitute Yoga practice. Krishna states that of the sacrifices (Yajnas), he is the repetition of mantra (Japa-Yajna), most specifically the single syllable mantra or Oṁ.[93] Yet mantra has an application in action, which is ritual or karma. Vedic Mantra Yoga has its corresponding Karma Yoga. The *Vedas* outline the original rituals behind the practice of Karma Yoga, which in India today still extensively employs Vedic fire offerings. Mantra is meant to teach Dharma or the laws of life. The *Vedas* encourage sacrifice, giving, and helping others that is the basis of Seva or service, another important aspect of Karma Yoga.

Ritual can be defined as a way of sacred action in which we use name and form to approach the nameless and the formless. Vedic fire rituals are not done simply to produce heat or cook food but to carry messages to the higher worlds. The implements and materials used in the ritual are not employed for their literal or practical value. They indicate movements and offerings of the heart. Ritual is way of bringing the sacred Brahman into action. When that ritual action is turned within, it becomes Yoga.

> *Brahman is the offering ladle. Brahman is the offering that is offered by Brahman into the fire of Brahman. One goes to Brahman, by this ritual of samadhi or mergence in Brahman.*[94]
>
> *Bhagavad Gita IV.24*

The inner sacrifice involves the offering of speech, prana, and mind to the deity within the heart. Yoga can be traced to this inner sacrifice (antaryaga) that works through mantra, pranayama, and meditation. The *Gita* is not stating anything new here but making clear the older Vedic approach.

The Vedic Yoga and Other Yoga Teachings

Yoga is a common topic in all Hindu teachings, whether *Tantras, Puranas, Mahabharata*, or *Vedas*. The *Mahabharata*, which includes the *Bhagavad Gita*, contains long sections on Yoga. The *Upanishads* teach the principles of Vedantic philosophy and the Samkhya system that the *Yoga Sutras* uses.[95] They explain in detail the Yogas of Knowledge and Devotion. The *Upanishads* deal with the themes of Yoga as Oṁ, mantra, meditation, control of the mind, the nature of prana, and knowledge of the Purusha that are reflected in the *Yoga Sutras*. Many Upanishadic sages like Yajnavalkya, the main teacher in the *Brihadaranayaka Upanishad*, were regarded as great yogis. In addition, there is a whole set of *Yoga Upanishads* that arose at a later period.

The Vedic Yoga is arguably the origin and seed of the other Yogas. The *Rigveda* with its thousand hymns is one of the longest Yogic texts and reflects the teaching of the greatest number of Yoga teachers. Many yogic and Vedantic teachings, starting with the *Upanishads*, look back to Vedic teachings, and quote or paraphrase them.

The *Mahabharata*, the great epic in which the *Bhagavad Gita* occurs, contains many explanations of Vedic teachings in its *Moksha Dharma* section, which like the *Gita* deals with the highest Self-realization. The *Bhagavad Gita* contains many allusions to the Vedic Yoga, recast in a later language around the figure of Lord Krishna. Krishna states says that he taught the original Yoga to Vivasvan, who in turn taught it to Manu.[96] This specifically identifies Krishna's Yoga with the Vedic Yoga, as Manu is the original founder of all the Vedic teachings.

Among the seers, Krishna says he is Ushanas, who is the foremost among the seer-poets or Kavis.[97] This statement of Krishna looks back to the greatness of Ushanas in the *Rigveda*, as revealed in this following verse:

> *Rishi, seer, guide of men, skillful, wise, Ushanas by his seer power, he found that which was hidden, the secret hidden Name of the rays (or cows of light).* [98]
>
> *Ushana Kavya, Rigveda IX.87.3*

Ushanas' great discovery is of the Divine Name or nature hidden in the spiritual heart, which he accomplishes by his seer power. It is not a matter of mere cows but the inner light of our soul that has been hidden in the darkness of ignorance.

Shaivite Yoga can be traced back to Rudra and the Maruts in the Vedic teachings. Rudra appears as the personification of the Vedic Yajna, as in the famous Rudram chant of the *Krishna Yajur Veda*.[99] Shaivite Yoga was earlier called the "Pashupata Yoga" in the *Mahabharata*, from Shiva as Pashupati or the "Lord of the wild animals." This goes back to the Rudra Yoga or Yoga of the Maruts in the *Rigveda*, an important formulation of the Vedic Yoga. Classical Yoga rests upon the figure of Hiranyagarbha, who is connected to Vedic mantras in the *Mahabharata*, as we will examine in a later chapter.

Vedic Yoga and the *Yoga Sutras*

Yamas and Niyamas

Among the most obvious connections between the Vedic Yoga and classical Yoga can be found in the *yamas* and *niyamas*, the yogic principles and life-style practices that constitute the first two of the eight limbs of Raja Yoga. The *Vedas* are first of all an attempt to embody and teach Dharma. Classical Yoga, as a Vedic tradition, rests upon the dharmic foundation of the yamas and niyamas, the yogic principles of dharmic living. The yamas and niyamas of Yoga are a summation of Vedic Dharmic principles found throughout older Vedic texts. The yamas and niyamas reflect the Vedic idea that one must have a dharmic foundation in daily life in order to truly approach the spiritual path.

Kriya Yoga of the *Yoga Sutras* consists of the three niyamas of *tapas, svadhyaya,* and *Ishvara pranidhana*,[100] which form the foundation of the five niyamas. *Tapas* is perhaps the key principle of Vedic practice, relating specifically to Agni, the basis of the Vedic Yoga and is often identified with the Yajna or the Vedic sacrifice. Ganapati Muni identifies tapas with Yoga. The *Rigveda* states that it is through tapas that the universe is created.[101] Agni gives us the power of tapas, self-discipline, aspiration, will-power, and inner heat. Agni is related to Tapo Loka or the realm of tapas, in Puranic thought.

Svadhyaya commonly means study of the *Vedas* in Vedic texts up to the *Upanishads*.[102] It does not simply refer to Self-study in a general sense but to the study of the specific Vedic teachings that were part of one's family background or given by one's guru. The fruit of Svadhyaya as explained in the *Yoga Sutras* is the vision of the Ishta Devata,[103] or chosen form of the Divine that one worships. These were the prime Hindu Gods and Goddesses of Shiva, Vishnu, Brahma, Surya, Ganesha, and the many complimentary forms of the Goddess and Divine Mother.

Perhaps the most important connection between Patanjali Yoga with the Vedic Yoga is the emphasis on *Ishvara pranidhana*.[104] Ishvara pranidhana involves surrender to the Divine as the supreme inner power, which is reflected in the Vedic Bhakti Yoga that involves surrender to the deity in the form of the Vedic Deities like Indra, Agni, and Soma. "Ishvara," or the Lord, is a synonym for Indra, the ruler of the Vedic Gods. Ishvara pranidhana can be defined primarily as *Indra pranidhana* in Vedic terms, as Vedic Indra and later Ishvara have the same basic meaning.

Relative to Ishvara Pranidhana, Patanjali emphasizes the importance of Pranava or primal sound, the main form of which is the seed mantra Oṁ.[105] As the *Vedas* are a development of Pranava, he is referring not just to the chanting of Oṁ but also to the study of the *Vedas*. This makes sense as Patanjali was also a famous Sanskrit grammarian. Sanskrit grammar (Vyakarana) is said to develop from Pranava or Oṁ. It is one of the Vedangas or limbs of the *Vedas*.

The Yamas are common dharmic principles in Vedic texts. *Ahimsa* or non-violence is a key principle of Yajna or sacrifice, and is commonly extolled in the *Bhagavad Gita* and *Mahabharata*. Yajna does not mean harming other creatures. It means offering everything to God. Even the rare animal sacrifices that were performed in Vedic times, like Native American ritual killing of the buffalo, were mainly for people who depended upon animals for food.

Satya or truthfulness is one of the main principles of Vedic thought. In the *Rigveda*, the Vedic Gods are called *Satya*, particularly Indra. "Indra, we affirm you as truth (Satya), but never as untruth."[106] *Ṛtam*, which is a synonym for Satya as a truth, is lauded throughout the *Rigveda*, often in the form of *Ṛtam Bṛhat* or the "Vast Truth."

> *The thousand stream bull who increases by the juice, beloved for the Divine birth, who born of the truth increases by the truth, the Divine King, the Vast Truth.*[107]
>
> *Gauraviti Shaktya, Rigveda IX.108.8*

Brahmacharya is a key Vedic principle, meaning "dwelling in Brahman," and is equated with the Vedic Yajna or sacrifice in the *Upanishads*.[108] *Shaucha* is an important Vedic principle of cleanliness, particularly various forms of ritual bathing (snana) that were done on a daily basis.

Pranayama and Meditation

The dominant deities of the *Vedas* are those of the Pranic sphere like Indra, Vayu and Vata, Rudra, the Ashwins, and the Maruts. Indra as the Supreme Deity of the *Vedas* is first of all the cosmic and supreme prana. He is the lord of the air and atmosphere. While we do not find specific pranayama practices detailed in Vedic texts, we do see many hints about them, as well as a frequent extoling of the power of prana and Vayu.

The *Vedas* deal with meditation and samadhi. The *Rigveda* speaks of various states of bliss, spiritual intoxication or the flow of Soma. These are not simply drug-based inebriations but a poetic rendition of the Vedic experience of *samadhi* that is the goal of all the teachings embodied in the Soma hymns.[109]

Tantric Yoga and Hatha Yoga

Traditional Tantric Yoga employs ritual, mantra, pranayama, and meditation, much like the Vedic approach, recognizing Agni and Soma or the cosmic fire and nectar powers. Agni relates to the Kundalini Shakti and the three lower chakras that are the seat of Agni or fire in Tantric thought. Soma relates to the nectar of immortality or the Moon in the crown chakra and the three higher chakras in general. In this way, Tantric Yoga develops from the Agni-Soma Yoga of the *Rigveda*, but recasts Agni as the Goddess and Soma as Shiva as its dominant symbolism. The inner Vedic Yoga of Agni and Soma could easily be called "Vedic Tantra" and supplements the practices of Tantric Yoga, which reflects secret Vedic practices. Tantric Yoga rests upon the mysticism of the Sanskrit alphabet whose roots are in the *Vedas*. It includes a number of Vedic chants like the *Gayatri Mantra*.

The main difference between Vedic and Tantric Yogas is that the Vedic Yoga rests upon a symbolism of light, whereas the Tantric reflects a more anthropomorphic symbolism of male and female energies. This gives Tantra an iconic presentation, whereas the Vedic is naturalistic. But even here there is considerable overlap.

It is easy to see the Vedic basis of traditional Hatha Yoga, because Hatha Yoga is first of all a Yoga of the Sun and the Moon, which are Agni and Soma. Hatha Yoga looks at the Sun and the Moon through the solar and lunar nadis or the Ida and the Pingala. It regards Agni as Kundalini and the digestive fire, and Soma as the crown Chakra.

Primary Practices of the Vedic Yoga

Vedic Yoga like classical Yoga is a complex and many-sided discipline designed to address the needs of different levels and temperaments of individuals. Vedic Yoga addresses all of life and works with all of nature, like a symphony using many instruments, with many movements, scales, tones, and harmonics. Though it has its practical methodology and precise application, Vedic Yoga cannot be reduced to a simple pattern, formula, or method. One could compare it to a great banyan tree, with roots in both the air and on the ground, and many trunks and branches, on which many creatures live and find nourishment. Its very complexity is daunting as it reflects the teachings of numerous seers over many centuries.

Beyond its seemingly immense intricacy and labyrinthine maze of forces, however, Vedic Yoga follows a coherent and structured process that unfolds in each individual human being in a similar manner. Though we are all different at one level, at another level, we are all part of the same species, the same life and consciousness, following the same rhythm of action and expression. In our inmost souls, we all reflect the Divine Will to reach the Supreme, which has its own law and follows its own seasons. Once we understand the basic principles of the Vedic Yoga, we can discern how its apparently discrete elements fit together into an integral and organic whole. That is why in the end, whatever Vedic deity is followed, one merges the deity into light, bliss, oneness, and transcendence.

Vedic Deity or Devata Yoga

The Vedic is a "Deity Yoga," or *Devata Yoga*, as is common in Hindu, Buddhist, and native traditions. Vedic Yoga requires that we awaken the deities within our own minds and hearts and learn to work with them through the forces of the universe. The *Rigveda* in particular is the Vedic book of the deities or Devatas, revealing their names, natures, and functions. It is through these Divine powers that the Vedic Yoga and Vedic Dharma proceeds.

Mere practice of Vedic mantras and techniques is not enough to constitute a complete Vedic Yoga. Vedic deities are the agents and instruments of the Vedic Yoga, not we ourselves, our ordinary minds and human personalities. To understand the *Vedas*, we must understand the meaning of the Vedic deities and come to a living experience of their manifold powers.

Each Vedic deity represents an important approach to inner knowledge, energy, and delight. It is both a reflection of the Supreme Godhead and a way to its realization. We can experience these Vedic deities like Indra and Agni as vividly as any other Divine form or manifestation. Ultimately, the Vedic Yoga requires that we understand the deities or cosmic powers behind all that we do. This begins with the biological forces behind our body, breath, and senses, and extends to the spiritual principles behind the cosmos.

Vedic Yoga as Rishi Yoga

The Vedic Yoga is a Rishi Yoga, a Yoga of the seers. It requires a seer-vision in order to fully apply it. Something of the Rishi consciousness is necessary in order to appreciate the Vedic Yoga, or understand the intricacy of the Vedic language. The Vedic Yoga is not for those who cannot discern the inner meaning of words, images, symbols, and aspirations. The Vedic mantric language is the language of the Rishis and cannot simply be approached as any ordinary form of discourse.

Vedic Yoga aims at turning us as human individuals into Rishis. For this we need to awaken the seed of Rishi consciousness within our own hearts and nourish it with Yoga, sacrifice, search, and devotion. Vedic deities are the cosmic counterparts of the Rishis. The Rishi is the one with the power to invoke the deity, and the deity is the means through which our Rishi consciousness is energized at a cosmic level.

Agni, Awakening the Soul's Search for Divinity Through its Many Lives

The first step of Vedic Yoga consists of awakening the soul or the deeper consciousness of immortality within us. Yoga in the inner sense is a process for the soul or our eternal being to unfold. Yoga is not for the profit or entertainment of our transient personality caught in the illusions of this present birth. Yoga's purpose is to develop the greater potentials of our inner being, of which our outer personality and self-image are but a veil. One must first be willing look beyond the ego-self, its urges, demands, and expectations to be able to approach Yoga in the classical sense of the term.

In yogic thought, what could be called the soul or inner being is the individual Self, our internal or core consciousness that persists throughout the karmic cycle of birth and death, the *Jivatman* of Vedantic thought. The soul has many bodies, lives, and personalities. Yet behind these outer formations, the soul has an inherent sense and sure awareness of its own immortality, its Divine purpose, and goal. For Yoga to be an authentic spiritual practice, it must be done by the soul. Yoga done by the ego or by the mind is a Yoga done in the shadows, not in the light of higher awareness. Our practice of Yoga must be a practice of the heart beyond social, commercial, personal, and cultural concerns. This Yoga of the heart is not a Yoga of the physical, emotional, or psychological heart. It is a Yoga of our immortal essence as an eternal soul, whose true labor in its many lives is Yoga, the search to realize its divine and cosmic Self.

Awakening the soul of Yoga requires bringing our inner fire or soul flame forward as the guide and master of our being. It means awakening to our inner guru and linking up with the inner tradition of truth. This usually requires the light of the outer guru, teaching, and tradition, in one form or another, to help us. Lighting our inner fire and keeping it burning throughout all our states of consciousness as waking, dream, and deep sleep, is the foundation of all deep Yoga and meditation. This "Yoga of the Inner Fire," or *Agni Yoga*, consists of the cultivation of higher awareness through mantra, inquiry, and meditation. For this there is a wonderful Vedic verse that Sri Aurobindo emphasized:

> *The mantras love him who remains awake. The harmonies come to him who remains awake. To him who remains awake the Soma says, "I am yours and have my home in your loving friendship".*
>
> *The fire remains awake, him the mantras love. The fire remains awake, to him the harmonies come. The fire remains awake, to him the Soma says, "I am yours and have my home in your loving friendship."*[110]
>
> *Avatsara Kashyapa, Rigveda V.44.14-15*

At first, this Agni or sense of God-consciousness is but a spark, a flicker or a small flame hidden deep in the subconscious mind, a mere latent possibility. The Vedic Yoga rests upon a surrender to that fire and a cultivation of it, until it can guide us back to the universal light that is its origin and goal. Yoga consists of various offerings of body, speech, senses, mind and heart into that inner fire. The fire in turn grows with each offering, granting us greater illumination, understanding, and well-being.

Eventually that small spark becomes a mighty flame that consumes all impurity – then expands into a great spiritual Sun within us, full of truth and light, with unlimited powers of illumination. The power of Agni, its *tapas-shakti*, purifies, heats, ripens, transforms, and delivers us from the darkness to the light. We cultivate that fire through right intention, consecration, mantra, inquiry, and meditation. This inner fire develops through a higher power of the will, higher values, and a deeper search and inquiry in life. Through it, all the other Divine powers have a place to manifest within us, according to their nature and their qualities.

Developing Indra, the Master Force of Self-realization

Once the flame of the soul is awakened and has come forth to guide our development, manifesting the Gods or Divine powers, we must soon contact and set in motion the master force, the Divine consciousness, in order to achieve the ultimate goal. The Vedic God Indra represents the cosmic consciousness that descends into the human being as the lightning flash of direct perception that reveals the highest truth. This descent of grace from above links up with the ascending power of our soul fire from below. Indra is the God-consciousness within us that carries the cosmic and supracosmic Divine in seed form. As ascending and descending forces, Agni and Indra complement one another and comprehend the yogic quest.

This Indra consciousness enters through the fontanel and takes its seat in our heart along with Agni. Indra manifests through the perceptive power of the higher or great prana (Maha Prana), the master life-force behind the universe that is ever seeking greater self-expression, self-mastery, and self-realization—ever marching forward to the goal of realizing the entire universe within the mind. These two great powers of Indra and Agni, enlightened prana from above and awakened will-power from within, overcome all obstacles and manifest all the Gods or truth principles.

The cultivation of the master force consists of pranayama, discriminating insight, and deep meditation. It involves a revolution at the core of our consciousness itself. This means an inner battle between the powers of light and darkness, a movement from the darkness to the light, in which we can no longer accept anything limited and superficial into our being. Indra is the spiritual warrior who causes us to see the supreme. Though the Indra force begins to manifest at an early phase of the Vedic Yoga, it is only when the Yoga is complete that his full power can be known. Otherwise that Indra energy must face various obstacles and opposition, the various enemies that he must defeat and conquer along the way.

Developing Surya, the Enlightened Awareness

There are many Vedic Sun Gods called *Adityas*, which mean "powers of unbounded energy and forces of primal intelligence," sons of the great Goddess Aditi of boundless space. The Adityas represent the different powers and principles of the illumined mind and heart. Following a solar symbolism, they are said to be seven or twelve in number. The Adityas reflect the principles of Dharma and modes of conduct. Each indicates a teaching that is necessary for our higher realization.

Most important of the Adityas are the pair Varuna and Mitra, who much like Soma and Agni – which they are often identified with – represent the overall cosmic duality. Varuna and Mitra are great Lords of Dharma and instill in us Dharmic values, allowing us to lead a Dharmic life. Varuna, which means "the vastness," represents the discrimination between truth and falsehood, the recognition of karma and the necessity for purification. There is something stern about our meeting with Varuna, who effaces the ego into the higher truth. Yet Varuna protects the Soma principle or cosmic waters, which his grace releases once we have purified ourselves. Along with Varuna is Mitra, who is the deity of compassion and love, complementary to Varuna's stern judgment. Mitra, which means friend, is the Divine Friend who leads us like a friend and causes us to seek friendship and harmony with all. Mitra connects us to Agni as the principle of light and the inner guide.

Along with Mitra and Varuna, Aryaman is the third Aditya, the one who holds the power of nobility and refinement (Arya). Aryaman represents law and force in action, the ability to help, mediate, and harmonize. Mitra, Varuna, and Aryaman govern the three higher luminous heavens (rochanas) beyond the ordinary three realms of earth, atmosphere, and heaven.

The fourth Aditya is Bhaga, who holds the supreme power of bliss and delight. He resembles a masculine counterpart of the Goddess Lakshmi, granting not only worldly wealth, but also spiritual abundance and the richness of devotion. Mitra, Varuna, Aryaman, and Bhaga form the four kings or great rulers of Dharma. Bhaga is associated with Savita, the transformative aspect of solar energy, which represents the ascending Divine will in creation.

Our Agni, the flame of our inner mind, develops the truth principles and dharmic powers represented by the Solar Godheads. There is a progressive development and expansion of the light of truth from this inner flame to the universal Sun. The Sun Gods complement the master force and insight of Indra, adding various powers of knowledge and illumination. The Yoga of the higher mind involves meditation on the Adityas and awakening their powers within us. Indra is present behind them as their ruling force.

Developing Soma: The Ecstasy of Samadhi

Yoga is a methodology of achieving the state of samadhi, the level of bliss or Ananda, in which the mind is absorbed in God or in the Self that is its origin. Soma is the Vedic deity of samadhi, in which all the Vedic deities merge. Soma is lauded as the king of the Gods. All Vedic deities drink the Soma, are energized by the Soma, and are themselves manifestations of the Soma power of bliss. This Soma or bliss is the creator of all but also the goal of all.

Agni is enkindled in order to prepare the Soma. Indra reaches its fullness of power by the Soma or ecstatic essence of delight of which he is the main drinker. It is his drinking of the Soma that energizes Indra and affords him his master power. The Sun as an enlightenment force exists to take us to the higher bliss of Soma. Soma is the food, milk, and lifeblood of all the Vedic deities. It is the unfoldment of the inner Soma that makes one into a Rishi or a seer and gives great creative powers. Vedic Yoga reaches its culmination in the free flowing of Soma that is the highest samadhi. In samadhi one learns to drink the immortal Soma that is the consciousness of immortality.

Other Vedic Deities

The many deities lauded in the Vedic hymns also have their roles in the Vedic Yoga, generally defined relative to the sphere of the main deity that they relate to as earth (Fire or Agni), atmosphere (Indra), and heaven (Sun or Surya).

There are many forms of Surya or the solar force of light and the world of heaven. Along with the many *Adityas* or the Sun Gods, are the Universal Gods or *Vishve Deva* that reflect the universal light. There is also Ushas as the Goddess of the Dawn. The many deities of the atmosphere are connected to Indra. These include Rudra and Brihaspati who govern over sound and mantra, and deity groups like the Maruts, Rudras, and Ashvins that reflect prana and energy. Agni and Soma do not have as many associated deities in their respective spheres but have many names and forms of their own. Agni is associated with a group of deities called the Vasus. With Soma are watery deities and Goddesses.

The Yoga of Light

The Vedic deities are forms of light, with four forms being most prominent: Agni or fire, Soma or Moon (reflected light), Indra or lightning, and Surya or the Sun (illumination). These aspects of light function in the outer world and in the inner world. In the psyche, Agni or Fire is speech and motivation, Soma or Moon is the reflective aspect of mind and emotion, Indra or lightning is the energetic aspect of the mind as the power of perception, Surya or the Sun is the illuming power of the mind as awareness. These are the four related light centers in the subtle body:[111]

Surya - Sun	Spiritual Heart	Awareness
Soma - Moon	Crown chakra	Reflection
Indra - Lightning	Third Eye	Perception
Agni – Fire	Root	Speech

Through understanding these four energy centers, we can see that the subtle body and its chakra system was well known to the Vedic seers and integral to the Vedic mantras. The Vedic Devatas or Godheads of light reflect the deepest energies of our own consciousness and their integral development

Shvetashvatara Upanishad: The Vedic Link

To show how Vedic Yoga relates to classical Yoga, let us look to an important older *Upanishad*, the *Shvetashvatara*. It is one of the early *Upanishads* to emphasize the term Yoga, though Yoga, particularly as knowledge or devotion, is common to all the *Upanishads*.

Most significant for our current discussion is that this *Upanishad* quotes specific Vedic verses for explaining the practices of Yoga, revealing the yogic implications of Vedic deities, which can be equated with Ayurvedic principles. The *Shvetashvatara* is regarded as the most important *Upanishads* for the worship of Lord Shiva, who is the deity of Yoga, particularly in the traditions of Hatha Yoga and Siddha Yoga.

This great *Upanishad* begins with a discussion of the wheel of the cosmos and speaks of the great sages who "having achieved the Yoga of Meditation (Dhyana Yoga) have perceived the Shakti of the Divine Self hidden in its own qualities."[112] Then it explains the realization of the Self: "As sesame oil in sesame seeds, as ghee in cream, as water in the channels, as fire in the fire sticks, thus the Self is grasped in the Self, by him who through truthfulness and tapas perceives it."[113]

In the second of its six chapters, this *Upanishad* outlines the main practice of Yoga, starting with five verses from the *Shukla Yajurveda* that this particular *Upanishad* relates to, including two verses from the *Rigveda* that are part of these. Note that many of these verses are to the deity Savita, the transformative aspect of solar energy who is the deity of the Gayatri mantra, and sometimes called *Hiranyagarbha* or the golden fetus, a name for the founder of the Yoga Darshana tradition.

Shvetashvatara Upanishad Chapter II

1. *Yoking first the mind, having extended the intelligence, discerning the light of the fire, the transformative Sun Savita brought it forth from the earth.*[114]

The verb "yuj," or "yoking," from which the term Yoga arises, is here used in a verbal form relative to the mind or manas, along with extending the higher intelligence, meditative mind, or Dhi. The idea of Yoga here is a control of the lower mind, much as in the *Yoga Sutras*, and an awakening of the higher intelligence.

The light of the fire that comes out of the earth here suggests the Kundalini fire that arises from the root or earth chakra. The connection of Agni with the digestive fire occurs in the *Rigveda*,[115] as it is in yogic thought, where it is connected to the Kundalini, which like Vedic Agni is a power of speech and mantra.

The transforming Sun, Savita, is the deity of the famous Gayatri mantra. He represents the guiding Divine intelligence within us, the seed of our higher yogic evolutionary potential. He is one of the solar powers behind the greater yogic process. He governs transformations in the cycle of time, like sunrise and sunset.

2. *With a yogically controlled mind in the impulse of the Divine transforming Sun, may we have the power to reach the world of light.*[116]

Yukta manas, or the "yogically controlled mind," is the basis of all Yoga practice, as in the *Yoga Sutras*. This control is not by the personal self but according to the impulse, energy or motivation of the Divine, through our surrender within or Ishvara pranidhana. It takes us to the higher realms of the light of consciousness.

3. *Having yoked by the mind the Gods that lead to the world of light, by the power of insight to heaven, creating the vast light, the transforming Sun impels them forth.*[117]

The Gods here are our own heaven moving powers and faculties, starting with our mind and senses turned within in pratyahara, by the power of the Dhi or buddhi. Once we turn our attention within, our own faculties guide us to their deeper perceptions and the higher truth.

4. *Seers of the great illumined seer yogically control the mind and intelligence. One only he ordains the invocations of the Gods. Great is the affirmation of the Savita, the Divine creative Sun.*[cxvii]

The verbal root "yuj" for "yoking" is used here again. The seers, *vipra*, yogically control the mind or manas and higher intelligence or Dhi, as mentioned in verse one. Savita here indicates the Divine will toward union or Yoga inherent within us. This is the basis of all the manifestations of the Gods or Divine powers within us. This is a verse from the *Rigveda*.

5. *I yogically unite by the power of surrender to your ancient Brahman. May this chant go forth by the path of the Sun. May all the sons of immortality hear it, those who dwell in celestial domains.*[119]

Bhakti Yoga or the Yoga of Devotion is indicated here, through another verbal derivative of the noun "Yoga." The path of the Sun is the path of light up the spine or Sushumna to the light of the Self. This is a verse from the *Rigveda*. It is attributed to the Sun God Vivasvan, who is traditionally the father of Manu. It is to Vivasvan that Krishna says in the *Bhagavad Gita* that he taught the original Yoga.[120]

6. *Where the fire is enkindled, where the wind is controlled, where Soma overflows, there the higher mind is born.*[121]

This is perhaps the key verse here helps us understand the yogic implications of the main Vedic deities. Agni, Vayu, and Soma as the great Vedic deities of Fire,

Air, and the Moon refer to their internal counterparts of will, prana, and mind and are indicative of the practice of Yoga.

The Fire is the Kundalini fire. Control of wind refers to pranayama. Soma here is the bliss of meditation or samadhi. In these the higher mind or consciousness is born. Agni, Vayu, and Soma here also relate to Pitta, Vata, and Kapha doshas, the biological fire, air, and water humors of Ayurvedic thought.

7. *By the impulse of the creative Sun, honor the ancient Brahman. Make your source there. Then your merit will never be lost.*[122]

The solar urge towards light and enlightenment unfolds the yogic path to the supreme truth. Following that motivation is our guide to the highest. Clearly the Sun in this teaching is the higher awareness, not just the light in the sky!

8. *Making straight the three places, balancing the body, merge the senses along with the mind into the heart. By the boat of Brahman the knower should cross over all the channels that bring us fear.*

The three places are the navel, heart, and head, indicating a straight spine in a balanced sitting pose, delineating the basics of asana practice. The channels that bring us fear are the nadis of the subtle body that keep our energy caught in duality, particularly the lunar and solar or Ida and Pingala nadis. One crosses over them to the central channel or Sushumna that takes us beyond the fear of death. The boat of Brahman is the power of the chant or the higher knowledge.

9. *Merging the pranas here, with controlled action, when the prana is withdrawn, one should exhale through the nostrils. As a chariot with difficult to control horses, the knower should concentrate the mind (dharana) without any distraction.*

Here pranayama, pratyahara, and dharana are indicated, including the practice of Kevala Kumbhaka or entering into the breathless state. This occurs when the inner unitary prana is awakened. One then relaxes through exhalation and enters into the higher awareness.

10. *One should practice in a level pure place, devoid of rocks, fire or insects, and free of people, sound, water, and houses, pleasing to the mind, and not disturbing to the eyes, secret, and free of wind.*

General indications of the right type of place for Yoga practice, emphasizing nature and solitude.

11. *Like mist, smoke, the Sun or Fire, like a firefly, lightning, sparks or the Moon. These signs are precursors of the realization of Brahman in Yoga.*

Similar to the outer light forms in nature, inner light forms manifest in the mind during meditation indicating a growing direct contact with the deity and higher light.

12. Earth, water, fire, air, ether arisen in a fivefold form proceed in the qualities of Yoga. He has no disease, no old age or death, who has gained the body created by the fire of Yoga.

The five elements here refer to the five chakras that are the sites of the cosmic elements, which open and are dissolved during Yoga practice. The fire of Yoga is the Kundalini Shakti. The body gained through the fire of Yoga is the purified subtle body that is beyond all the limitations of the physical body.

13. Lightness, health, lack of instability, good complexion, good speech, good fragrance, reduction of the amount of urine and feces, these are among the first signs of progress in Yoga.

Such statements of purification of the body occur in many later yogic texts as well.

14. Just as mirror tainted by dirt shines brightly when purified by water, so having perceived the truth of the Self, the One, the master of the body, having achieved his goal becomes free of sorrow.

Such statements of purification of the mind occur in later Yoga texts.

15. Who by the truth of the Self, like a lamp, self-controlled sees the truth of the Brahman here, the eternal unborn transcending all cosmic principles; knowing that deity, one is released from all bondage.

The language is now abstract and the symbology of the Vedic deities is not used, but we can still infer this deeper side to their meaning.

16. He is the Deity who is in all directions, born before all, he stirs within the child. He is what has been born and what will be born. He stands before all men whose face is to every side.

This verse reflects the immortal Self in all human beings that pervades the entire universe. Within the child or fetus, garbha, is also within the small space within the heart.

17. Which Deity is in fire and in the waters, which has entered into the entire universe, which is in the plants and in the trees, to that Deity we offer our surrender.

Here the Vedic surrender or namas to the deity is indicated. This Deity is our Self that pervades all of nature. Fire and water or Agni and Apas here do not just indicate the outer elements but their inner counterparts as well.

****

This *Upanishad* introduces Yoga as another definition of the Vedic practice of working with the elements and deities of nature. The *Upanishad* reminds us of a verse from the *Yajurveda*:

> *That is Agni, That is the Sun, That is Vayu, and That is the Moon. That is the luminous, That is Brahman. These are the waters. He is the Lord of Creation.*
>
> *All winkings of the eye were born of the Lightning Person (Vidyut Purusha). No one has grasped him, above, across or in the middle.*[123]
>
> *Shukla Yajurveda XXXII.1*

In these *Yajurveda* verses, it is not just the outer Fire, Sun, Wind, and Moon that are indicated, but both their inner and cosmic forms. That or "Tat" is the supreme Self. The Purusha is both the outer and the inner Fire, Sun, Wind, Moon, and Waters. The lightning Purusha is the Vedic Indra who is the supreme Seer, with his Vajra or thunderbolt. In other words, the practice of Yoga is hidden in the very concept of the Vedic deities as powers of light and aspects of Yoga practice.

Hiranyagarbha, Patanjali and the Vedic Basis of Classical Yoga

May we know the inspirer of the higher mind; May we meditate upon Hiranyagarbha; May the power of Yoga direct that towards us.

Swami Veda Bharati, Hiranyagarbha Gayatri[124]

Many people today look to Patanjali, the compiler of the famous *Yoga Sutras*, as the father or founder of the greater system of Yoga. While Patanjali's work is very important and worthy of profound examination, a study of the ancient literature on Yoga reveals that the Yoga tradition is much older than Patanjali – and that its main practices existed long before his time. Patanjali was a compiler, not an originator of the Yoga teachings.

Traditional Yoga, meanwhile, is more than the Yoga Darshana system that Patanjali is part of, but extends to all branches of Yoga as Knowledge (Jnana), Devotion (Bhakti), Works (Karma), and many others. In addition, the traditional founder of *Yoga Darshana*, or the Yoga system of philosophy that the *Yoga Sutras* of Patanjali represents, is said to be *Hiranyagarbha*. It is nowhere in classical Yoga literature said to be Patanjali. The *Mahabharata*, the great ancient text in which the *Bhagavad Gita* of Sri Krishna occurs and which is sometimes called the "fifth Veda," states: "Kapila, the teacher of Samkhya, is said to be the supreme Rishi. Hiranyagarbha is the original knower of Yoga. There is no one else more ancient."[125]

Elsewhere in the *Mahabharata*, Krishna states, identifying himself with Hiranyagarbha: "As my form, carrying the knowledge, eternal and dwelling in the Sun, the teachers of Samkhya, who have discerned what is important, call me Kapila. As the brilliant Hiranyagarbha, who is lauded in the verses of the *Vedas*, ever worshipped by Yoga, so I am remembered in the world."[126] Note that Krishna identifies yogic Hiranyagarbha with the deity of the same name in the *Vedas* that is identified with the Sun. Krishna also speaks of his different names mentioned also in the *Rigveda, Yajurveda, Atharvaveda, Samaveda, Puranas, Upanishads,* Jyotisha (Vedic astrology), Samkhya, Yoga Shastras, and Ayurveda, showing the antiquity and interrelationship of these Vedic traditions.[127]

Other yogic texts like the *Brihad Yogi Yajnavalkya Smriti*[128] similarly portray Hiranyagarbha as the original teacher of Yoga, just as they do Kapila as the original teacher of the Samkhya system. So do commentaries on the *Yoga Sutras*. Vijnana Bhikshu, the great Samkhya teacher in his *Yogavartika* commentary on the first sutra of the *Yoga Sutras*, explains Hiranyagarbha as the *Adiguru* or primal guru of Yoga, quoting the *Yogi Yajnavalkya.*[129] While the depth, clarity, and brevity of Patanjali's compilation is noteworthy, it is the mark of a later summation, not a new beginning.

The vast literature of the *Vedas*, *Mahabharata*, and *Puranas* speak of numerous great yogis but does not mention Patanjali, who was of a later period.[130] Even Yoga literature that is later in time than Patanjali, like that of Kashmir Shaivism, Siddha Yoga or Hatha Yoga, does not make Patanjali central to its teachings, though they may mention him, but rather emphasize the deity Shiva as *Adinath* or their original guru.[131]

Several *Upanishads* like the *Katha, Kena,* and *Shvetashvatara* are called Yoga Shastras, besides numerous later *Yoga Upanishads*. They do not mention Patanjali and have Yoga taught by a variety of teachers, including famous Vedic figures like Yajnavalkya and Shandilya. The *Puranas*, which are large encyclopedic works of traditional knowledge going back to medieval and ancient periods, contain many sections on Yoga but do not give importance to Patanjali. When such texts teach Yoga, they often use quotes from the older Vedas, like the *Shvetashvatara Upanishad* that we discussed in the previous chapter of this book.

The *Bhagavad Gita* is the primary text lauded as a *Yoga Shastra* or 'definitive Yoga teaching' in the ancient literature. This Yoga connection can be carried to the *Mahabharata* as a whole, in which the *Gita* occurs. Bhishma in the *Mahabharata* speaks of a Yoga teaching "established in many Yoga Shastras."[132] The *Anu Gita* section of the *Mahabharata* has an interesting section that begins, "Thus I will declare, the supreme and unequalled Yoga Shastra,"[133] and describes Yoga as Self-realization.

The topics addressed in the *Yoga Sutras* from yamas and niyamas to dhyana and samadhi are already taught extensively in the older literature. In the *Mahabharata*, the sage Yajnavalkya relates the description of Yoga after that of Samkhya.[134] The *Shandilya Upanishad* refers to an eightfold or Ashtanga Yoga, which it describes in great detail, but does not mention Patanjali.[135]

Patanjali in the *Yoga Sutras* is referred to as a compiler, not as an inventor of the Yoga teachings. He himself states, "Thus is the teaching of Yoga."[136] This is quite unlike Krishna, the avatar of Yoga, who states, "I taught the imperishable Yoga to the Sun God Vivasvan. Visvasvan taught Manu. Manu taught Ikshvaku, thus handed down by tradition, the royal Rishis know it. That Yoga by the long course of time has been lost. That ancient Yoga I have declared today.[137]

Patanjali is sometimes regarded as a devotee of Vishnu/Narayana, whose main human avatar is Krishna. This suggests that Patanjali himself was a devotee of Krishna. Traditional Sanskrit chants to Patanjali laud him as an incarnation of Lord Shesha, the serpent on which Lord Vishnu/Narayana resides. This Shesha attribution links Patanjali to Krishna/Vishnu. Yet others view Patanjali as a Shaivite Yogi, for his emphasis on Ishvara and Oṁ, which are more commonly associated with Shiva than any other deity.

The earlier Yoga literature before Patanjali can perhaps be better called the *Hiranyagarbha Yoga Darshana* as it is said to begin with Hiranyagarbha. In fact, most of the Yoga taught in *Vedas, Upanishads, Bhagavad Gita, Mahabharata,* and *Puranas* – which is the main ancient literature of Yoga – appears as of this Hiranyagarbha tradition. This means that the Patanjali Yoga Darshana is a later subset of an earlier *Hiranyagarbha Yoga Darshana*. It is not a new or original teaching meant to stand on its own.

While no Hiranyagarbha Yoga Sutras text has survived, a number of the teachings of the Hiranyagarbha tradition have remained. In fact, the literature on the Hiranyagarbha Yoga tradition may be as large as that of the Patanjali Yoga tradition, which itself represents a branch of it. This means that we cannot speak of a Patanjali Yoga tradition as apart from an older set of Yoga teachings rooted in the Hiranyagarbha tradition. The Patanjali Yoga teaching occurs in the context of a broader Yoga Darshana that includes other streams. This Yoga Darshana existed long before Patanjali and was taught in many ways. It is the Yoga Darshana originally attributed to Hiranyagarbha and related Vedic teachers.

Yet this Yoga Darshana that is connected to the Samkhya system, also called the 'Samkhya-Yoga darshana', is not the only line of Yoga. The *Mahabharata* and other ancient texts speak of the Vaishnava Yoga that relates to Krishna and of the Shaivite or Pashupata Yoga that goes back to Shiva. Indeed the main Yoga traditions in India are largely Shaivite and use the *Yoga Sutras* only in a secondary manner. Shaivite Yoga includes the traditions of Hatha Yoga and Siddha Yoga (which has its own Raja Yoga), which are more rooted in Shaivite Yoga texts than in the *Yoga Sutras*. While we should certainly honor the Samkhya-Yoga tradition, we should also remember the greater diversity of yogic paths.

Parallel With the Samkhya Tradition

A similar situation, in which the main Sutra text of a Vedic philosophy is later in time than its original teachings, occurs relative to Samkhya. The main sutra text on Samkhya philosophy is the *Samkhya Karika* of Ishvara Krishna. Ishvara Krishna (who is not the Krishna of the Gita) is a figure of the early centuries AD who debated with Buddhist teachers near the time of Vasubandhu, the main teacher of Yogachara Buddhism. Ishvara Krishna is a much later teacher than the original founder of the Samkhya system, the sage Kapila, who is regarded as legendary even at the time of the Upanishads and *Bhagavad Gita*. Ishvara Krishna is more recent than Patanjali, though Patanjali Yoga rests upon the Samkhya philosophy.

There are many Samkhya teachings in the Vedic and Puranic literature older than the *Samkhya Karika*. The *Samkhya Karika* has its prominence as a late and clear compilation of an existing tradition, not the original presentation. This means that there is no need to regard the main text on a particular Vedic darshana as the oldest teaching, or its compiler as the founder of the tradition.

Hiranyagarbha and Vedic Yoga

Who then was Hiranyagarbha, a human figure or a deity? The name Hiranyagarbha, which means "the gold embryo", first occurs prominently as a Vedic deity and form of the Sun God, which has many names involving *hiranya* or gold. There is a special Sukta or hymn to Hiranyagarbha in the *Rigveda*, which is commonly chanted by Hindus today in their daily rituals, in which Hiranyagarbha refers to the Supreme Being or Ishvara, "who among the Gods is the One God."[138]

The *Mahabharata* speaks of Hiranyagarbha as he who is "lauded in the Vedic verses and taught in the Yoga Shastra."[139] As a form of the Sun God, Hiranyagarbha is related to other Sun Gods (Adityas) like Savita, to whom the famous Gayatri mantra used in many Yoga traditions is addressed, and is important in many early Yoga teachings. Therefore, the Hiranyagarbha Yoga tradition appears to be a Vedic tradition rooted in the use of Vedic mantras. We could accurately call it the *Hiranyagarbha Vedic Yoga* tradition. The medieval Sanskrit commentator Uvata speaks of the entire Vedic tradition as going back to Hiranyagarbha, not just the Yoga portion of it.[140] This statement shows that even in much later times the unity of Yoga and Veda was well known.

The *Mahabharata* identifies Hiranyagarbha, as other texts do, with Brahma or Prajapati, the creator among the Hindu trinity, who represents the *Vedas* and is the source of all higher knowledge.[141] Most of the Vedic sciences are first taught by Lord Brahma, who represents the cosmic mind. The *Mahabharata* also identifies Hiranyagarbha with the Buddhi or Mahat, the higher or cosmic mind and Brahma (also called Virinchi).[142]

Hiranyagarbha appears more as a deity than a human figure, though it is possible that a teacher of that name once existed. The chief disciple of Hiranyagarbha in the ancient texts is said to be the Rishi Vasishtha, the foremost of the Vedic seers (seer of the seventh book of the *Rig Veda*), who passed on the Yoga teachings to Narada.[143] Vasishtha teaches the Yoga Darshana in the *Mahabharata*: "The Yoga Darshana has so been declared to you by me according to the truth."[144] Vasishtha passes on his knowledge to his son, Parashara, in whose line was born Veda Vyasa, who compiled the *Vedas* and wrote the *Mahabharata*.

Vasishtha is also the primary early teacher of other Vedic disciplines like Advaita Vedanta (the tradition of Jnana Yoga or the Yoga of Knowledge), and carries on the Yoga teachings of the deities Shiva and Vishnu as well as that of Hiranyagarbha. There are several important Yoga texts in the Vasistha line like the *Vasishtha Samhita* and *Yoga Vasishtha*, the latter of which is often considered to be the greatest work on both Yoga and Vedanta. While these texts derive from a later time period than the Vedic Vasishtha, they do show a continuity of tradition. Vasishtha is related to the Rishi Agastya in the *Rigveda*, who is said to be his older brother.[145] Agastya is very important in South Indian Yoga traditions, which through him may be connected with Hiranyagarbha as well.

The original Yoga darshana tradition appears not as the Patanjali tradition but the Hiranyagarbha tradition. Its teachings are found not only in the *Yoga Sutras*, but also in the *Mahabharata*, and *Bhagavad Gita*, *Moksha Dharma Parva* and *Anu Gita* sections, which contain extensive teachings on Yoga. These in turn connect to the *Vedas, Upanishads, Puranas* and *Tantras*, which address Yoga in many forms like mantra, ritual (Karma Yoga), knowledge (Jnana Yoga), and devotion (Bhakti Yoga). Samkhya, Yoga, and Vedanta – the three main Vedic philosophical systems – are presented as interrelated aspects of the same tradition in the *Mahabharata*. Ayurveda and Vedic astrology are set forth important aspects of its outer application.

The Hiranyagarbha Yoga tradition appears to be a Vedic Yoga tradition. The Patanjali Yoga tradition arises as an offshoot of it or a later expression of it. If we want to go back to the traditional roots of Yoga and restore the original teachings of Yoga, we should examine the Hiranyagarbha Yoga Darshana. In addition, we should look to its Vedic connections and its associations with all Yoga paths and branches. This will take us back to the original Vedic Yoga that encompasses all the Vedic deities.

Misinterpretations of the *Yoga Sutras*

Modern Yoga often projects a misinterpretation and misunderstanding of the *Yoga Sutras*. The first problem is that many people look at the *Yoga Sutras* as an original text that stands in itself, when it is a later compilation that requires knowledge of its background in order to make sense of it. This causes people to separate Yoga from the earlier Vedic tradition that forms the context of Patanjali's teachings, which is why the Hiranyagarbha tradition is little known in the world of Yoga today.

The second problem is that the *Yoga Sutras*, consisting of short aphorisms, can be slanted in different directions according to the inclinations of the interpreter, particularly if one does not give credence to classical commentaries and connections to earlier teachings. This causes people to imagine meanings in the *Sutras* that may actually not be there in the original.

Third, the Yoga Sutra tradition has been made into something sectarian, for example, opposing Yoga and Samkhya as competing philosophical systems to Vedanta. This causes people to separate Yoga from related Vedic traditions that also employ Yoga practices.[146] This complication is not something of the modern age only, but also occurs in debates between Indian philosophical systems in the Middle Ages, a time in which precise logical analysis was often emphasized over any broader synthesis. The original Hiranyagarbha Yoga teachings, such as we find it in the *Mahabharata*, is presented as in harmony with Samkhya and Vedanta. The synthesis of these three systems is as old as Krishna, who relates his teachings back to Manu, the founder of the Vedic Dharma, and also one of the earliest teachers of Yoga.

Such an older integral Yoga as in the *Bhagavad Gita* is of the same general type of integral Yoga as the Yoga-Vedanta taught by great modern Yoga gurus of India like Vivekananda, Yogananda, Aurobindo, and Shivananda – the teachers who first brought Yoga to the West over the last century. They teach the *Yoga Sutras*, the *Bhagavad Gita*, and the *Upanishads* as part of the same broader tradition, often adding Shankara's Advaita Vedanta. Such teachers regard the philosophical differences between Samkhya, Yoga, and Vedanta as minor variations within the same greater teaching.

So, how can we best approach the *Yoga Sutras* in order to understand its real intent? It is arguably best to do so in the context of the older and broader Yoga Darshana. There is one greater Yoga Darshana that exists like a thread through all the texts and traditions of Yoga. There is no Patanjali Yoga Darshana as an entity in itself apart from the older Hiranyagarbha Yoga Darshana, nor is the Hiranyagarbha tradition rigidly delineated from other Yoga teachings and approaches, including the Shaivite systems.

If we want to understand the meaning of the technical terms in the *Yoga Sutras*, we should do so with recourse to the older literature, not by inventing our own meanings, or by trying to make these terms unique to the *Yoga Sutras*. Whether it is the yamas and niyamas (particularly tapas, svadhyaya, and Ishvara pranidhana), the different types of samadhi, or the different aspects of Yoga practice – such terms alluded to briefly in the *Sutras* can be found explained clearly and in detail in the older and broader Vedic literature.

In addition, we should look at the *Yoga Sutras* in light of Vedanta, not only the *Bhagavad Gita*, but also the *Upanishads*, which the *Yoga Sutras* as a Vedic philosophy accept as authoritative. While Patanjali emphasizes Purusha rather than Brahman (the Absolute), we must remember that the Hiranyagarbha tradition gives Brahman its place, and that Brahman and Purusha can be synonyms. We can look to Vedanta for a greater description of Ishvara or God, which Patanjali only alludes to, but which Vedantic texts examine in great detail. This includes both non-dualistic (Advaita) and dualistic (Dvaita) traditions of Vedanta, which have their own important Yoga teachings.

We should discriminate between the greater tradition of Yoga, which includes all branches and types of Yoga, and Patanjali's *Yoga Sutras*, placing the latter in the context of the former. We should not limit Yoga to the *Yoga Sutras* but use the *Sutras* to connect us with the greater Yoga tradition. This includes both the ancient Yoga literature before Patanjali and the later Yoga literature after him – the various lines of Vaishnava, Shaivite, Shakta, and Vedantic Yogas, regardless of their philosophical variations.

Besides looking at Patanjali in a new light, we should work to restore the teachings of the Vedic Hiranyagarbha Yoga Darshana. These can be compiled from the *Mahabharata*, *Upanishads*, and other ancient Vedic teachings. Through the Hiranyagarbha tradition, we can reconstitute the Vedic Yoga that was its basis.

Asana and Exercise in Classical Yoga

Asana is the visible face of Yoga in the modern world. For most people today, Yoga first of all means asana or Yoga postures. If they are looking for a Vedic Yoga, they are probably first looking for a Vedic way of performing asanas. However, asana is the aspect of Yoga least emphasized in Vedic and Yogic texts. Sometimes little more about asana is said than the need to sit straight (*Bhagavad Gita* and *Upanishads*), or to maintain a comfortable pose (*Yoga Sutras*).

This lack of attention to asana in older yogic teachings has led some people to think that active asana approaches and exercise movements, such as are popular with many modern Yoga groups, were not part of the older Yoga traditions or not known in India at all. To adequately approach this issue, we must first examine the exercise traditions of India and Vedic martial arts. We must understand how Yoga asana and exercise relate, their similarities and differences, and their respective places in Indian culture. Classical Yoga was oriented primarily towards meditation rather than exercise, but related martial arts covered all aspects of exercise and were part of monastic traditions and yogic paths in India.

Asana and Exercise Traditions: Related but Different

There has been a tendency to look at asana or Yoga postures as the main exercise system practiced historically in India, with more active exercise approaches like calisthenics and weight lifting, being perhaps a recent borrowing from the West – or something not particularly Indian, with Indians being more mental than physical types. This plays into stereotypes of India as not having strong martial or military traditions, arising perhaps from the recent emphasis on Gandhian ahimsa in the country.

First of all, Yoga asana, as part of classical Yoga traditions like the *Yoga Sutras*, was never meant simply as an exercise or fitness system. Asana in Sanskrit means a 'chair' or a 'seat', and in terms of bodily postures implies a seated pose, and by extension any pose assumed or held for an extended period of time. Asana in classical Yoga was not a term for physical exercise, called *vyayama* in Sanskrit, but as part of Yoga practice, called *sadhana*, a spiritual discipline resting upon the ability to sit or be still for long periods of time to support the practice of meditation. Traditional Yoga asana was not meant as a workout in the modern sense of the term. We must recognize, however, that other exercise traditions did exist in India besides Yoga asanas that were more active in nature, and which did include asanas along with other stronger practices.

Yoga asana could be used as part of other Indian exercise approaches, for example, serving as preliminary warm ups or stretches. In these cases, such asana practice was not regarded by itself as Yoga, which implies a spiritual path, but as a means of bodily health and strength. In other words, asana as part of exercise approaches did exist in older India, but as a different orientation from asana in classical Yoga, whose main concern was a seated posture for meditation. This use of asana in exercise approaches should be discriminated from its role in meditation approaches, though some overlap naturally exists.

India as a vast subcontinent and ancient civilization has had its own ancient and diverse traditions of exercise, martial arts, gymnastics, and dance that cover the full range of exercise practices, along with every sort of callisthenic. India did not require the Europeans in order to bring the idea of physical fitness or healthy exercise into the region. The same situation existed in China and the rest of Asia that had slower or more internalizing forms of exercise like Yoga or Tai Chi, which did not mean that they did not also have stronger exercise approaches as well.

Martial Arts and Indian Exercise Traditions

The *Vedas* speak of the unity of *Brahma* (spiritual) and *Kshatra* (warrior) traditions, and the need to honor both.[147] India has a long history of its Kshatriya, martial, military, aristocratic or princely class. It is among India's traditional martial arts, sustained mainly by the Kshatriyas, that we find the most diverse and extensive traditions of exercise. Hindu warrior traditions continued and developed along with changes of warfare through the centuries.

The *Vedas* contain a special tradition of martial arts called *Dhanur Veda*, which is one of the four *Upavedas* or secondary *Vedas*. Such Vedic martial arts like *Kalari* remain popular in South India to the present day, though many others have been lost in the course of time. Dhanur literally means a bow, so archery was central to these martial arts. Yet India has a tradition of sword fighting as another important martial art.

The most famous ancient guru of the martial arts or *Dhanur Veda*, who is mentioned in the *Ramayana* teaching the martial arts to Rama and Lakshman, is the Vedic Rishi Vishvamitra, a famous Rajarshi or royal sage, who combines both Kshatriya and Brahmin lines. Vishvamitra is the seer of the third book of the *Rigveda* and the seer of the famous Gayatri Mantra, the most widely used Vedic mantra for all Hindus.

The Hindu *Puranas* contain extensive king lists and accounts of ancient warriors along with their great victories. The *Vedas* contain many verses in praise of ancient kings and their martial exploits, like Trasadasyu who is lauded as a demigod,[148] with a few Vedic hymns composed by such royal sages like Sudas or Mandhata. Great warriors like Arjuna or Rama, mentioned in the epics of the *Mahabharata* and *Ramayana*, had special weapons created through the power of mantra and meditation, used to harness the forces of nature.

Hindu monastic traditions have martial lines, like the famous Naga sadhus who wield tridents or Trishulas, leading the marches of monks for the great Kumbha Mela gatherings. A Hindu monastic order today is called an "akhada," which also means a gymnasium (much like the Greek Academy). These monastic orders prescribe asanas, exercises, and martial arts, in part to keep the monks active and physically fit. Some Hindu monastic orders served as warriors and defended temples during the Muslim invasions of the Middle Ages.

Hatha Yoga itself arose as part of a martial and monastic approach to Yoga. The term Hatha means 'force' in Sanskrit. Martial arts are well known in Buddhist monastic traditions of China and Japan. Buddhist martial arts are attributed an Indian origin to Bodhidharma, who came from the famous city of Kanchipuram, not far from modern Chennai, and who also brought the practice of Zen.

The Indian warrior class used mantras and called upon deities for success in battle, like the battle cry "Jai Sri Ram", still used by the Indian army of the state of Uttar Pradesh. The Goddess Durga was said to have given the royal sword to the kings, including such figures as Shivaji of Maharashtra, Guru Gobind Singh and Ranjit Singh of the Sikhs.[149]

The colonial British army owed its prowess largely to its Sikh and Gurkha soldiers from India and Nepal. Gurkhas mainly worship the Goddesses Kali and Durga, Hindu martial Goddesses, and claim connection to Siddha Gorakhnath, the main Nath Yogi behind Siddha Yoga and Hatha Yoga traditions. Their war cry is "Jai Ma Kali!"

Weight Lifting, Weapon Lifting, and Physical Development

Indian martial arts involved the use of heavy weapons, including swords and the mace (gada). Bhima, one of the five Pandavas and companions of Lord Krishna, was famous for his use of the mace and defeated Duryodhana in a mace fight. Hanuman also was famous for his mace. Such heavy weapons served like weight-lifting training.

The use of the bow, particularly the long bow that we find in depictions of Lord Rama, requires a lot of muscular strength in order to wield. Only Rama had the power to string the bow of Lord Shiva as it was very difficult to bend. All the other princes tried and failed. Rama gained Sita as a wife as his reward.

India has extensive traditions of wrestling. Lord Krishna was a great wrestler and defeated his enemy Kamsa in a wrestling match. Such wrestling traditions employed different exercise approaches than Yoga asana and resembled wrestling from throughout the world.

India has a long tradition of depiction of athletes and warriors, as do most of the cultures of the world. Lord Rama is the foremost of these, portrayed carrying a long bow and having a strong physique. Hanuman, his monkey companion, is a kind of Indian superman, noted for his muscular strength and miraculous powers, particularly his ability to make himself either as small or as large as he wants. Bhima, one of the five Pandavas, and the strongest warrior in the *Mahabharata*, is another such figure. Another is Parashurama, who precedes Rama as an avatar of Lord Vishnu, who wielded an axe to conquer the deviant Kshatriyas or unrighteous kings. Modern Hindu Yogis have not simply been emaciated ascetics; many show great physical strength. Hindu deities like Shiva are not portrayed weak in form or stature, but as physically strong.

Hindus have had their own armies up to modern times. It was primarily the armies of the Hindu Marathas that brought down the powerful Mogul empire in the eighteenth century, taking control of most of India before the British arrived, and then becoming the main enemies of early British rule. Such warrior traditions have deep roots in India.

The Kshatriyas had their own approach to ahimsa, which was to reduce the amount of harm in the world, not simply to avoid any violent confrontations. The *Mahabharata*, though lauding ahimsa as the supreme principle, also states that if the King does not have clear rules of law and punishment (the danda or staff), then there is likely to be no peace in his kingdom.[150] Even in Buddhist countries from Tibet to Japan, ahimsa was not employed as a state policy but only for personal practice, and Buddhist martial arts were prominent.[151]

The Kshatriyas had their own Yoga approaches, which blended with the martial arts. Many monastic traditions arose from the Kshatriya class as an extension of military discipline. Buddhism is a good example of this.

Gymnastics and Dance

India has similarly had a long tradition of gymnastics. This is best revealed by the circuses in India, which remain popular today, and have a great antiquity. The gypsies, who originated in India, brought these gymnastic traditions to Europe, along with their circuses.

India has many traditions of classical dance like Kathak, Bharat Natyam, Odissi, and Kathakali. Each region of India has its own type of dance. These require strength and include gymnastic movements of various types. Indian dancers use asanas in order to gain flexibility. Shiva is not only the Lord of Yoga and the Lord of Asana, he is also the "Lord of Dance," *Nataraja*. The 108 dance poses of Lord Shiva include many exercise movements and vinyasas (movement based asanas).

Older Vedic Origins

We find a number of ancient Indus or Harappan seals with figures in various Yoga postures, sitting, and stretching.[152] Many Vedic deities like Indra, Agni, and Soma have warrior characteristics and are portrayed as possessing great physical strength. They use a variety of weapons and have various magic powers. Indra and Rudra among the Vedic deities are referred to as dancers. Rudra, who is later connected with Lord Shiva, is a famous archer in Vedic texts, bringing in *Dhanur Veda*.

Conclusion

Callisthenic practices tend to be alike worldwide because they work with the same human body and its range of movements. Similarities in active exercise approaches between India and the West does not necessarily prove that India had no such traditions before the modern period. This is not to say that there has been no borrowing of exercise methods, but that similar exercise practices existed in India, just as in other Asian countries like China. Modern Yoga in the West does include influences from western exercise, massage, and bodywork practices. But this does not mean there were no strong exercise approaches in older India, or that anything of this type that one may see in recent India must reflect recent western origins.

Asanas have long been part of exercise traditions in India, just as part of meditation traditions. This is a different application of asana, however, and included other active forms of exercise. We must discriminate between these two different usages, rather than think that one necessarily excludes the other. It would be good if there were more research on the exercise, martial arts, gymnastic, and dance traditions of India, and the place of asana within these. No doubt much is yet hidden, not only in Sanskrit, but also in the local dialects of India that have their own long literary histories.

The active Yoga commonly practiced in the West today does have antecedents in India, but it was not always called Yoga, a term used more specifically for meditation traditions. Such more active asana approaches were commonly part of Indian martial arts, dance, and gymnastic traditions. They were part of India's Kshatriya or warrior traditions along with the use of various weapons. Such stronger exercise approaches did extend to India's monastic and sadhu communities that also had a martial side. One could call these Indian martial arts a kind of Yoga, as they were often performed with mantras and devotion.

Classical Yoga was not in itself a fitness system, but asana was employed as part of other Indian fitness systems, particularly the martial arts, even when the rest of Yoga practice was not brought along with them. Hatha Yoga crosses over both these realms of exercise and Yoga sadhana, having a connection to the martial arts, but primarily using asanas to prepare the body for meditation.

Part III

Foundations of the Vedic Yoga

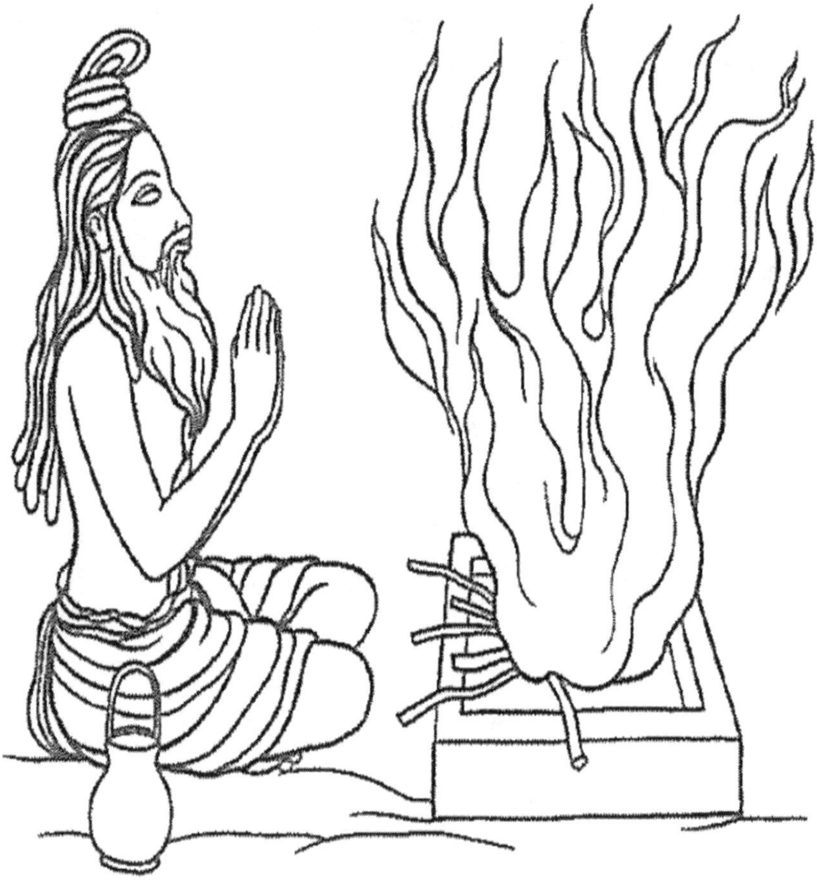

SECRET KNOWLEDGE:

Traditional Levels of Vedic Interpretation

How do we approach cryptic mantras from ancient cultures, which are said to require special initiations in order to understand them? Can we assume that their evident meaning according to our present mindset of several thousand years later should be accurate? So far, that has been the case with most who have tried to interpret the *Vedas*. Yet if we look at the *Vedas* with a greater poetic and yogic insight, cosmic dimensions emerge in almost every verse of this great compilation of seer wisdom.

One of the most common statements in later Vedic texts extending to the *Upanishads* is "*Parokṣa priya hi devāḥ,*"[153] which means "The Gods are fond of indirect statements." The Vedic language is a paroksha language, referring to one of implied meanings rather than evident statements. This statement in itself should be enough for us to look at the Vedas with a deeper vision.

Good poetry is based upon presenting word and image plays that hold several different levels of meaning, weaving together nature, human experience, and yet deeper connections. A degree of subtlety and multiplicity of indications is the basis of good poetry in the first place. The great scriptures of the world, which reflect a deep poetic vision, similarly claim several levels of meaning – including meanings that are hidden or esoteric, or very different than their literal import. The *Vedas* as mantric poetry should be looked at in the same way, containing secret implications, in which ordinary objects can take on cosmic connections. The *Rigveda* itself mentions four levels of speech, three of which are hidden in secrecy.

> *Four are the levels of speech that are measured, these the wise sages know. Three hidden in secrecy, they cannot manipulate, only with the fourth level of speech do humans talk.*[154]
>
> *Dirghatamas Auchatya, Rigveda I.164.45*

Agni as the Vedic sacred fire is commonly identified with the power of speech. He is said to be the child of seven voices or seven forms of speech, which suggests a system of seven levels of interpretation for the Vedic mantras.

> *Eternal here the youthful sisters with a common origin, the seven voices conceive a single child.*[155]
>
> *Gathina Vishvamitra, Rigveda III.1.6*

The Main Traditional Levels of Vedic Interpretation

As part of such secret meanings, the *Vedas* have several well-defined traditional levels of interpretation that we find mentioned in later Vedic texts. These reflect such multiple types of meaning that exist simultaneously. Each Vedic deity has different roles and functions according to the level of approached involved. The three most important are:

- Adhyatmic – Relating to the Self or the individual being, the psychological level
- Adhidaivic – Relating to the Gods, deities or cosmic powers
- Adhibhutic – Relating to the Elements of nature

We can find these three mentioned in many traditional texts of Vedic interpretation from the *Brahmanas* and *Upanishads* to the *Bhagavad Gita*.

Let us take Agni, which is generally identified with the natural phenomenon of fire to the modern mind. At the Adhyatmic or individual level, Agni is identified primarily with speech (vak), our main form of expression. At the Adhidaivic or cosmic level, Agni is primarily the Sun, the light of heaven, not merely as a material force but as the Divine light. On the Adhibhutic level, Agni is fire as an element, and the fire we use in our daily lives.

Adhyatmic – Psychological

The Adhyatmic level begins with a recognition of three primary aspects of our individual nature as speech (vak), prana, and mind (manas). In addition to these can be added a fourth level as the Jivatman or embodied soul, and a fifth as Paramatman or the Supreme Self.

The Adhyatmic approach takes us back from our individual powers of speech, breath, and mind to the higher Self that is their true reality: the speech of speech, the mind of mind, the prana of prana as the *Upanishads* say.[156] The Adhyatmic level does not reflect just our ordinary faculties. It recognizes the reality of the Divine word, Divine life, and Divine mind and strives to connect us with these.

When Agni is invoked in the *Vedas*, it is as the Divine speech within us that calls the Gods or cosmic powers. When Indra is invoked, it is as the Divine immortal prana, not our mere creaturely breath. When the Sun is invoked, it is as the illuminating power of Divine consciousness, not simply the outer mind. These inner faculties come into function only when our outer faculties are brought into a silent state, the stillness of Yoga practice.

Adhidaivic – Theological/ Ontological

The Adhidaivic level recognizes three powers of light at the three levels of the cosmos as Agni (fire – earth), Vayu (lightning/air – atmosphere), and Surya (sun – heaven). These are the three forms of Ishvara (the cosmic Lord) who is the fourth factor, with Brahman or Paramatman, the Absolute, as the fifth.

The Adhidaivic approach is concerned with worship of God (Ishvara) to lead us to Brahman. It recognizes the reality of the Divine fire, Divine spirit (wind), and Divine light (Sun). The Adhidaivic approach can be called *Adhibrahman* as its goal is Brahman or the Absolute. It is a theological approach in which we honor the Divine ruling powers of the universe, which are the forces of Being, Consciousness, and Bliss.

These two levels, Adhyatmic and Adhidaivic, are the most important. Their conjoined purpose is to link the individual Self or Atman (Adhyatmic Satya or individual truth) and the Supreme Being or Brahman (Adhidaivic Satya or cosmic truth).

Adhibhutic – Elemental

The elemental recognizes the five elements as the main factors behind our outer world experience. Earth, Water, and Fire are part of the earth realm ruled by fire or Agni. Air is of the atmosphere belonging to air of Vayu. Ether is heaven ruled by the Sun or Surya. The fourth beyond these three is the higher space of the soul, and the fifth is Brahman or Atman, the Absolute as the supreme space beyond. Atma-Bhuta (Self-nature) or Brahma-Bhuta (Absolute Nature) refer to this highest state of the elements.

The elemental approach means to merge the elements by stages from earth to ether into Brahman, reflecting the chakra system of Tantric Yoga that leads us from the root chakra and Earth element to the crown chakra or thousand petal lotus and the Supreme Self. This elemental approach has spiritual implications and is not merely a recognition of the outer forces of nature in a materialistic sense.

We can equate these three levels with the three worlds. The Adhibhutic or elemental level is that of the earth (nature), the Adhyatmic or individual level that of the atmosphere (the human being), and the Adhidaivic or cosmic level that of heaven (God). There is much crossover between their energies and influences.

The Yajna as the Fourth Level

Adhiyajna – the Ritual Order

A fourth level is often added to this primary three, which is Adhiyajna or relative to the Vedic sacrifice. The Vedic Yajna or way of worship is twofold as outer (bahir yajna) and inner (antar yajna).

The outer sacrifice offers certain items, like wood, cow dung or ghee, into the sacred fire along with devotional worship of Ishvara. It can be performed as a type of Bhakti and Karma Yoga. Each Vedic deity relates to a power or priest in the inner and outer sacrifice that constitutes both the cosmic and psychological order.

The inner sacrifice is a yogic practice in which we offer speech, breath, and mind through mantra yoga, Prana Yoga and meditation, into the Divine presence and supreme Self that is the ultimate goal. The *Bhagavad Gita* outlines such Yoga practices as pranayama, pratyahara, and meditation as Yajnas.[157]

There is a tendency among scholars to regard only the Adhyatmic level as a spiritual interpretation and the others as having only outer meanings. This does not look deeply into all the implications involved. All these methods of interpreting the *Vedas* can be spiritual or yogic in nature and indicate different approaches to Atman or Brahman. Adhidaivic brings in theology, a recognition of a single cosmic light or reality, which as a power of consciousness is the cosmic Lord. Adhibhutic brings in the Self as the subtlest of all the elements (Sarvabhuta-antarātman). Adhiyajna brings in Yoga as the inner sacrifice, in which we offer speech, prana, and mind into the Divine presence within.

Different Levels Relative to Agni

To understand how these different levels work, let us examine how Agni is portrayed according to them. In the individual, Agni is mainly speech, but not simply the vocal organ, all powers of speech and articulation. At the cosmic level Agni is the Sun or the supreme light. In the material world, Agni is the element of fire. In the Vedic sacrifice Agni is the priest of the invocation or Hota, who calls the Gods. In the inner sacrifice, Agni is the soul that brings the Divine into us.

Adhyatmic	Adhidaivic	Adhibhutic	Adhiyajna
Speech	Sun	Fire as an element	Hota-Invoker, the soul or Jiva

Yet these multiple correlations are only the beginning of a broad range of associations extending to the entire universe. They have additional ramifications and cannot be reduced to a few mechanical constructs. They reflect languages and paths to the spiritual reality. Their application can constitute different forms of Atma-Vichara (Self-inquiry) and Brahma-vichara (Inquiry into God or the Absolute). They use the various factors of our life experience to arrive at the higher truth. There are additional approaches that we find in Vedic texts, but are not as specifically defined:

Adhiloka – relating to the worlds, generally reflecting the Adhidaivic level of the deity that rules a particular world, like earth and Fire, but correlating outer worlds with inner worlds like earth and the body, atmosphere and the prana, and heaven and the mind.

Adhijyotisha – Relating to light. Much like Adhidaivic as Vedic deities are primarily light forms. Tracing the forms of light to pure consciousness.

Adhikala – Relating to time. Reaching the eternal through the movement through time, with the day symbolizing the physical, the month indicating the astral, and the year indicating the causal realm.

Adhiganita – Relating to numbers. Reaching either the One or the infinite through an examination of sacred numbers. Often the numbers of the Vedic meters are used in this way or the numbers of Vedic deities, like the 33 prime Devas.

Adhimantra – Using mantra as a way of understanding Self and universe, returning everything to the Divine word Oṁ.

Adhichhandas – Using the meters as a way of understanding Self and universe, with each meter signifying a certain deity or Loka.

Taking a subtler vision, one can go deeper into any of these areas. For example, at the level of Adhyatmic or the inner Self, Agni has many forms, not just Vak or speech. There is also the digestive fire, the pranic fire, the eye, the fire of intelligence or buddhi, the fire of consciousness, and the fire of being itself (Brahmagni). Relative to the worlds, Agni is not only fire and the Sun, but also lightning, the Moon, and the stars – whatever reflects light and heat, extending to the cosmic light of consciousness.

Our modern mind is usually content to find one level of meaning in ancient texts and stop there. To understand the *Vedas*, we must universalize the Vedic principles to link all levels of our experience together in the unity of consciousness.

The *Vedas* and Theological Views of Monotheism and Polytheism

The Vedic view is of a multi-leveled universe with a parallel development inner and outer, higher and lower, individual and cosmic. Such a view cannot be reduced to a simple theology of God as being One or Many, as monotheism, pantheism or polytheism as exclusive views.

The *Vedas* honor the Divine as One, recognizing a common Self and being in all beings. Yet the *Vedas* also honor the Divine as many, seeing the many as different forms and functions of the One. The *Vedas* honor the Divine as both pervading all nature (pantheism) and as transcending all manifestation in time and space (as the Absolute). The Vedic view has a place for monism (unity of all), monotheism (oneness of the creator), polytheism, pantheism, and other approaches to truth. Yet it cannot be defined according to any one of these alone.

Modern scholars generally regard the *Vedas* as a type of polytheism with hints of the monism of the *Upanishads* and Vedanta, which they see only in a few late Vedic hymns like the *Purusha Sukta*. This apparent Vedic polytheism, we should remember, is not different from the apparent polytheism of the later Hindu *Puranas*, with their trinity of Brahma, Vishnu, and Shiva, and their many Gods and Goddesses, which can individually or collectively be equated with the Supreme Divine or Brahman, and reflect Vedantic philosophies of Self-realization and God-realization.

The Hindu view is similar to the theology of ancient Egypt, where a recognition of the unity of the Divine light existed behind an apparent diversity of deities. The term "henotheism" was invented by modern scholarship to explain this view where a single deity can be lauded as the supreme, which they saw as a confusion of multiplicity and unity, not their integration. The term only shows our modern inability to see unity behind multiplicity.

Vedic polytheism would be better called "Vedic pluralism," an approach to the One Divine that accepts many different angles and perspectives. Vedic deities are described as our friends, with whom we have a relationship of kinship, equality and unity. All the deities are to be honored, none is to be denigrated in the name of only one as supreme.

> *None of you are small, Devas, none of you are childish, all of you are great.*[158]
>
> *Manu Vivasvan, Rigveda VIII.30.1*

Yet each deity is part of the same One Reality. Each deity represents an important and integral aspect of the cosmic truth and reality. That vast truth, Ritam Brihat, is more than any single deity and constitutes the essence of all both individually and collectively.

> *That which is the One Being, the seers describe in various ways.*[159]
>
> *Dirghatamas Auchatya, Rigveda I.164.46*

The *Vedas* approach unity through a comprehensive vision of the sacred presence pervading all of life. The *Vedas* emphasize wholeness and completeness, not singularity and exclusion. Their supreme deity is not a one God opposed to other Gods, but a unity of truth that encompasses all Divine powers and principles – and is both behind all names and forms and beyond all names and forms. These Vedic deities can be equated with one another, but have specific roles as well. They represent a difference of function, not one of reality.

The Vedic Godheads represent an interdependent reality, where all is One and One is All as various manifestations of the same light and consciousness. The formed world is a symbolic or visionary manifestation of the formless world. That is why the main Vedic deities are powers of light and only vaguely anthropomorphic in their attributes. The human side of their imagery is outweighed by their other natural correspondences. They are universal forces, not simply a projection of the human psyche onto the realm of nature.

VEDIC DEITIES: GUNAS, ELEMENTS, AND DOSHAS

The *Vedas* present a vast pantheon of deities (Devatas), sometimes said to be infinite in number, relating to all aspects of life and the vast universe around us. Clearly the ancient seers saw the world from a very different angle than we do and were overwhelmed by a sacred presence from every side. We can easily become bewildered by this abundance, though we can also find great depths within it, if we examine it carefully.

To simplify matters, this classification of deities is a matter of cosmic mathematics, reflecting the symbolic language of numbers. For the ancients, numbers also constitute a mystical language. Numbers were Gods or Devas and Devas had their numbers. Vedic numbers relate to Devas, Rishis, the meters of the chants, as well as the divisions of time, space, the movement of heavenly bodies, and the structure of the different worlds. Such diverse levels of numerology can be correlated in various ways in order to unlock the secrets of the universe. This extends to the numbers inherent in the body and its different limbs, parts of the hand, or numbers of bones. The numerical divisions of the individual parallel those of the universe and cosmic person (Purusha), and can unlock the secrets of life.

For a specific number, the Vedic Gods or Devatas are said to be 3339 in total.[160] This is clearly a play on the number three, the prime number behind all universal forces. Not surprisingly this number is reduced to 333, 33, to 3 and then to 1.[161] One of the main classifications of the Vedic Gods is to reduce them to the three prime deities or light forms relative to the three main worlds of our life experience. The Devas are the principles of light and energy that operate within the worlds as their fields of activity. Agni or Fire on earth (Prithivi), Vayu/Indra or Wind in the atmosphere (Antariksha), and Surya or the Sun in heaven (Dyaus).

The hymns of *Rigveda* are organized in a corresponding threefold manner with the hymns to Agni coming first, then the hymns to Vayu and Indra, and finally the hymns to the Sun. The *Brihaddevata*, the late Vedic work, which correlates the Vedic deities, follows the same approach.[162]

Each of these three realms of earth, atmosphere, and heaven in turn is said to have eleven main deities, making a total of 33 in all. This is the basic system. However, this classification is general. Sometimes earth is said to have 8 deities, the Vasus, the atmosphere 11, the Maruts, and heaven 12, the Adityas or Sun Gods, with the 2 Ashvins making 33 deities total.

There are higher realms beyond the ordinary three worlds. Yet these, like the three luminous heavens (tri rochana), also follow a threefold organization. The three times three or nine worlds can eventually extend into three times seven or twenty-one. For example, there are three times seven or twenty-one names or planes of the Mother or World principle.[163]

The three main Vedic deities of Agni, Vayu, and Surya are not separate deities but three aspects of the One Deity or Purusha, the higher Self whose nature is pure light. We can equate Agni with heat, Vayu with electrical force, and Surya with pure light as illumination. These three aspects of light represent the inner lights of consciousness, the three aspects of the cosmic person, with Agni or fire as speech (vak), Vayu or wind as breath (prana), and Surya or the Sun as the perceptive aspect of the mind (manas and buddhi).

All Vedic deities are reducible to One deity, often identified with the Sun, not as a material principle but as the light of consciousness. However, any single Vedic deity can represent all deities and function as the supreme Divinity. Agni can be Vayu and Surya as well. Vayu as lightning is the atmospheric form of fire, while Surya as the Sun is the heavenly form of fire. Surya can be Agni or Vayu. Agni or fire is the earthly form of the Sun, while Vayu or lightning is the atmospheric form of the Sun.

Indra, the king of the Vedic Gods, most commonly assumes this supreme role (though Indra is sometimes seen as the deity of the atmosphere like Vayu). Fire is the lord or Indra of the earth, Vayu the lord or Indra of the atmosphere, and the Sun the lord or Indra of heaven. Indra represents the master power of light and consciousness in the universe behind all the Devas. For this reason he is commonly coupled with the deities of the three realms as Indra-Agni, Indra-Vayu, and Indra-Surya.

The Three Gunas

Most Yoga students are aware of the three gunas of *sattva, rajas,* and *tamas*, the cosmic forces of balance, movement, and inertia, and their profound levels of meanings. The three gunas are one of the keys for understanding Vedic cosmology and the Vedic Yoga. In the philosophy of classical Yoga, reflecting Samkhya and Vedanta, all matter in the universe is reducible to one primary substance or ground of experience called *Prakriti*. Prakriti literally means the original power (pra) of action (kriti) and indicates process. It is characterized by constant change and shifting of qualities.

Prakriti does not refer to substance in the physical sense but to the root power from which all forms of matter, energy, and mind arise, and to which they must eventually return. Prakriti is the original state of potential energy out of which all things become possible. Prakriti is the latent state of substance, like the seed that holds the pattern for a great tree. It is the root power of the world of which matter, energy, and mind are manifestations. Prakriti, we could say, is the causal or original form of all substances, from which their subtle and gross forms arise. Yet Prakriti has no form of its own and is known only by its manifestations. Prakriti is a composite of three prime qualities of sattva, rajas, and tamas.

- Sattva is the power of harmony, balance, light and intelligence – the higher or spiritual potential.
- Rajas is the power of energy, action, change and movement – the intermediate or life potential.
- Tamas is the power of darkness, inertia, form and materiality – the lower or material potential.

Perhaps the simplest way to understand the three gunas for the modern mind is as matter (tamas), energy (rajas), and light (sattva), the three main factors of the physical universe. The three gunas reflect the three worlds of Vedic thought.

- Earth is the realm of tamas or darkness, gross, solid, or physical matter.
- The atmosphere, also called rajas in Vedic thought, is the realm of action and change, symbolized by the storm with its process of lightning, thunder, and rain, but it indicates energy or subtle matter on all levels.
- Heaven or the sky is the realm of harmony and light indicated by the Sun, Moon and stars, sattva guna. Heaven indicates light as a universal principle that is the causal or original basis of the gross and subtle elements.

The entire universe consists of light (sattva) that moves in the form of energy (rajas) and becomes densified in the form of matter (tamas). The three Vedic deities of light as Agni, Vayu, and Surya or Fire, Wind, and Sun also relate to the gunas.

- Agni is the form of light in the sphere of tamas, the fire that is hidden in darkness.
- Vayu is the form of light in the sphere of rajas, light in its active and energetic mode as lightning or electrical force.
- Surya is the form of light in the sphere of sattva, light as pure illumination.

The movement from tamas to sattva is a movement from earth to heaven. It occurs through bringing the light out of the earth (Agni) and raising it to heaven as the Sun (Surya) by crossing the atmosphere and using its forces (Vayu). It reflects the movement from body (tamas) to prana (rajas) to mind (sattva). In Yoga practice, this is the movement from the root chakra or seat of fire, through the heart chakra, the seat of Vayu or air, to the crown chakra or thousand petal lotus or the light beyond space.

The Vedic deities of Agni, Vayu, and Surya represent the powers of light or pure sattva behind the three gunas of sattva, rajas, and tamas. They constitute a pure or transcendent form of sattva that can bring the light out of rajas and tamas. We should not equate them with the lower gunas that they work through and help us master.

The negative power of rajas is represented by the Asuras or anti-Gods who fight the Devas for power in the universe. The negative power of tamas is represented by negative forces like Rakshasas that seek to prevent all positive action from occurring. Vedic stories of the wars between the Devas and Asuras symbolize the struggle within the gunas that occurs both at cosmic and individual levels.

The Threefold Purusha

The three Vedic forms of light are the three forms of the Purusha or the higher Self that is defined in terms of light. The three visible lights are manifestations of the invisible divine light of consciousness that illumines all things, including visible light and darkness. The three gunas and three worlds exist within us, as do their light forms as powers of our own awareness.

Agni – Earth	Tamas – matter	Body – speech (vak)
Vayu – Atmosphere	Rajas – energy	Breath (prana)
Surya – Heaven	Sattva - light	Mind (manas)

These three aspects of the Purusha or consciousness principle reflect the three aspects of Prakriti or the material principle. The Purusha is threefold in its human manifestation as speech (body), breath, and mind, just as Prakriti or the world is threefold as earth, atmosphere, and heaven or as matter, energy, and light. This Vak or speech Purusha, Prana Purusha, and Manas Purusha is the embodied soul that is a reflection of the unmanifest Purusha or higher Self.

Agni represents light or the Purusha in the realm of matter or the earth and holds the presence of consciousness in the material world. Vayu is light or the Purusha in the realm of energy of the atmosphere. It holds the presence of consciousness in the realm of energy. Surya is light or the Purusha in the realm of light or heaven. It holds the presence of consciousness in the realm of light. In the Vedic view, the Purusha or consciousness principle is not limited to embodied creatures but pervades these great forces of nature as well. These light forms that relate to the gunas help us not only to understand Prakriti, but also to approach the Purusha. The Vedic Yoga works with these three light reflections of the Purusha in order to master and transform the three forms or aspects of Prakriti.

The Threefold Vedic Yoga of Agni, Vayu and Surya – Speech, Prana, and Mind

The Vedic Yoga is threefold in its basic formulation. First is *Agni Yoga* or Fire Yoga. It consists of developing the powers of speech on all levels up to the Divine Word. It leads to mantra and silence. Through the inner power of speech and fire we can purify the body and the subconscious mind. Entering into the fire as a cosmic force, we can travel through all the kingdoms of nature on earth and understand all their secrets. Fire's main work is to purify, which includes removing the darkness or tamas within us.

Second is *Vayu Yoga* or Air Yoga. It consists of developing the power of prana on all levels up to the Divine Prana. It works mainly through pranayama and pranic based meditations. Through the power of prana we can purify our vital urges, instincts, and desires. Entering into prana as a cosmic force we can travel into space and cross the atmosphere to worlds beyond. Vayu's main work is to energize, which includes spiritualizing the force of rajas within us.

The third is *Surya Yoga* or Solar Yoga. It consists of meditation and moving in space (heaven), unfolding the Divine light on all levels up to the Divine mind. Through the power of the concentrated mind we can purify our minds and senses. Entering into the cosmic mind we can perceive the entire universe within ourselves. The Sun's main work is to illumine, spreading the light of sattva with us.

Table of Vedic Deities and Gunas

Agni – Fire				
Body	Faculty	Yoga	Guna	Constituents
Physical body and internal organs	Speech	Mantra Yoga	Tamas - matter	Five gross elements
Vayu – Wind				
Body	Faculty	Yoga	Guna	Constituents
Vital body and motor organs	Prana	Prana Yoga	Rajas – energy	Five pranas
Surya – Sun				
Body	Faculty	Yoga	Guna	Constituents
Mental body and sense organs	Mind	Dhyana Yoga	Sattva – light	Five sense qualities

Agni as the power of speech is the means of purifying and controlling both the physical body and physical matter, and mastering the guna or quality of tamas. Through it we can control our internal organs and the gross elements. The Yoga of speech involves chanting, singing, internal repetition of mantras and meditation on mantras.

Vayu as the power of the breath is the means of purifying and controlling the vital body and the realm of energy and mastering the guna of rajas. Through it we can control our motor organs and the five pranas (five motor actions). The Yoga of the breath involves pranayama and pratyahara or the internalization of prana. Through it we gain control of our emotions and pranic impulses.

Surya as the power of thought is the means of purifying and controlling the mental body and the realm of light and mastering the guna of sattva. Through it we can control our sense organs and the subtle elements. The Yoga of the mind is meditation. Through it we can gain control of the rational mind and open a higher intuitive perception.

The Three Gunas and the Threefold Vedic Yoga

Whenever any one of the three gunas is in ascendancy within us, we fall into its sphere of influence and forget the action of the other two gunas. We compartmentalize ourselves according to the dominant guna. For example, when we are in a depressed or tamasic state of mind, we forget both our active or rajasic moments and our clear or sattvic moments. If we could but bring our sattvic moments into our tamasic moments they would dissolve.

An important part of the Vedic Yoga is transforming the gunas. This requires bringing sattva (light) into rajas (energy) and tamas (matter). It means becoming aware of the light or fire hidden in matter, recognizing that all contracted mental states are simply fuel for the fire of awareness. This is part of Agni Yoga. It means contacting the light of awareness within us that persists even through tamasic states of sleep, death, or unconsciousness. This transforms tamas into sattva.

Similarly, mastering the gunas means seeing the light of awareness that underlies all states of change and movements of energy, as in rajasic moments of breathing, discharging vital urges, or immersing ourselves in action. This is part of Vayu Yoga or Indra Yoga, contacting the light of awareness that gives power to all energy. It transforms rajas into sattva.

The Four Vedic Godheads and the Five Elements: The Ayurvedic Key

Perhaps the most important theory in all the Vedic sciences is that of the five great elements (Mahabhutas) of earth, water, fire, air, and ether. The five element theory is found in all Vedic disciplines of Yoga, Ayurveda, and Vedic astrology. It is shared by Greek thought and many other systems. While appearing simple, it is profound.

The five element theory occurs in the *Rigveda*, which is perhaps its oldest existing formulation. The five elements form an important factor for understanding the Vedic deities and their functions. However, the five element theory is not obvious to a superficial reading of the *Vedas*, but part of symbolic indications.

The five elements represent the five densities of matter as solid, liquid, radiant, gaseous, and etheric. The elements are not a chemical theory, nor are they limited to physical matter. The five elements indicate the five basic levels or "strata" of all substances in the universe from the gross to the subtle.

We can observe this "principle of stratification" in all aspects of nature. We can see the strata in the different layers of rock on a cliff, the different layers of clouds in the atmosphere, or the different layers of galaxies in the greater universe beyond. We can observe the stratification of our own bodies with their different tissue layers.[164] The universe follows a principle of "stratified organization" with different levels of subtlety and density reflected in the five elements. The universe is an evolution from the subtle to the gross and back again, from space to earth and earth to space. The five elements reflect the nature of reality from gross matter to pure spirit.

The five elements not only represent different levels of matter or substance, they also represent different forms and frequencies of light. Space, we could say, is the field of light. Air is electrical energy or lightning. Fire is the heat and color-producing aspect of light. Water is reflected light. Earth is shadow. In the Vedic view, light is consciousness or the Purusha, which is the original light of self-awareness. As forms of light, the five elements symbolize powers of mind and consciousness, aspects of the Purusha at an inner level, just as the elements comprise aspects of Prakriti or nature at an outer level.

As powers of mind, the five elements have corresponding sensory qualities with earth as smell, water as taste, fire as sight, air as touch, and ether as sound – which are identified as the subtle elements. As powers of prana or vital energy, the five elements have counterparts in the motor organs as well, with ether as the voice, air as the hands, fire as the feet, water as the organs of emission, and earth as the organs of reproduction.

We can correlate the five elements with the three gunas, with the gross elements (earth, water, fire, air, and ether) corresponding to tamas or inertia, and the five sensory qualities (smell, taste, sight, touch, and sound) as corresponding to sattva guna or the quality of light. Rajas relates to the motor organs and the pranic connections of the elements.

On a higher level, the five elements represent different aspects of consciousness with space as the space of consciousness, air as the energy of consciousness, fire as the light of consciousness, water as the delight and nourishing power in consciousness, and earth as the stability or coherence in consciousness.

The Three Main Elements of Water, Fire, and Air

The five element theory pervades the *Rigveda*, but three elements predominate: these are Agni, which is fire, Indra (also called Vayu or Vata), which is air or wind, and Soma, also connected to Apas as the waters or moistening energy. These three are the most important Vedic elements because fire represents the soul in the body, air represents the cosmic spirit or God, and Soma or water represents their union or delight. Water, fire, and air constitute the three mobile or active aspects of the five elements, which work in the atmosphere, and are responsible for life in the manifest world, making them very important at both biological and psychological levels.

In addition to these three elements, the *Vedas* mention heaven and earth as the father and mother of all creatures. Sometimes heaven and earth are called the two mothers. Heaven can be identified with the element of space and earth with the element of earth. The mobile elements of water, fire and air occur between these two as powers of the atmosphere, their children or the Gods that arise between heaven and earth.

Vedic Deities and the Purusha Consciousness-Principle

In the *Vedas*, Agni, Vayu, Surya, and Soma constitute the four main manifestations of the Purusha, defined in terms of light. The Vedic Godheads are not forms of the elements, rather the elements are vehicles for the Devas to manifest. Indra is not air but the Divine motivating power that works through the air element. Vedic Sun Gods like Mitra and Varuna are not the Sun in the outer sense, but the powers of truth and Dharma that manifest through it. Soma is not water in the outer sense, but the watery essence of delight that manifests through the worlds as a whole, and particularly through the water element. Agni is not fire as an element, but the Divine light hidden in and working through the material world and the physical body.

The Four Vedic Deities of Light

The four primary deities (Devatas) in the *Rigveda* as Agni, Indra, Surya, and Soma, outwardly relate to fire, wind, the Sun and water (or the Moon). Here the Moon or Soma relates to the fourth world of the waters (cosmic space) or to the watery aspect of heaven, while Fire is the deity of earth, Indra or air of the atmosphere and the Sun of heaven. We find in these the three mobile elements of fire, air, and water, with light (Surya) as the fourth principle.

To grasp these four Vedic light forms, we find a helpful key in Ayurveda. Ayurveda, of all the Vedic disciplines, has best preserved the name, form, and function of the older Vedic Deities. We can use the physical understanding of the Vedic Gods in Ayurveda as a foundation to incorporate their deeper psychological and spiritual meanings.

The Three Doshas of Ayurveda

Vedic Yoga as Inner Doshic Balancing

Ayurveda's biological theory of life revolves around the three *doshas* or biological humors of *Vata*, *Pitta*, and *Kapha*, which relate to the elements of air, fire, and water and their attributes and actions. The three doshas are the main forces at work in our bodies, with Vata as the basic motivating energy of the mind and nervous system, Pitta as the transformative power of the digestive system, and Kapha comprising the main bulk of the body that is watery in nature. Ayurveda goes into great detail into the locations, functions and subtypes of the doshas, along with their impact on the processes of growth, health, and disease within the organism. It classifies foods, herbs, lifestyle, and environmental factors relative to their doshic effects.

Though dominant in one element, each of the doshas is more specifically defined relative to two of the five elements, with Kapha as earth and water, Pitta as water and fire, and Vata as air and ether. One element serves as the basic force of the dosha, the other as the field in which it acts. Kapha is water moving in the field of earth. Pitta is fire operating in the field of water (the blood). Vata is air operating in the field of ether or the spaces within the bones and joints.

We can use the Ayurvedic two-element model to approach the Vedic deities. Each primary Vedic deity just like each dosha reflects two of the five great elements of earth, water, fire, air, and ether. Each contains two adjacent elements, which represent its states of motion and rest. This provides a simple and easy correlation between three of the four main Vedic deities and the three doshas. Indra in the *Rigveda* is called Vata and Vayu. Vata in Ayurveda is also called Vayu. Pitta in Ayurveda is closely connected to Agni.

- Indra or Vayu is the air element that moves in the field of ether and indicates Vata dosha.
- Agni is the fire element that moves in the field of water (or oil) and indicates Pitta dosha.
- Soma is the water element that moves in the field of earth and indicates Kapha dosha.

This scheme leaves us with Surya or the Sun as the fourth prime Vedic deity unaccounted for. If we examine the Ayurvedic scheme we see doshas for earth-water, water-fire, and air-ether, or a sequence of one dosha per two adjacent elements. One set of two elements is left out, which is fire-air. This can be associated with the Surya or the Sun, the fourth main Vedic deity.

Ayurvedically, we can associate the Sun as a gaseous fire to the breath, fire burning in air, as opposed to Agni or the digestive fire, the fire burning up solid and liquid food. This would make for two forms of Agni, a digestive earthly fire and a pranic or breath air-based fire. Surya would then be prana, or the subtler form of Agni. It would fall under the sphere of Pitta, as the airy or Vata form of Pitta, with Agni or the digestive fire and its watery (oily) aspect as the watery or Kapha form of Pitta.

Surya or the Sun can be identified with prana as a force of positive health. One is reminded of ancient Greek medicine and its fourth, airy or sanguine humor that is a force of positive health, suggesting a similar scheme. In Vedic thought, Surya is often prana, just at other times it relates to mind, perception or Self.

Deity	Elements	Doshas	Cosmic
1. Indra /Vayu	Air and Ether (air that moves in the ether)	Vata	Energy
2. Surya	Fire and Air (fire that moves in the air or gaseous fire)	Pitta/Vata	Light
3. Agni	Fire and Water (fire that burns in water or oil)	Pitta/Kapha	Heat
4. Soma	Water and Earth (water that moves on earth)	Kapha	Matter

The Four Vedic Deities and the Doshas

We can divide these four into two groups. The first or lower pair—Agni-Soma or fire and water— reflects the lower, form-based or material worlds. They symbolize the individual soul (Jivatman) embodied within the worlds and bound to the cycle of rebirth. The second or higher pair—Indra/Vayu-Surya or air and fire—reflects the higher, formless or spiritual realms. They symbolize the universal self (Paramatman) which manifests through the worlds as Ishvara, the creator, preserver and destroyer of the worlds, God as the universal lord.

The higher or heavenly order has two aspects as Vayu and Surya or wind and the sun. Wind symbolizes the formless spirit that energizes all things but itself cannot be seen. This is far beyond air as a material element. The Sun symbolizes the light of consciousness that transcends all material forms. This is far beyond the Sun as the luminary of our solar system.

Sometimes these four are reduced to two sets: earth, water and fire, lauded mainly as Agni (Fire). Fire, air and ether, lauded mainly as Surya (Sun). Here Agni refers to the material fire of fire, water, earth, while Surya indicates the spiritual fire of fire, air, and ether. The movement of spiritual practice is to progress from the material fire to the spiritual Sun, from the limited light of the brain to the higher light of cosmic intelligence. The four Vedic light forms have specific interactions in various dual forms, in which their influences combine.

Through working with the Vedic deities, we can practice an Ayurvedic Yoga of Inner Doshic Balancing, using the energies of these four main Vedic light forms. We can expand our Ayurvedic practice from the physical to the psychological and the cosmic.

The Three Vital Essences of Prana, Tejas and Ojas

The Three Doshas, which are usually described as disease-causing factors in Ayurvedic medicine, have their internal counterparts that are factors of positive health. These are called *Prana*, *Tejas*, and *Ojas*. Prana is the health-giving aspect of Vata or air. Tejas is the health-giving aspect of Pitta or fire. Ojas is the health-giving aspect of Kapha or water. The three Vedic deities of Indra, Agni, and Soma represent Prana, Tejas, and Ojas. We could say that they are a deeper level or application of Prana, Tejas, and Ojas for the internal yogic alchemy of self-realization.

Indra in the *Rigveda* is the main drinker of the Soma and power of Ojas. He indicates the highest Prana at an inner level, which arises from Ojas and holds the power of Tejas as well. Soma provides the Ojas for the powers of Tejas and Prana. Tejas is twofold as Agni and Surya. Agni or fire is Tejas at the level of willpower. Surya is Tejas at the level of Prana or vital energy. Sometimes Agni is more specifically called Tejas, which implies heat, and Surya is called Jyoti, meaning light in the sense of illumination.

Chanting or listening to the Vedic mantras to Indra, Agni, Surya, and Soma respectively can aid us in the development of Prana, Tejas, and Ojas. This is one of the simplest ways to benefit from their Vedic healing application. For example, the Gayatri Mantra to the Sun helps develop the higher powers of Tejas. Note the following prayer of the *Shukla Yajurveda*, which shows that these inner powers are gained through the Vedic mantras.

You are Tejas, place that Tejas in me. You are heroic strength, place that heroic strength in me. You are power, place that power in me. You are Ojas, place that Ojas in me. You are spirit, place that spirit in me. You are the force, place that force in me.[165]
Shukla Yajurveda XIX.9

The Vedic Godheads and the Three, Four or Seven Worlds

The underlying threefold Vedic symbolism has variations. The first is that the three worlds are not always earth, atmosphere, and heaven, but earth, heaven, and the atmosphere or the realm of the cosmic waters. This relates to the threefold order of speech, mind, and prana, with prana rather than mind as the supreme principle. Prana here does not mean breath but rather Spirit. In the *Upanishads*, prana is often lauded as the Supreme principle beyond the mind.[166]

Earth	Agni	Body	Waking state
Heaven	Surya	Mind	Dream
Atmosphere/Waters	Indra/ Vayu	Prana	Deep Sleep

- Agni as the fire in the earth is the awareness that persists in our physical state of consciousness or waking state.
- Surya or the Sun is the light of the mind that lights up the dream state.
- Vayu as the wind or lightning is the life-force that dominates our state of deep sleep in which both body and mind are in a state of rest.

Sometimes this third realm is the realm of the Waters, Apas, or the Moon. This formulation has three light forms as Agni/Fire-earth, Surya/Sun-heaven, and Soma/Moon-waters. The waters can stand for the waters of space in which all the worlds are located, the *prima materia* or higher material principle connected to the Moon. Yet sometimes the waters refer to the atmosphere (Antariksha) as the intermediate world (source of the rain), other times they refer to the realm of space as the world beyond the Sun. Again the Vedic formulation is variable and creative.

Four and Seven Lokas

The threefold Vedic view is the basis of other numerical correlations. Sometimes a fourth world is added as a higher heaven. This fourth principle is sometimes the unity or original basis of the three. It is most commonly represented by Indra as the overall Divine ruling power. It is related to the higher heaven (Svar), the higher atmosphere (air and space among the stars) or the higher waters (Apas). Sometimes there are three luminous heavens (tri rochana) beyond the ordinary heaven.[167]

Vedic deities relate to the seven worlds or cosmic principles of later Vedantic thought. This is a general adaptation as Vedic deities have actions in all the lokas.

1. Anna	Food or physical	Agni	*Bhūr Loka*	Material Realm
2. Prana	Breath or energy	Vayu	*Bhuvar Loka*	Atmosphere
3. Manas	Emotional mind	Soma	*Suvar Loka*	Lower Heaven
4. Vijnana	Intelligence	Surya	*Mahar Loka*	Higher Heaven
5. Ananda	Bliss or Love	Soma, higher aspect	*Jana Loka*	Realm of Creation
6. Chit	Consciousness	Agni, higher aspect	*Tapo Loka*	Realm of Tapas
7. Sat	Being	Indra, Vayu, higher aspect	*Satya Loka*	Realm of Truth

Surya or the Sun is the central principle, the supreme Godhead that carries both the lower three worlds of outer manifestation and the triple absolute of Sacchidānanda or Being-Consciousness-Bliss. We could consider all seven lokas to be rays created by this central Sun. All the Vedic Godheads are truth principles or formations of Sat. They are connected to Satya, Ritam, Dharma and Brihat, the Vedic principles of truth, law, harmony, and vastness. Indra is most commonly the Lord of Sat. Such approaches have an integrative function, and do not aim to set up rigid structures, which is why they have variations.

VEDIC MANTRA YOGA: THE WAY OF THE CHANT

Most of us first contact the power of the *Vedas* through hearing the power of Vedic chanting. Vedic mantras have an extraordinary calming effect upon the mind and heart, extending through the prana into the cells of the body itself. They awaken our inner consciousness and subtle senses, drawing us into the inner worlds, allowing us to feel the Divine powers at work behind the manifest universe. To hear the *Vedas* chanted properly, or to participate in that chanting, is one of the most elevating experiences possible in Yoga.

Vedic Yoga is rooted in mantra and is, first of all, a type of Mantra Yoga, though of an intricate nature. Vedic chants are metrically based verses or longer mantras, not simple seed syllables like Oṁ. They reflect the power of sound on many levels, including the power of the Sanskrit letters, which remain alive and vibrant as the root sounds of the Vedic language. Vedic chants reflect the power of meaning as well, having indications on all levels of the universe, without and within.

Perhaps the best way to understand the Vedic mantra is as an effort to translate the Divine Word into cohesive sound and meaning patterns devised to enlighten the human mind to the nature of cosmic reality. The *Veda* can be defined as a scripture in the sense that it is a manifestation of the Divine Word, which is the core vibration of consciousness in the hearts of all beings. The *Veda* is a mantric and symbolic revelation of the great truths or dharmas of the cosmic mind. Yet this Vedic mantric revelation does not promote any particular person, organization, or belief. Its aim is to awaken the Divine Word within us, so that we can experience the entire universe as sacred.

To receive the Vedic mantra, the Rishi had to enter into a superconscious state of samadhi and contact the inner vibration behind the manifest worlds. Vedic mantras are an effusion of the heart of the Rishi as he returns to the origins of the universe and beyond to the timeless Absolute. The Rishi is first of all a seer of the mantra as a cosmic power, not a creator of the hymn in the ordinary human sense of the word, as a product of the human mind or intellect. The Rishi learns the cosmic language of consciousness, which is mantra, and reflects that back into our human world. The Vedic hymn is born of this mantric epiphany.

Vedic mantras reflect the process of cosmogenesis, the process of the unfoldment of the universe through the power of light and sound. This is mirrored in our own minds and hearts, forming the structure of the subtle body of the soul. The Vedic mantra projects the vibratory force, the causal and archetypal patterns hidden behind the form-based world in which we live. The Vedic mantric process pervades all of nature and manifests through both light and sound, not as mere sensory qualities but as cosmic principles. Sound projects energy and meaning and is itself a manifestation of the light of consciousness. Light is the perceptual power of consciousness and has its sound vibrations.

Oṁ and Primal Sound

The Vedic language is rooted in the syllables of the Sanskrit language, which are based upon cosmic qualities. These sacred sounds ultimately resolve into one syllable, described as *Pranava*, primal sound, or Oṁ. The Vedic term for letter or syllable, *akshara*, also means "that which is imperishable," reflecting the eternal power of the Word to create and dissolve all things. There is a famous Vedic verse, frequently quoted by Maharishi Mahesh Yogi.

> *The Vedas rest in the imperishable syllable in the supreme ether (of the heart). Those who do not know that, what can they do with the Veda? Those who know that are gathered here.* [168]
>
> *Dirghatamas Auchatya, Rigveda I.164.39*

This verse reflects the heart connection with the Divine Word necessary for us to enter into the Vedic language and perceive the inner dimension of the Vedic Yoga.

Ganapati Muni teaches that Pranava or primal sound is the basis of time and is not different from Prana.[169] Pranava is the unmanifest sound that is inherent in the supreme space, not manifest sound which is its production. When unmanifest sound becomes manifest through the movement of time, it is the basis of all creation. Such unmanifest sound, which is the root state of all mantras, carries all knowledge and all powers in seed form. The *Vedas* connect time, light, prana, and mantra and find a cosmic equivalence between them in the presence of space and consciousness. The Rishi has an understanding of how to work with all these forces in an integral manner.

The *Upanishads* describe the 'small space within the heart' in which the entire universe dwells.

> *In this space within the heart are contained both heaven and earth, both Fire and Air, both Sun and Moon, lightning and the stars, what is here and what is not all that is contained there.*[170]
>
> *Chandogya Upanishad VIII.1.3*

The Divine Word is self-manifesting and self-effulgent. It does not rest upon sound as a material or energetic phenomenon. It arises of itself from the highest space, which is the unmanifest space that exists before all time. It is the unstruck (anahata) and unending cosmic vibration.

The *Vedas* take these root sound vibrations, which are the basis of the Sanskrit alphabet, and develop them as broader statements that unfold our relationship with the cosmic powers. In this regard, Vedic hymns reflect the language of the crown chakra or thousand petal lotus of the head, which contains all possible sound combinations and the deepest level of meaning. Single syllable bija mantras like Oṁ vibrate behind it. The Vedic language takes the supreme level of speech indicated by Oṁ but as projected in the realm of detailed expression.[171]

Vedic Mantra Yoga, therefore, is not a matter of ordinary speech or poetic expression. Nor is it simply another form of religious mysticism and devotion. It arises through the Divine silence that holds all manifestation in a single vibration. To understand it requires that we silence our outer speech and mind and become aware of the inner vibrations of the Absolute. To practice Vedic Mantra Yoga, we must awaken the flame of the soul within us and let its Divine Voice, which is a seeking of the Divine, come forth. This requires stillness in the outer aspects of our mind and body, our sensory and motor organs, the practice of pratyahara in the yogic sense. The Vedic language is rooted in silence and meditation. To approach it we must be able to control our speech and calm the mind and heart.

Vedic Mantra Yoga is the basis of Vedic Bhakti Yoga or the Yoga of Devotion, which is the main yogic approach that occurs based upon the chant. The Yogas of Knowledge (Jnana), Service (Karma), however, and the great variety of yogic methods and techniques extensively employ mantra and chanting. Mantra is the language through which all the Yogas proceed. Mantra is the language of Yoga. The *Rigveda* constitutes the oldest language of Yoga. This is not simply a spoken language but the language of the universal sound.

Vedic Chanting Today

Vedic mantras pose a problem for us today, as few of us are trained in Vedic Sanskrit and know how to read, pronounce, and chant these mantras, or understand their meaning. There is a new movement in Vedic chanting and several Yoga groups teach Vedic chanting, however, not only in India but also in the West. For some of these groups, the mantras are pronounced in a modern style (as in the modern kirtan movement), for others a strict traditional pronunciation is used.

Modern Vedic chanting uses Vedic mantras primarily for their sound value and does not extensively explore their meaning, which is very hard to access. In the Vedic view, the sound of mantras has a value and power of its own, even if we do not know their meaning. The Vedic mantra becomes more powerful, however, if do we know its meaning and take time to meditate upon it. This is not a simple matter of knowing the dictionary meaning of Vedic terms, it implies being able to connect to the Vedic deities to whom the mantras are directed. While learning the correct pronunciation of Vedic mantras is essential, it should include a deeper study of their meaning and application.

Vedic and Classical Sanskrit

Vedic Sanskrit is different than classical Sanskrit in several ways and poses challenges even for those who may know classical Sanskrit. Vedic Sanskrit is more fluidic overall and not fixed into terms of grammar or meaning. Words are living and adaptable, reflecting different levels of applications and different contexts of associations.

The sound forms of Vedic words is not simply limited to their roots, which dominates classical Sanskrit, though these are important. The same word can be divided up in different ways, with each syllable having its own indications.[172] This makes Vedic Sanskrit at times difficult for those trained in classical Sanskrit and expecting the same precision of grammar and etymology. Those trained in classical Sanskrit can misinterpret Vedic statements by interpreting them strictly according to later grammatical rules. One needs a particular flexibility of mind in order to uncover all the levels of meaning, symbol, and association contained in the Vedic hymns.

Rishi, Devata and Chhandas

Each Vedic hymn has three factors crucial for its proper usage and understanding:

1. The Rishi (Ṛṣi) who saw the mantra, who is the subject of the mantra.
2. The Deity (Devatā) to whom it is addressed, the object of the mantra.
3. The Meter (Chhandas) in which it is composed, the energy of the mantra.

It is said that to be able to use the mantra fully one must understand all three factors of Rishi, Devata and Chhandas. Maharishi Mahesh Yogi has always emphasized this point.

Of these three factors, the Deity is the most important. Ultimately speaking, the Deity is Brahman or the Godhead behind nature, the Absolute. The Rishi is the Atman or higher Self within us, our awakened soul. The chhandas is the vibration of our own mind, the Brahma Vritti that connects our Atman with Brahman, which is also the state of samadhi.

Rishi

To connect with the Rishi, one must understand who the Rishi is and what the Rishi represents, which is revealed by his name and his family (gotra), as well as his symbolic reality. Agni is the primordial Rishi beyond all the human Rishis. Ganesha in the form of Brihaspati, or the Vedic lord of speech, is another formulation of the primordial Rishi or Sadguru. Yet many other Vedic deities are called Rishis or sages, including Indra, Soma, and Surya.

Some great human Rishis like Vasishtha and Vishvamitra have many stories about them, particularly in the *Mahabharata* and *Puranas*, which help us understand their energies and qualities. Their names contain certain meanings like Vasishtha, as the one with the greatest power of self-control, or Vishvamitra, as the universal friend, a form of Agni, and power of tapas. The Rishis have inner correspondences extending far beyond the human, like the seven Rishis and the seven sensory openings in the head, or as the powers of the seven chakras. They are part of different cosmic symbolisms.

Deity or Devata

To connect with the Deity, one must understand what the Deity represents both outwardly and inwardly. For example, to connect to Agni one must understand fire as a natural power and cosmic principle externally, and as a spiritual and psychological principle internally, from human speech to the Divine Word. Most importantly, one must understand the consciousness or Purusha factor inherent in the Deity. For example, one must experience fire as a form of consciousness or the Self, not merely as an outer element, in order to appreciate the Vedic Agni.

One should respectfully address and actually communicate with the Deity as with another person. The Vedic chants are primarily directed to the deities. They are rarely statements or instructions for other human beings. You must think about the deity that you are wishing to invoke, rather than thinking of yourself as one who is doing the chanting, much less any audience that you might be chanting for! The true Rishi is one who can call down the deities or bring them into manifestation in our minds and into our worlds. He or she is a conduit for the Divine. We must learn to invoke the Vedic deities within our own psyche as the powers through which the Vedic Yoga proceeds.

Meter or Chhandas

To recite the mantra properly one must understand the meter (chhandas) in which it is composed, which includes all factors of sound, pronunciation, and rhythm. Each Vedic meter has a mathematical pattern according to the number of its syllables. These relate to various cosmic laws, through the movements of time and prana.

Among the Vedic deities, Soma relates most to the meters, which reflect the Soma energy of delight. Yet different Vedic meters relate to different deities. Relative to the three most common meters, the Gayatri meter, with eight syllables per line, relates to Agni and to the eight Vasus or eight earth deities. Trishtubh meter, with eleven syllables per line, relates to Indra and the eleven Rudras or Maruts, the eleven atmospheric deities. Jagati meter, with twelve syllables per line, relates to Surya or the Sun, and the twelve Adityas, the heavenly or solar deities.

Relative to the seven main Vedic meters, an important hymn of the *Rigveda* relates the seven Vedic meters a specific deity. [173] We can equate these with the seven chakras.

Earth or Root chakra	Gayatri, 24 syllables	Agni, Fire
Water chakra	Ushnik, 28 syllables	Savita
Fire chakra or navel	Anushtubh, 32 syllables	Soma
Air or heart chakra	Brihati, 36 syllables	Brihaspati
Ether or throat chakra	Pankti, 40 syllables	Mitra-Varuna
Third eye	Trishtubh, 44 syllables	Indra
Crown chakra	Jagati, 48 syllables	Vishvedevas, Universal Gods

Agni here relates to the root chakra as the Kundalini fire. Indra as the power of perception relates to the Third Eye. The crown chakra or thousand petal lotus relates to the Vishvedevas or the Universal aspect of the Vedic deities. The Vedic meters are forms of Soma or food for the Devas, connecting it to the navel chakra. Brihaspati is the lord of the Divine word that connects to the heart.

One must be able to put one's consciousness in the rhythmic, musical or vibratory mode of the chant. Different meters have their powers to connect with the Divine forces both within and around us. They represent the vibratory power of creative intelligence. It is the meter that takes us to the deity. In this regard, the meters represent the worlds or planes of experience (lokas).

Sacred Use of Name and Form

As a sacred language in which everything is symbolic, Vedic statements can go against the common-sense meaning of words. Vedic words are not mere words. The Vedic cow or *gau* is seldom only a cow. It is a symbol of expression, nourishment, or knowledge at various levels, including indicating the mind and sense organs. The horse or *ashva* is seldom a horse. It is a symbol of energy, effort, movement, or change at various levels, including prana and the motor organs. Vedic terms are intimations of something beyond words. This is why they are paradoxical or indicate something supernatural.

What binds us to the illusory world of Samsara is the material, literal or particularized usage of name and form – which is how we ordinarily use language. This is the realm of outer meanings in which everything is taken as it appears to be, in which we take the outer world as real in itself, and our bodily identity as who we really are. The sacred usage of name and liberates us from this limited outer application of words. The realm of the Vedic mantra is the realm in which everything is an intimation of a higher reality in which its separative, utilitarian, or personal meaning loses significance. The outer form is but a shape that carries the inner light. That is why all Vedic deities eventually blend into one another and cannot be rigidly defined or distinguished.

All Vedic names we could say are intimations of the nameless. They do not indicate separate entities but the different qualities, energies and aspects of the nameless Deity. The nameless is the content of all names but also transcends them all. The nameless is the true subject that is the giver of all names.

All Vedic forms are similarly suggestions of the formless. The formless is the content of all forms but is not limited by any of them. It is like the water that is the content of all the waves but not limited to any particular wave. For this reason the forms of Vedic deities are types of light or energy more so than specific objects in the external world.

Names and forms are reality or Brahman at a symbolic or indirect level. What they are at a visible or perceptive level is only Maya or a relative appearance. We must take name and form, not as they appear to be, but for what they intimate, not for their practical reality but for their spiritual aesthetic. This is the Vedic way of ritual and meditation.

Types of Vedic Mantras

Vedic mantras are of different types, mainly according to the deity that is invoked and the way in which it is called down.

Stuti – the power of praise

Vedic chants consist primarily hymns of praise to the deity, a practice called stuti in Sanskrit meaning affirmation. This is not a matter of praising an external deity but of invoking the Deity or Divine power within ourselves. The easiest way to influence a person is through praise. The easiest way to encourage a person to grow is to praise what is good in them. Praise has a great power to persuade and to ennoble, if used sincerely.

By seeing the good in others, the good in ourselves naturally grows. By honoring the Divine in others and in nature, the God in us also develops. By affirming Divine qualities, those qualities within us grow. By praising God, we can become humble and create the space for God to come into us. Without humility it is not possible to discover our true Divine Self, which otherwise will get confused with the ego.

Namas – the power of surrender

Along with stuti or praise of the deity comes *namas* or *namaskara*, offering reverence to the deity. On an inner level, this means devotional surrender of one's heart or soul to the deity. Namas is the inverse or complement of stuti, the inner humility that reflects the giving of praise. We will discuss this factor in detail in the next chapter, as it is the basis of the Vedic Bhakti Yoga.

Āvāhana – direct invocation of the deity

Some mantras are used specifically for calling down the Deity. This is necessary for the deity to manifest, bless us, teach us, or perform what other actions inwardly or outward that we may seek from them. Vedic mantras possess a special power to call down the deity, and to awaken the Rishi consciousness within us. This bringing down of the deity is an extension of stuti and namas, or affirmation and surrender.

Prārthana – the power of prayer

A number of Vedic chants consist of prayers or wishes. The deity blesses the sincere worshipper with its grace, help, and guidance. The *Vedas* call upon the deity to grant various spiritual and material wishes. Material blessings may be for longevity, wealth, progeny, protection from enemies, or victory in our struggles. Spiritual blessings are for peace, knowledge, freedom from sorrow, and union with the deity.

Svastivācana, Śāntipaṭha – chants for well-being and peace

These are specific forms of blessings. Vedic mantras are used for seeking good fortune (svasti), well-being, and peace (śānti) for ourselves and for all beings.

Upadeśa – instruction

Vedic mantras are formulated to teach, guide, enlighten, and promote us along the path of dharma. Such hymns may consist of questions and answers. This Vedic instruction is mantric and symbolic, seldom in an evident language, and can be hidden under other forms of expression. It requires an inner vision to entirely discover. As the purpose of the *Vedas*, which mean knowledge, is to promote knowledge, a factor of instruction can be found in all Vedic hymns, reflecting the deepest application of Vedic mantras. The Vedic Deities are primarily powers of cosmic knowledge and Self-knowledge, which is their primary gift to us.

Usage of the Different *Vedas* and their Branches

The *Rigveda* as the largest or core *Veda* contains all other applications that we find in the other *Vedas*. The greatest power of the Vedic mantras resides in the mantras of the *Rigveda*, starting with those to Agni that are necessary to invoke the other deities. The *Rigveda* primarily reflects the power of the deity and how to invoke it.

The *Samaveda* primarily reflects the power of devotion and inspiration, as it consists primarily of selected hymns of the *Rigveda* placed in a more musical chant. We could regard it as a more energized application of the *Rigveda*, enhancing its powers. That is why it is sometimes said to be the highest of the *Vedas*. Krishna in the *Bhagavad Gita* states that among the *Vedas*, he is the *Samaveda*.[174]

The *Yajurveda* reflects primarily the power of ritual, which may be outer, a seeking of material blessings, or inner, a development of yogic practices and inner offerings. Yet it does contain very powerful chants like the Rudram that are not found in the *Rigveda*. Oṁ as a primary mantra arises in the *Yajurveda* in this Rudram chant.

The *Atharvaveda* contains many original hymns of its own, which form a kind of appendix to the *Rigveda* covering a greater variety of subjects and supplementary concerns. That is why the *Vedas* are sometimes counted as only three. The Atharvaveda shares a number of hymns with the *Rigveda* and a few with the *Yajurveda*.

The *Brahmanas* of the different *Vedas* reflect more the ritualistic meaning of the Vedic mantras but in a more detailed matter than the *Yajurveda*, though they do have a special powerful mantras of their own. The *Upanishads* reflect more the spiritual and yogic meaning of the Vedic mantras and teach the main principles of Vedic and Vedantic philosophy. This includes teaching several Vedic mantras like Gayatri and bija mantras extending to Oṁ. The *Aranyakas* fall in between the *Brahmanas* and *Upanishads* in their usage, with a more internalized ritual, including special mantras. But there is a considerable cross over between all the different aspects of Vedic literature and no rigid demarcation or division exists between them.

Application of Vedic Mantras

Vedic mantras can be recited in several ways from strong outward recitation to deep silent meditation. Generally one starts with chanting the mantras out loud, then a soft whispering of the mantra, then using the mantra along with the breath, and finally a silent repetition combined with meditation.

1. Vocal Chanting

One usually begins with a vocal or out loud recitation of Vedic verses and mantras. There are several styles of Vedic recitation, with slight variations. One can begin with a monotone or single tone rendition of the chant. Most classical Vedic chanting uses three tones – *anudātta, udātta,* and *svarita* – which literally mean "low," "high," and "resonated," but these are intoned differently in different Vedic chanting styles. *Svarita* is usually the highest tone in terms of pitch, with *anudātta* at the lowest level and *udātta* in the middle.

There is a special *Rigveda* variation of Vedic chanting that is not commonly heard. In it all accented long vowels are drawn out two beats. In addition, there are variations in the metrical count of certain syllables in the *Rigveda* hymns, with long vowels counting as more than one syllable in places. There are traditional *svaras* or melodies for Rigvedic mantras marked in the text, though I have never heard these chanted.

Most commonly heard is *Krishna Yajurveda* style chanting, which is mainly from South India. Some people consider that this is the correct or only style, but it is one of several kinds. It commonly adds a kind of "goom" sound after certain letters. In the north of India one hears mainly the *Shukla Yajurveda* or *Sanatani* style that differs from the *Krishna Yajurveda* style in a significant manner, not only in chanting but also in the pronunciation of certain letters. For example, "sh" in Purusha is pronounced "kh" or "Purukha" in the Sanatani style. The *Samaveda* as the Vedic of music and chanting contains more elaborate chanting styles, with a greater variety of melodies and intonations.

Only a few *Upanishads* have chanting marks, notably the *Taittiriya* and *Mahanarayana Upanishads*, which follow the *Krishna Yajurveda* style of chanting. Some *Upanishads* like the *Brihadaranyaka* have only two tones.

2. Muttering or Whispering of Mantras

This consists of chanting the mantra softly and gently, whispering it along with the breath, rather than a strong vocal intonation. It helps us to carry the vibration of the mantra within.

3. Mantra Pranayama

This consists of chanting the mantra mentally along with the practice of pranayama. For example, one can repeat the first eight syllables of a Gayatri meter chant on inhalation, the second eight syllables on retention, and the third eight upon exhalation. One uses the mantra to measure the breath. The different numbers of the Vedic meters provide a variety of ways of counting the breath. Yet one should hold the deity of the mantra in one's mind during the practice.

4. Mantra Meditation

This consists of silently repeating the mantra along with meditation upon its Deity and its Rishi. One tries to feel the resonance of the chant's meter, and align one's thought vibration according to it. This Vedic mantra meditation is probably the most important as well as the easiest to practice for an extended period of time. A single Vedic verse can be used for this purpose, an entire hymn, or several hymns to a particular deity. One can hold a particular Vedic mantra, name of Vedic deity, or Vedic verse in one's mind throughout the day.

Like any other prayers or mantras, Vedic mantras should be repeated many times in order to properly energize them within our deeper awareness. Usually one should repeat a verse like Gayatri at least a thousand times in order to get a sense of its power. More than ten thousand repetitions may be required in order to energize it. One hundred thousand times is ideal for truly awakening the power of the mantra.

Generally one begins with a single verse of a Vedic hymn, and chants it a certain number of times each day, like a hundred times, for a certain period of time, like a month or forty days. One can only do an extensive repetition of a few Vedic verses as there are ten thousand verses in the *Rigveda* alone.

Another chanting method is to do a *parāyana* or recitation of particular Vedic texts, reciting each hymn only a single time and going through an entire *Veda* or a book (mandala) of the *Rigveda*. It is best if one knows the meaning of the words in the hymns, or knows the nature of the deities that one is invoking. Listening to Vedic chanting, particularly done by well-trained Vedic priests, is another helpful method but should not be a substitute for our own mantra practices. One can get the audio versions of the *Vedas* and listen to them. It is best to read or recite the mantras along with the playing of the recording.

A similar method is *adhyayana*, which is a study and silent reading of certain Vedic hymns. One may go through a single book of the *Rigveda*, like the ninth or Soma mandala, or the hymns of a particular Rishi (like the hymns of Parashara), or the hymns of a particular Rishi family to a particular deity (like the Atri hymns to Agni). Translation of Vedic hymns can be another form of *adhyayana*, particularly if it is done from a yogic perspective.

For purposes of simplicity, it is often recommended to repeat the Gayatri mantra of the Rishi Vishvamitra (*Tat Savitur vareṇyam*) in place of reciting the *Vedas* overall.[175] This is a good place to begin any Vedic chanting. The Gayatri mantra is said to be the essence of the *Vedas* and the Mother of the *Vedas* (*Veda Māta*). Another verse to the Sun also as *Savita* that is used in a similar manner is the *Ghṛṇi Sūrya Āditya Oṁ* mantra, which comes from the *Brahmanas*[176] and is mentioned in the *Upanishads*.[177] It is also said to be the essence of the *Vedas*.

A simpler way to gain the essence of the *Vedas* is to chant Oṁ. Usually a mental repetition of Oṁ ten thousand times is a good place to begin. Another way is to take the name of a Vedic deity and repeat it, generally with *Oṁ* and *namas* like *Oṁ Indrāya namaḥ*, or to combine it with seed mantras like *Oṁ Krīm Indrāya Namaḥ*.

I personally have spent more time reciting, reading, and translating the *Rigveda* as a whole, rather than chanting any single Vedic verse. This has allowed me to cover the entire *Rigveda* many times and significant portions of other Vedic texts. I have taken a few special Vedic verses to repeat regularly.[178]

Vedic Bija Mantras and Short Mantric Phrases

The Vedic language is called *chhandas* or meter, out of which the hymns are composed. Yet the *Rigveda* does recognize the importance of akshara or the single letter of the chant. Such bija mantras, particularly Shakti bijas like *Hrīṁ* and *Śrīṁ* can be found better explained in the *Tantras*. These bija mantras are hidden in the root sounds of the Sanskrit language, such as also occur in the *Rigveda*. For example, the Shakti mantra *Krīṁ* or Kriya shakti relates to the Sanskrit and Vedic root sound 'kri' meaning 'to do', such as we find in many Vedic terms like karma, krita, and kratu.

There is no overt listing of the letters of the Sanskrit alphabet in Vedic texts, though numerical lists of Vedic deities may relate to them, as the Vedic deities are powers of the Divine Word. The *Rigveda* does speak of the Vedic letters or aksharas as developing from one to one thousand, showing as in later times how, from a single syllable, the entire universe develops. The thousand syllables relate to the thousand syllables of the thousand petal lotus of the head that contains all the other sounds of the chakras.

> *The female cow has bellowed, fashioning the waters. She has become onefold, twofold, fourfold, eightfold, ninefold, and a thousand syllables in the Supreme Ether.*[179]
>
> *Dirghatamas Auchatya, Rigveda I.164.41*

> *Noble men, sages go to you, O Agni, with their insights for the victory, and to the Goddess of a thousand syllables.*[180]
>
> *Maitravaruni Vasishtha, Rigveda VII.15.9*

This idea is clarified in a later Vedic text, the *Taittiriya Aranyaka*, in which the number of vowels and consonants is counted as 360 each, and another 360 for their combinations, or 1080 total.[181] Another portion of the text identifies the consonants (sparśa) with the earth, the sibilants (s and h sounds) with the atmosphere, and the vowels (svara) with heaven. This indicates a cosmic symbolism for the letters.

In addition, the *Vedas* contain a number of shorter mantras and phrases used for special emphasis like bija mantras, which we will examine below.

- *Oṁ/Aum* – The seed mantra *Oṁ* first overtly occurs in the *Yajurveda* and becomes dominant in the *Upanishads* and *Mahabharata* as the prime syllable of the Divine Word or cosmic sound vibration (Pranava). The *Mandukya Upanishad* focuses upon its meaning in both the individual soul and the cosmic spirit. A related term "Oma" for protector occurs in the *Rigveda.*[182] It is connected to the term "ava" meaning grace and protection. Another related term is ether as *Vyoma*, which refers to wide (vi) space of protection (oma). It is in the supreme ether that the Divine Word or Akshara dwells in the *Rigveda.*[183] Oṁ is used along with the Gayatri Mantra and considered to be its essence.

- *Īm* – The mantra *Īm* (pronounced 'eem') is the most common seed mantra of the *Rigveda*, commonly used as a particle giving emphasis in a sentence, just as Oṁ is used in later Sanskrit. It is also mentioned in the *Yajurveda.*[184] Rishi Daivarata, following the teachings of Ganapati Muni, calls Īṁ the secret Pranava or Divine Word of the *Rigveda*, equating it with Oṁ as a word of power.[185] Īṃ is the mantra that connects us with the Divine as the cosmic lord (Ishvara or Indra) and with the ruling powers of the universe.[186]

> *Who resonates the imperishable word Īṁ and sounds forth by the word of Brahman, who is the Supreme Brahman, who practicing tapas according to the secret primal sound (gupta Praṇava), I choose that Indra for the realization of peace.*[187]

Īṁ grants the deeper perception, light, and electrical energy, as Oṁ gives the power of hearing, sound, and prana. Īṁ connects to Shakti as Oṁ connects to Shiva. Īṁ is the central mantra of the Sri Yantra and represents the bindu or primal point focus behind and beyond the manifest universe.[188] Oṁ represents its full expansion. Daivarata has given us the great Vedic mantra *Īṁ Oṁ Śrīḥ. Īm* focuses our energy. *Oṁ* expands it. *Śrīḥ* turns it into splendor.[189]

- *Hīm* – A term indicating Indra's vajra or thunderbolt and the direction of energy or Shakti. Useful for breaking through obstacles and destroying negative energy. It indicates *Ha* plus *Īm*, or adds the power of prana (ha) to Īm. It indicates prana as a force of energy and perception, as well as a weapon.

- *Sīm* – A term indicating concentration of energy, the summit or the ultimate. It helps stabilize and concentrate our energy to a point of pure awareness. It indicates *Saḥ* or Purusha together with *Īṃ*, the power of Speech or Shakti, the Self or pure being (Sat) in its own nature before the manifest speech of creation.[190]

- *Namas/Namaḥ* - The common Vedic term for devotion, adoration or surrender to the deity, used along with Divine names since the *Rigveda*, like *Oṁ Indrāya Namaḥ* or *Śivāya Namaḥ*!
- *Śam* – The common Vedic bija for peace and well-being, frequently used in the *Rigveda*, used for asking the grace of the Vedic deities. It is the basis of Shiva's names as Shankara and Shambhu. Often used as *Śam Yoḥ*.
- *Kam* – A common Vedic mantric interjection for bliss, happiness or well-being, water, and prana. A common particle in the *Vedas* indicating emphasis or energy.
- *Sat* – A Vedic single syllable word for being, existence or reality, the eternal and enduring, from which Satyam or truth arises.
- *Tat* – A Vedic single syllable word for consciousness and infinity, that which is extended, symbolically a pillar.
- *Śrī* – A Vedic single syllable word for beauty, splendor or delight, particularly relative to Soma.
- *Hrī* – A single syllable word in the *Rigveda* for light and power, used along with Shri, relative to the power of the day.
- *Śānta/Śānti* – The term for peace, repeated like *Śam* in various Vedic peace chants.
- *Svasti* – A common Vedic term for well-being, su-asti. Related to the swastika as its emblematic or symbolic representation.
- *Svāhā* –The Vedic term for offerings into the sacred fire or Agni, regarded as the wife or spouse of Agni. Often used instead of namas for this purpose or for a stronger energization of the mantra.
- *Svadhā* – The Vedic term for Soma offerings, also indicates the Self-nature.
- *Hari* – Hari as in Hare Krishna is a Vedic term meaning golden or delightful.[191] It is a development of the mantra Hrīṁ.
- *Hamsa* – A Vedic term for the sunbird, not simply the swan as in later times. Its mantric value was recognized relative to light and prana. The s and h-sounds are identified with prana in Vedic texts like the *Aitareya Aranyaka*.[192] There is a longer Vedic verse that is associated with the Hamsa that occurs in the *Upanishads*.

The Hamsa who dwells in the world of light, the indwelling power in the atmosphere, the invoker at the altar, the guest at the home, who dwells in the soul, who dwells in the supreme, who dwells in truth, who dwells in space, who is born of the waters, who is born of the light, who is born of truth, who is born of the mountain, who is the supreme truth.[193]

Vamadeva Gautama, Rigveda IV.40.5, Mahanarayana Upanishad 12

Hamsa is the sound of prana that is born in the spacc of consciousness. It is identified with Sun as the source of life and light. The mind itself breathes. Our outer breath is the manifestation of an inner breath, which is the breath of the mind and the breath of light. This mantra of the Rishi Vamadeva from the *Rigveda* occurs in the *Upanishads*.

The Three or Seven *Vyāhṛtis* from the *Yajurveda*

These are special short mantras often added to Vedic verses like the Gayatri or Mrityunjaya (Tryambakam) mantras. They are said to be the sounds through which the different worlds or lokas are created.

The Three Main *Vyāhṛtis*

Bhūr - Vedic mantra for the earth or the realm of manifest form.

Bhuvaḥ - Vedic mantra for the atmosphere or moving energy.

Svaḥ or *Suvaḥ* - Vedic mantra for heaven or the realm of light.

The Seven Extended *Vyāhṛtis*

Mahar - The great or the vast.

Jana - The creative or generating power.

Tapa - Tapas or fire purification.

Satyam - Truth or being.

The Extended Gayatri Mantra

Oṁ Bhūḥ! Oṁ Bhuvaḥ! Oṁ Suvaḥ! Oṁ Mahaḥ! Oṁ Janaḥ! Oṁ Tapaḥ! Oṁ Satyam!

Tat Savitur vareṇyam bhargo devasya dhīmahi, dhiyo yo naḥ pracodayāt,

Oṁ apo jyotirasomṛtam brahma bhūr bhuvas suvar Oṁ!

> *Oṁ Earth! Oṁ Atmosphere! Oṁ Heaven! Oṁ the Vast! Oṁ the Creative! Oṁ the Radiant! Oṁ the Truth! We meditate upon the supreme Light of the Divine solar creator that he may direct our insight. Oṁ the waters, the light, the essence immortal, Brahman, Earth, Atmosphere, Heaven, Oṁ!*[194]

This set of verses shows how the Vedic mind connected the worlds of the cosmos along with the Vedic chant, drawing us to the universal truth and the supreme light. These worlds represent aspects of our own deeper nature as a soul, but beyond our ordinary creaturely concerns. Here water and light are not simply outer factors, but the eternal essence that is Brahman.

Dhi Yoga: The Vedic Yoga of Meditation

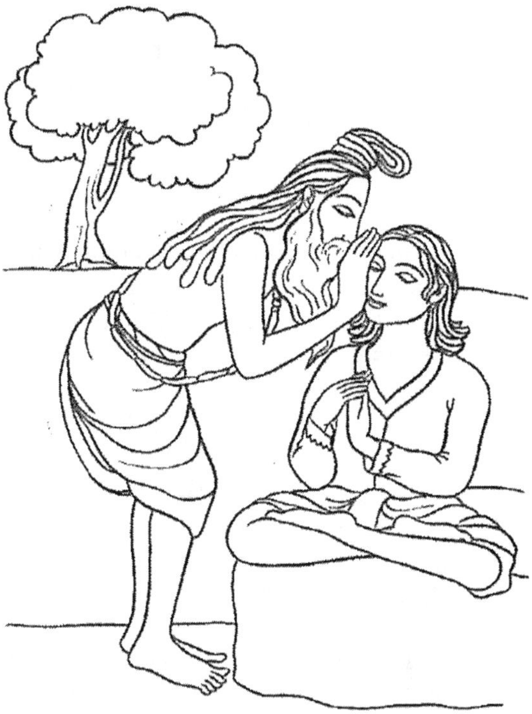

Central to the Vedic Yoga, just as that of classical Yoga, is the Yoga of Meditation. Meditation is the main method of coordinating and integrating our faculties in order to arrive at the ultimate state of unity and peace. Meditation is the key to both the Yogas of Knowledge and Devotion, and the foundation of all other Yogic techniques using body, prana, senses, and mind. Meditation is the state of mind that mantra brings us to.

The main faculty of the reincarnating soul (Jivatman) is the inner intelligence or natural wisdom called *Buddhi* in Vedanta, the power of cognition, or *Dhi*,[195] the power of reflection in Vedic thought. *Dhi* or Buddhi is our ability to discern truth from falsehood, right from wrong, reality from illusion, being from non-being, our true Self from outer appearances. Dhi aligns us with the Divine will towards spiritual and yogic evolution.

The *Vedas* discriminate between *manas*, a general term for the mind in its outer action through the senses, and Dhi, the more specific faculty of internal perception and judgment. Dhi, or intelligence, is the meditative part of the mind that is detached from the senses. Awakening the Dhi requires controlling the manas, or yogically mastering the outer mind. Buddhi in Vedantic philosophies has a similar distinction from manas in its functioning.

The Vedic Yoga can be overall described as *Dhi Yoga*, consisting of harnessing or controlling the mind, senses, and pranas – for which the verb "yuj," meaning "to yoke" is used, from which the term Yoga originally arises.[196] The Vedic Yoga is evidenced through the different types of Dhi or meditative intelligence mentioned in Vedic texts. It includes various aspects of higher knowledge, reflecting many other Vedic terms for knowledge, truth, or discernment.

Dhi Yoga reflects all the Yogas of knowledge, devotion, mantra, and prana. It has different applications relative to the main Vedic deities or light forms of Agni, Soma, Indra, and Surya – Fire, Moon, Lightning, and Sun. Both Ganapati Muni and his disciple Brahmarshi Daivarata, emphasize the Vedic Yoga as Dhi Yoga.

Classical Yoga seeks to develop the buddhi as the sattvic aspect of the mind. Control of the mind is only possible from the development of the buddhi.[197] Buddhi Yoga is one of the main yogic approaches of the *Bhagavad Gita*, which emphasizes its development through balanced awareness.[198] Buddhi Yoga is the Yoga of the intelligent mind, of right judgment, balance, and moderation. It teaches a discriminating approach in everything that we attempt, including a proper understanding and right usage of the body, prana, and mind. Yet Buddhi has an inspirational side, which is to search out the Divine essence in everything, to refine our feeling nature into an awareness of unity and peace. The *Gita* and Upanishadic Buddhi Yoga is a continuation of the Vedic Dhi Yoga, in a different language.

Dhi is related to the term Dhyana for meditation, which rests ultimately on the root 'dhi' meaning 'to hold or reflect'.[199] Dhi is the reflection of the Divine light into our human consciousness and carries the flame of our aspiration as a soul. Dhi is the higher intelligence that is the yogic mind or the enlightened mind. For it to manifest, we must bring calm and silence to the outer mind[200] and remove its distortions and fantasies.

Reorienting our Intelligence Within

Ordinarily we use our intelligence in an outer sense, seeking to define the names and forms of external reality so that we can be more successful in our activities in the outer world. This outer intelligence proceeds through measurement and categorization of external objects and energies, most notably through the naming process. The outgoing intelligence creates the realm of science and its development through technology, which are mathematically based.

The outer use of the mind to understand the external world has its place and is necessary for our practical functioning in life. It provides useful skills and information on many levels. Yet this outgoing intelligence is not the appropriate means for directly knowing reality or our true Self, which is the witness of the mind, and cannot be examined as an object for the mind's analysis.

In the yogic approach, a different movement of thought and attention is required than what we ordinarily do with the mind. Yoga asks us to turn our intelligence within – to look beyond the names and forms of the outer world to the essences and energies, the light consciousness hidden behind them. The *Vedas* reflect an inner directed intelligence, which is not the intelligence of the brain but that of the spiritual heart. It does not belong to the mind or the ego but to the soul and higher Self.

There are three types of knowledge that we have:

1. **Direct perception (Pratyaksha)**: knowledge allied with the senses through which we can perceive the outer world. Various instruments that extend the powers of the senses are part of this.
2. **Intuition (Paroksha)**: knowledge based upon intuition that comprehends the inner powers or Divine energies at work behind the worlds. This includes an ability to perceive the cosmic links between things, which has its own rationality.
3. **Direct unmediated experience (Aparoksha)**: knowledge based upon the nature of awareness itself, not through the senses, reason, or any instruments, and beyond the mind. This is our intrinsic knowledge of the Self or pure being, the inner light that makes all other forms of knowledge possible. It is sometimes referred to as the higher *pratyaksha* because it is a kind of direct perception through consciousness itself.

Vedic thought has a common statement that can be applied to its entire approach to language and knowledge. "*Parokṣa priya hi devāḥ*," meaning that the Gods or sages prefer what is *paroksha*, what is cryptic, symbolic, indirect or intuitive, while they dislike *pratyaksha*, what is direct, evident, obvious or based upon the senses.[201] That is why the *Vedas* resort to mantras, symbols, and paradoxes, and veil their meaning with outer life indications. As the Vedic is a paroksha or intuitive language by its own implicit declaration, we cannot expect it to contain pratyaksha or direct statements of outer knowledge, or try to interpret it literally – though that is what most scholars attempt to do anyway.

The Vedic language is not about the practical facts of the outer world, and is very different from a modern rationalist or journalistic approach. In the modern world, we are used to having everything spelled out in black and white, along with simple instructions and clear illustrations, so that what is meant is obvious to everyone at a quick examination. The best example of this is the Power Point computer presentation that passes on distinct information bits in a clear and precise manner. This direct information approach, however helpful in its own sphere, will not take us very far into the Vedic world, where what is meant is very different than what appears to be said.

The *Vedas* exist to stimulate our deeper intuition, not to pass on readymade answers to our outer minds. Simple verbal answers may satisfy our outer intelligence but do not bring us any closer to the great mystery and marvel of existence that transcends all words and expressions. The Vedic language is meant to promote our inner experience of the Divine, not to allow our ordinary mind to feel comfortable that it knows what God is through words, thoughts, or emotions.

Often when asking a question of the Vedic teacher – such as we find in the *Upanishads* – the student may be told to go off into the forest and practice meditation for a year, and then come back for the answer. This is obviously not the instant information approach of our current civilization, and would not sit very well with most people today. It is a different type of knowledge that is aimed at, which we must understand in order to appreciate the Vedic methodology. The year in the forest is part of gaining the answer and requires a sadhana during that period. It is not just a time of waiting for the guru's favor!

In some instances, the Rishi would give to the student – who might not be ripe for the real truth – the answer he wanted to hear, even if it was not correct. When Indra, the king of the Gods, and Virochana, the king of the Asuras, came to the Creator Prajapati and asked what the true Self was, the Creator replied that the true Self was the body. Virochana went home happily getting the answer he wanted to hear and continued with his life of enjoyment. Indra went away briefly but further doubts arose in his mind. "How could the true Self be this transient body?" he thought, as the body is mortal and subject to disease, decay, and death. He returned to the Creator who then taught him by stages the deeper truth of the Self as pure consciousness.[202]

In the Vedic tradition, the student has to question the teacher and probe deeply in order to receive the right answer. The teacher will not disclose the higher truth to an unprepared student, as the answer would be purely verbal in nature, not experiential. Vedic knowledge is sacred, not commercial or mundane. It cannot simply be given by request, much less by demand, or made evident to anyone who might be able to read the texts at a verbal level. Certain Vedic Vidyas or ways of knowledge were kept intentionally hidden. Some teachings were preserved in oral traditions only and not written down. Vedic intuitive knowledge is based upon an opening of the inner eye and the leading of a Vedic lifestyle.

Advaita Vedanta emphasizes *aparoksha* knowledge, which is direct experiential knowledge of the Self.[203] What convinces the ordinary mind about the reality of the external world is the directness and vividness of the information provided through the senses, which affects us at a physical level, especially the sense of touch. Yet more primal and important than the knowledge gained from the senses is the sense of Self, what could be called the "sixth sense" or "direct sense of being." That sense of self is common to and pervades all the movements of the mind and senses. Advaita Vedanta emphasizes meditation that cultivates this sense of self-being, dwelling in which the external sensory world gradually fades and is revealed as an illusion.

The intuitive (paroksha) approach of the *Vedas* is closely linked with the direct experience (aparoksha) approach of Vedanta. The Self or pure being is the inner essence of all that we perceive and is not limited by any outer forms. The *Vedas* cultivate an inner perception of the Gods, the inner lights or powers of consciousness behind the external world that take us to the same essence of Being. The Vedic Devas are not seen with the light of the senses, rather, the light of the senses works through them. The Vedic/Vedantic method consists of no longer pursuing the seen but going back to the reality of the Seer who is pure light.

Ganapati Muni attributes an aparoksha or direct knowledge approach to the *Vedas* at a mantric level.[204] He regards the Vedic mantric revelation as the basis for the authority ascribed to the *Vedas* and the reason that the *Vedas* constitute the prime scripture or source teaching of the Vedic and Hindu tradition. According to his view, the *Vedas* convey direct knowledge in the form of mantra or svara (sound), drawing us into the Divine Word or Oṁ vibration that is unmanifest sound. Such mantric knowledge takes a different form than the philosophical aparoksha or direct knowledge approach of Vedanta but leads to the same goal. The Rishi is a seer of the higher truth, just as is the Jnani or Advaitic sage. The Rishi language, however, is a manifestation of cosmic sound, not philosophy or theology even of the highest type.

Cultivating this Vedic intuitive approach involves symbol, analogy, metaphor, and mantra. We could compare it to poetry in which indirect statements become a source of great meaning and beauty, and direct statements are avoided as unpoetic. When a poet using a paroksha or symbolic language lauds a woman's face as like the autumn moon, he is saying that she is beautiful. To reduce the statement to its literal meaning destroys its poetic value. We cannot find fault with a poet for deficient knowledge of astronomy because he compares a small human face with a planetary orb thousands of miles around! Clearly a *pratyaksha* (literal) approach to a *paroksha* (symbolic) language creates distortions. Yet we must also understand the symbols. The Vedic mantras are not simply artistic symbols but symbols of the highest consciousness.

Dhi Yoga, Speech and Mantra: Sarasvati and Brihaspati

The Vedic Dhi Yoga is intuitively based, connecting individual intelligence with cosmic intelligence (Mahat) that is mantric in nature. Dhi is a manifestation of cosmic speech (Vak) and expresses itself through the voice of the soul that arises when the outer mind is silent. Vedic mantras reflect the language of the Dhi, the intuitive language of the soul.

Dhi Yoga is *Vak Yoga* or Mantra Yoga, not as mere repetition of sounds but as deep contemplation and meditation through the power of the Divine Word. Dhi is the portion of the Divine Word or Logos that dwells within the human soul. It contains all the creative capacities of the cosmic logos. This Vak Dhi Yoga is revealed in the following verses to the Goddess Sarasvati:

> *Sarasvati like a great ocean gives awareness through her ray; she rules over all the powers of intelligence (dhiyo viśvā vi rājati).* [205]
> *Madhuchchhandas Vaishvamitra, Rigveda I.3.12*

> *Goddess Sarasvati with power full of all power, as the protectress of our intelligence, protect us (dhīnām avitryavatu).*[206]
> *Bharadvaja Barhaspatya, Rigveda VI.61.4*

Dhi, like Vak or speech, is a feminine term and is worshipped as a Goddess as *Devi Dhi*, as well as Sarasvati.

> *Sustain the Goddess of Wisdom (devīm dhiyam), fashion your speech in the Godhead (devatrā vācam).*[207]
> *Maitravaruni Vasishtha, Rigveda VII.34.9*

The Vedic Gods live in the mantra. The mantra brings them to life. This mantra is the word of Dhi or higher intelligence. All forms of the Vedic Yoga share the mantra or the Divine speech as their common basis and support. *Brihaspati* or *Brahmanaspati* is the Vedic deity who governs specifically over the Divine word and power of the mantra.

> *Brahmanaspati now speaks the mantra, the hymn, in which Indra, Varuna, Mitra, Aryaman, and the Gods make their homes.* [208]
> *Kanva Ghaura, Rigveda I.40.5*

This mantra connects to meditation, which is the vibration of the mantra within us. Brihaspati, or the lord of the Vast or Lord of Prayer, is another name for Brahmanaspati.

> *Brihaspati who has three stations, by his call has up pillared with strength the ends of heaven and earth. The ancient Rishis, the illumined ones, while meditating, first sustained him as the tongue of bliss.*[209]
>
> *Vamadeva Gautama IV.50.1*

Brahmanaspati or Brihaspati grants union with himself as the ruler of the Divine word.

> *Blessed, he flourishes in the bliss of the Gods, whomever Brahmanaspati makes one with him (yujam).*[210]
>
> *Gritsamada Shaunaka, Rigveda II.25.5*

The discovery of the higher thought or Dhi, which has seven heads, reflecting the seven worlds and seven chakras, is central to the Vedic Yoga. It grants to the great Angirasa Rishis, the understanding of the Yajna, sacred worship or Sacrifice that constitutes the nature of the cosmic reality. Brihaspati is the first of the Angirasa Rishis whose main disciple was Ayasya.

> *This insight which has seven heads (imām dhiyam saptaśīrṣṇīm), born from truth and vast, our father (Brihaspati) found. Generating a certain fourth that generates all, the seer Ayasya declared it as a hymn to Indra.*[211]
>
> *Declaring the truth, meditating straightly, the sons of heaven, the heroes of the Almighty, the Angirasa Rishis, holding the station of the seers, meditated out the original nature of the sacrifice.*[212]
>
> *Ayasya Angirasa, Rigveda X.67.1-2*

Other Important Rigvedic Knowledge Principles

Below are some of the main Vedic synonyms for Dhi, or higher intelligence, and its related faculties and functions.

Hṛd or *Hṛdaya* – the spiritual heart, as in the *Upanishads*, not simply the physical heart

Manas – mind, particularly in the contemplative and reflective sense

Mati – thought determination

Sumati – good thoughts, happy mindedness

Manīṣa – inspired mind, intuition

Mantra – the word as a formation of the higher mind

Medhā – deeper wisdom, sacred knowledge

Citta – mind in general

Kratu – will power, particularly the will to truth

Dakṣa – discernment, discrimination

Vāk – the word of command, guidance, teaching and power

Pracetas – profound in wisdom and consciousness

Vicetas – wide in wisdom and consciousness

Satyam – truth, reality

Ṛtam – truth, law, cosmic order

Bṛhat – the Vast or infinite

Dharma – natural law, laws of consciousness

Ṛṣi – seer, one who is inspired or has the power of the higher mind

Kavi – poet, one who has the design or ability to envision

Vipra – enlightened or illumined one

The Fourfold Dhi Yoga

In Vedic symbolism, the Yoga of meditation is the great Yoga of light that relates to the Vedic deities of light, truth, and consciousness. The different aspects of meditation are represented in the Vedic light forms of Agni, Soma, Indra, and Surya (Fire, Moon, Lightning and Sun). The Vedic Dhi Yoga as a Yoga of meditation is evidenced by such verses as the Gayatri Mantra, which is said to be the essence of the *Vedas*:

> *May we meditate upon the supreme light of the Divine creative Sun, that he may direct our intelligence (dhī).*
> *Gathina Vishvamitra, Rigveda III.62.10*

This Vedic mantra to the Divine Sun for the illumination of the inner intelligence summarizes the entire Vedic teaching and its Yoga of mantra and meditation.

Dhi or deeper intelligence holds the reflections of the three Divine lights of Being (Sat), Consciousness (Chit), and Bliss (Ananda), symbolized in the *Vedas* by the light forms of Indra, Agni, and Soma (Lightning, Fire and Moon), while the Sun

(Surya), as the fourth, represents the light of truth in general. The Sun, Lightning, Fire and Moon are the cosmic or Adhidaivic side of the four Atmic or spiritual lights that manifest through the Dhi or Buddhi. These are the powers of light inherent in the ether of consciousness.

- The reflection of this higher Sun, or light of truth reflected in the human being, is Dhi, or intelligence of the soul.
- The lightning, or Indra aspect of Dhi, is Sat-shakti, the power of direct perception and realization, arising from pure Being. This Vidyut shakti, or lightning, gives quickness of comprehension, cutting through all illusion and ignorance. It is the weapon of the Self to dissolve all falsehood.
- The fire, or Agni aspect of Dhi, is Cit-shakti, the consciousness power reflected through it, the enduring flame of awareness.
- The lunar, or Soma side of Dhi, is the Ananda, the joy or ecstasy aspect of the Self as working through it, including the power of devotion.

The Vedic Dhi Yoga becomes fourfold relative to the four main Vedic Devatas and the powers they represent.

- Surya Dhi– Solar meditation, illumined or enlightened solar intelligence, relates to comprehension and awareness – faculty of Divine intelligence.
- Indra Dhi – Lightning meditation, ruling lightning intelligence that destroys all obstructions, relates to perceptive mind – faculty of Divine Prana. Dhi and Prana or the soul's intelligence and immortal life power go together.
- Agni Dhi – Fire meditation, ascending or fire intelligence, relates to will power, mantra, and inquiry – faculty of Divine speech.
- Soma Dhi – Lunar meditation, descending joy or watery/lunar intelligence, relates to contemplative mind and to devotion – faculty of Divine mind. As Ananda, the Vedic Dhi Yoga is also Bhakti Yoga, Bhagavata Prema or Divine love.

The Vedic Dhi Yoga consists of harnessing or controlling the mind, senses, and pranas, for which the root "yuj," meaning to yoke, is commonly used. Unfortunately, many scholars have only looked to the term "Yoga," which is rare in the *Rigveda*, but have ignored other noun and verb forms of the root "yuj," which are common, from which it arises. Note such references in the discussion of Dhi Yoga below.

Agni is first of all the power of Dhi or luminous thought, through which all the other Divine powers are invoked and can manifest within us:

Thou, oh Agni, were the first thinker of this insight (prathamo manotāsyā dhiyo), the wonderful invoker.[213] *You shining lead the people through the luminous realms of heaven.*[214]

Bharadvaja Barhaspatya, Rigveda VI.1.1,7

Agni, who is made supreme by the insight or power of dhi, directs us to the "Yoga of truth" (ṛtasya yoge), the inner linking with the cosmic reality.

He was made supreme by the insight (dhiyā cakre vareṇyam). I have held the seed of all beings, the father of discernment in an extended form.[215]

I have placed you supreme, you who are made by strength, by the word of discernment, O Agni, shining brightly and inspired.[216]

The Fire, the controller, who crosses the waters, in the Yoga of truth (ṛtasya yoge), the sages enkindle you with power.[217]

Gathina Vishvamitra, Rigveda III.27.9-11

Indra, as the master power, directs the *Dhi Yoga*, through which we discover the original truth.

Without whom (Indra), the sacrifice of the enlightened one is not perfected, he directs the Dhi Yoga (sa dhinām yogam invati). [218]

Medhatithi Kanva, Rigveda I.18.7

Indra, that which is your newest blissful declaration is generated, you who are conscious, the insight of the mind (manasam dhiyam), the nectar of the original truth.[219]

Tirashchi Kanva, Rigveda VIII.95.5.

The Sun grants the power to yogically control Dhi and manas, the outer and inner aspects of the mind.

Seers of the great illumined seer, yogically control the mind and intelligence. One only he ordains the invocations of the Gods. Great is the affirmation of the Savita, the Divine creative Sun.[220]

Shyavashva Atreya, Rigveda V.81.1

The path of the Sun is the path to the Supreme reality, the pure light of awareness.

I yogically unite (yuje) by the power of surrender to your ancient Brahman. May this chant go forth by the path of the Sun. May all the sons of immortality hear it, those who dwell in celestial domains. [221]

Vivasvan Aditya, Rigveda X.13.1.

Soma, or the nectar of bliss, is developed through the intelligence that yogically controls the mind.

> *Thou, Soma, release the intelligence yogically linked to the mind (dhiyam manoyujam), like the thunder the rain. You nourish the treasures of heaven and earth.* [222]
>
> *Rebhasunus Kashyapa, Rigveda IX.100.3*

Yoga and the Yoking of the Vedic Chariot

Vedic worship or Yajna is compared to a chariot (ratha) or to a wheel (chakra). The Devas have their special chariots with magical powers, and their special wheels. These chariots symbolize the subtle body and its chakra system. Yoga can be defined as yoking our inner chariot, which is the mind, the senses, and the subtle body. The Ribhus lauded below are the magical craftsmen of the Gods, who fashion the chariot of the Gods.

> *Whose horse was not born, which has no reins, which is laudable, the chariot with three wheels moves around the atmosphere. Great is that declaration of the Divine, when Ribhus, you nourish heaven and earth.*
>
> *The easy turning wheel that does not waver that you made by the power of consciousness, from the mind by the power of insight (manasas pari dhyayā).* [223]
>
> *Vamadeva Gautama, Rigveda IV.36.1-2*

The Rishi Dirghatamas makes the yogic nature of the Vedic chariot clearer. This is just one of many verses that deal with the subject in a similar light:

> *Seven yoke the chariot that has a single wheel (sapta yuñjanti ratham ekacakram). One horse pulls it who has seven names; a wheel with three centers that is undecaying and cannot be overcome, in which all these worlds exist.*
>
> *This chariot where the seven stand has a sevenfold wheel and is pulled by seven horses. Seven sisters sing together where is hidden the seven names of the Cow of Light.* [224]
>
> *Dirghatamas Auchatya, Rigveda I.164.2-3*

The Rishi's chariot reflects the subtle body with its seven chakras or energy centers that are interlinked in various ways. It is hardly an actual chariot that is meant, and the mystical implications are hard to deny. A wheel or chakra in which all the worlds exist is an inner energy center of consciousness. Dirghatamas describes the Vedic horse in a similar cosmic symbolism. The horse is a symbol of prana or the soul. The Vedic concern is not simply with actual horses!

> *Three they say are your bonds in heaven, three in the waters, and three in the ocean. And you appear like Varuna (the Lord of heaven) to me, O horse, where they say is your supreme place of birth.*[225]
>
> *Dirghatamas Auchatya, Rigveda I.163.4*

The Ashvins, the magical twins and horsemen, have their magical chariot. It is yoked by the mind and travels over all the worlds.

> *Your chariot, which binds heaven and earth, is golden and moves by bull horses. Extending over the five worlds, with a threefold seat, may it come, yoked by the mind (manasā yuktah).*
>
> *Maitravaruni Vasishtha, Rigveda VII.69.1,2*

> *Nobly, wonder workers, by your mind-yoked chariot (manoyujā rathena), wide with power, Ashvins, you follow the Dawn Goddess.*[226]
>
> *Brahmatithi Kanva, Rigveda VIII.5.1*

The chariot of the Gods goes around the seven rivers that can be identified with the streams of the seven chakras of the subtle body. Of course, one could argue that the term yoke here has nothing to do with Yoga but only refers to horses and chariots. Yet given the fact this yoking involves mantra, meditation, and the power of the mind, it is difficult to deny any yogic connections.

> *In a single common yoke (ekasmin yoge samane), O Ashvins, you who move quickly, your chariot goes around seven rivers. Your fast and powerful horses yoked by the Gods (deva yuktā) do not waver as they carry you at the poles of the chariot.*[227]
>
> *Maitravaruni Vasishtha, Rigveda VII.67.8*

The Ashvins are especially connected to Soma and have the knowledge of the *Madhu* or honey-bliss that they share with the Gods. They represent the unity of all dualities and the balancing of all contraries through which the bliss of Soma flows. The *Upanishads* highlight the Ashvins in the important *Madhu Vidya* (honey-bliss doctrine) of the *Brihadaranyaka*, as quoted below.

This Self is the honey-bliss of all beings. All beings are the honey bliss of the Self. That which in the Self is the Purusha composed of light and composed of immortality, that which is the Self and the Purusha composed of light and composed of immortality, that is the Self, that is the immortal, that is Brahman, that is everything.[228]

That honey-bliss Dadhyak, son of Atharva, spoke to the Ashvins. That the Rishi Kakshivan, perceiving this said. "That twin lords for the victory, wonderful, and fierce I declare, like the thunder the rain. Dadhyak Atharvana declared that honey-bliss to Ashvins, through the head of the horse."

Brihadaranyaka Upanishad II.5. 14, 16, Kakshivan Dairghatamasa, Rigveda I.116.12

This Madhu Vidya, or knowledge of the honey-bliss of immortality, is the goal of the Vedic Yoga and Dhi Yoga. It is the supreme Ananda or bliss of oneness. Here the *Upanishad* again quotes the *Rigveda* for the highest knowledge. The Ashvins are great teachers of Ayurveda, as they have all magical curative powers, up to this knowledge of immortality. The horse's head, or Ashvins Nakshatra (constellation), is set in the sky and marks the beginning of the sign Aries, which also represents the head.

Vedic Bhakti Yoga, Namas and Nama: The Power of Surrender and Divine Names

Yoga, which means unity, depends upon an inner longing for oneness with divinity, which rests upon a certain receptivity of the heart. This inherent longing for union is devotion or Divine Love, called *Bhakti* in Sanskrit. Bhakti means to partake of and to commune with the beloved, the Lord or *Bhagavan*. Bhakti means to consecrate oneself to the Divine and place one's being within the Divine presence and power.

Vedic Yoga, like classical Yoga, reflects a path of devotion or Bhakti Yoga, as one of its main, if not its main path. The *Ishvara pranidhana*, or surrender to God of the *Yoga Sutras*,[229] follows older traditions back to the *Rigveda*. Devotion is the basis of all other Yogic attitudes and states of mind. Unless one has faith in a higher reality and love for it, one cannot seek to know or to realize it.

The feeling of devotion is probably the best and simplest way to approach Divine unity, as it reflects the deepest urges of the heart. But devotion must be cultivated through Yoga practice in order to constitute a Yoga path. Merely to have devotion is not enough for realization and can remain a conventional religious sentiment, bias, or attachment. Bhakti Yoga requires a sadhana or spiritual practice aimed at union with the Beloved, which implies a daily discipline of ritual, chanting, mantra, and meditation, honoring the Divine within ones own heart.

Vedic hymns consist primarily of the Rishis' dialogue with Divinity in various forms and attitudes, most commonly addressing the divinity as "Thou" (Tvam). The *Vedas* are essentially a "dialogue with God," seeking Divine grace, help, and guidance in all aspects and facets. The *Vedas* represent the word of the awakened soul as addressed to God. The *Vedas* are not primarily spoken to other human beings but to the Divine. It is not human language that the *Vedas* teach us but how to speak to God, with God, and in God, with the entire universe as God. They reflect the soul's movement toward God that culminates in realization of its own Divinity.

Devotion is the main attitude behind Mantra Yoga, as most mantras as utterances of the spiritual heart reflect a devotional attitude to the Divine. Mantra is the Divine language within us, our means of communication with the cosmic powers. Bhakti Yoga develops from and rests upon Mantra Yoga. The chant is the effusion of devotion.

Vedic Yoga is not accomplished by mere human effort but by calling on the Divine powers to help us in our work. This calling of the Gods through the chant is a form of devotion. It begins with Agni as the sacred fire that allows the Divine energies of light to enter into our human world through worship, enabling them to manifest and to raise us up to a higher level of existence. Agni indicates our ability to call upon the Gods and carries the power of our devotion, representing the flame of Divine love. The sacred fire that calls the Gods is the fire of devotion.

In Vedic Bhakti Yoga we call upon the Divine powers mainly as our friends, allies, and family. The relationship of the soul and the Divine is one of affinity, trust, kinship, and unity. The Divine is our origin, goal, center, and heart. A certain joyousness predominates in the Vedic hymns, culminating in the great Soma offering, which is also an offering of the nectar of devotion.

Vedic devotion, however, is not blind emotion but a Yoga of intelligence, insight, and meditation. Real devotion is born of insight, not simply of emotion – of seeing God, not simply of faith or belief that God exists somewhere. Real devotion is cultivated through deep meditation. Devotional meditation in the *Vedas*, as in later Yoga texts, consists of visualizing, and honoring the presence of the Divine within our own hearts and minds.

Namas and Stuti: Surrender and Praise

All devotional approaches follow a twofold movement of surrender and praise. In surrender, called *namas* in Sanskrit, one humbly offers oneself to the deity, with reverence, obeisance, and love. In praise, called *stuti*, one affirms and glorifies the deity, recognizing the primacy of the Divine reality, which is to increase the power of the deity within oneself. In Vedic thought, one surrenders to the deity as one's deepest Self, and one praises the deity as the supreme power and essence at work throughout the universe.

Namas Yoga: The Yoga of Surrender

Many Vedic mantras use the term "namas" both as directed to a particular deity and as a term for devotional worship. Namas is commonly used along with Divine Names like *Oṁ Nama Śivāya* (reverence to Shiva). This use of the term "namas" remains common in Hindu, Buddhist, and Jain traditions, extending throughout the whole of Asia. It reflects an older Vedic usage, though few scholars make this obvious correlation.

The standard Hindu greeting *namaste* means "reverence (namas) to you (te)." This offering of namas or reverence is the essence of Bhakti or devotion, which is part of a culture of honor, reverence, and respect. It is an old Vedic practice.

> *Surrender (namas) is powerful. Surrender I worship. Surrender upholds heaven and earth. Surrender to the Gods as surrender is their lord. Sin that has been committed by surrender is removed.*
>
> *Bharadvaja Barhaspatya, Rigveda VI.51.7-8*

In these Vedic verses, we see the essence of devotion. By surrender to the Divine powers at work in the world we gain the favor of all the Gods. By offering ourselves to the Divinity, we ourselves become Divine.

Namas and Dhi, surrender and insight, are closely related in Vedic thought from the first hymn of the *Rigveda*. This surrender born of insight is very different from simple worship or adoration. It is an inner recognition not simply an outer faith or belief. Real insight, similarly, is born of devotion or an inner connection to the reality.

> *To thou O Fire, day by day, by dusk and dawn, with our insight (dhī) bearing our surrender (namas), we come to you.*
>
> *Madhuchchhandas Vaishvamitra, Rigveda I.1.7*[230]

Devotional Attitudes: The Divine Father and Mother

The Vedic Gods are awesome forces in their cosmic nature and we must be careful and respectful in dealing with them, just as we are with approaching the power of lightning. However, they are also our own kindred and respond to love and friendship. We ourselves are akin to the Gods and can ourselves become Gods or Devas, once we understand our immortal nature. This lauding of the Devas as friends and family is common in the *Rigveda*.

> *Awaken, Indra, as our protector, as a friend, the well-wisher, the compassionate one among those who carry the Soma. Friend, father, most fatherly of fathers, create a wide space for those who worship you, as the granter of vitality.*
>
> *Among those who are friendly, as a friend, awaken as a protector. Lauded, Indra, to those who affirm you grant vitality.*[231]
>
> *Vamadeva Gautama, IV.17.17-18*

The main Vedic term for friend, *Sakhā*, implies more than just a casual friend, but as a dear friend and beloved, suggesting ultimate unity and equality with the Divine.

The essence of Bhakti Yoga, or the Yoga of devotion, consists of developing a personal relationship with the Divine. This involves looking upon God according to various human relationships as the father, mother, brother, sister, child, friend, beloved, master, or teacher. All these devotional attitudes (Bhavas) are found in the *Rigveda*, in which the Divine is frequently addressed in the most intimate and personal manner.

The main attitude of devotion is towards the Divine as our Father and Mother. The Divine as a higher power is like a parent to us. This is part of the Vedic view of our kinship with the Divine powers.

> *Heaven our father, and earth our mother, harmless Fire our brother, may the Vasus be compassionate to us. All the Adityas together with Mother Aditi, may they grant us an abundant peace.*
>
> *Bharadvaja Barhaspatya, Rigveda VI.51.5*

The *Vedas* present a devotional attitude towards the deities of light, starting with Agni or fire, which we would not ordinarily look upon with such emotion.

> *Agni, like a father to his son, be helpful to us, hold closely to us for our well-being.*
>
> *Madhuchhandas Vaishvamitra, Rigveda I.1.9*[232]

Agni is lauded like a father, with a paternal devotion in this very first hymn of the *Rigveda*. This sets the tone for the devotional attitude that the Rishis take with the Gods. Agni is also lauded like a brother, son, friend, and mother.

> *Thou, oh Agni, men with their wishes like a father, thou resplendent in body like a brother with peace, you become the son of him who worships you. You are the friend of good wishes and protect us unceasingly.*
>
> *Gritsamada Shaunaka, Rigveda II.1.9*

One may ask how can one possibly have devotion to a fire as if to a family member. Is this not superstition or barbarism? The answer is that the Vedic seers were not speaking of fire as a mere element or natural force but to the Divine fire or presence of the Divine within us, the Divine being or Divine child of light. Can one not adore it? The ancients could perceive the spirit, Self or Purusha behind the forces of nature. They were not trapped to an anthropomorphic vision as we are today.

Indra, though portrayed as a warrior and a male God, can be approached as either father or mother.

> *You are our father, pervasive lord, Shatakratu, you are our mother. As such, we seek your blessings.*[233]
>
> *Nrimedha Kanva, Rigveda VIII.87.11*

In fact, the mother is regarded more highly than the father for devotional purposes, as she gives without expecting anything else in return.

Indra, you are greater than my father or a brother who is not liberal. You appear equal to my mother, oh liberal lord for the most generous wealth.
Pragatha Kanva, Rigveda VIII.1.6

The *Vedas*, though not having many hymns overtly to female deities, honor the Mother principle as the highest form of devotion.

They (the seers) meditated on the first name of the Mother Cow (prathamam nāma dhenos). They found the seven times three supreme planes of the Mother (triḥ sapta mātuḥ paramāṇi).
Vamadeva Gautama, Rigveda IV.1.16[234]

The Mother, or Mother Cow, is the power of light and mantra. Her three-times-seven or twenty-one planes are perhaps the three aspects of the seven chakras or seven lokas.

The Yoga of the Divine Names

"Name" in Sanskrit is "*Nāma,*" with a long a-vowel. Surrender or adoration in Sanskrit is *namas* but with a short a-vowel. The two terms sound alike and have a common usage, but are different.

The *Vedas* contain many Divine names. These begin with the names of different Vedic deities, which reflect their powers and qualities. Chanting the Divine name evokes the deity to come forth and manifest its energies, just as calling out a person's name draws their attention to us. Through the names of the Vedic deities, we can draw the Divine powers within nature and within our own consciousness to work with us.

The *Vedas* speak of the importance of Divine, or sacred names, in many hymns and there is a special set of Vedic chants called the *Nivids* that do this specifically. The use of Divine Names is part of Vedic chanting and Mantra Yoga. Often the deity is evoked with the mantra "namas" as devotion or surrender, and then its name, *Oṁ Indrāya Namaḥ*! Or "Reverence to Indra," for example.

Chanting of the Divine Name is one of the most important practices of Bhakti Yoga, lauded throughout yogic literature, whether it is the name of Krishna, Shiva, or Devi. It is common to many religious and spiritual traditions throughout the world. This practice is commonly met within the *Rigveda*, where the use of Divine names takes many forms. These names are sometimes said to be secret, "the secret names of the Gods (devānām guhyā nāmāni),"[235] referring to the secret cave of the heart, where we need to dwell in order to discover them.

> *Golden Soma flows along the path of truth, he raises the Word like a ship an oar. Divine, he reveals the secret Divine Names, to declare them on the sacred grass.*[236]
>
> *Praskanva Kanva, Rigveda IX.95.2*

The Seer must sometimes choose the right Divine name as part of the right path to follow.

> *Whose now, which of the immortal Gods, should we meditate upon his blissful name (cāru nāma)?*[237]
>
> *Ajigarta Shunashepa, Rigveda I.24.1*

Yet it is ultimately the One Divine Name that is behind the names of the different Gods. This Divine Name is the Divine nature of all deities, which is their unity in the Supreme.

> *They all worship the Divine Name (devatvam nāma), following the immortal truth according to their ways.*[238]
>
> *Parashara Shaktya, Rigveda I.68.2*

The deities have many names, meditating upon which we can commune with them and discover their essence and their qualities. The name is honored relative to all the Vedic Godheads, starting with Agni.

> *Mortals, of you the immortal, we meditate upon your many Names, of Agni, the Knower of all births, the sage.*[239]
>
> *Vatsa Kanva, Rigveda 11.5.*

> *Agni, Knower of all births, Divine Self-natured lord, many are the names of you the immortal; which Maya powers the lords of Maya, you as the friend of presence who energizes all, have established manifold in you.*[240]
>
> *Gathi Kaushika, Rigveda III.20.3*

> *The station of the Divine, encompassed by surrender, seeking knowledge they gained an inviolable knowledge. They held the holy names (nāmāni yajñiyāni). They took delight in your auspicious presence, O Agni*
>
> *Bharadvaja Barhaspatya, Rigveda VI.1.5*

This assuming of Divine Names for ourselves occurs as part of the process of spiritual rebirth. The name is ultimately the nature of the higher Self, which grants being to all that exists.

Indra, when you were born supreme from the supreme, you carried a revelatory name (śrutyam nāma) in the beyond. Then all the Gods were afraid of Indra when he won the waters that the restrainers had controlled.[241]

Babhur Atreya, Rigveda V.30.5

It is the very power of the Name that allows Indra to win the cosmic waters, the great forces of life and consciousness. Such names are not mere words to repeat but essential cosmic energies to contact and vitalize within us.

Shatakratu, with all our chants we implore your names, Indra, to overcome all opposition.[242]

Gathina Vishvamitra, Rigveda III.37.3

Self-glorious Indra, ever I declare your name.[243]

Maitravaruni Vasishtha, Rigveda VII.22.5

We can choose among these Vedic deity names those that we are drawn to for chanting or meditation purposes. We can repeat collections of Vedic deity names, or hymns in which several of their names occur. We must remember that the name is a vehicle to take us back to the Divinity within our own consciousness, not the name of an external deity. By the power of the name we invoke the same Divine energies within ourselves. Through the Divine Name we awaken the Divine Word and the Divine presence within our own minds and hearts.

The Vedic Yoga of Self-realization: Return to the Spiritual Heart

The Yoga of Knowledge (Jnana Yoga) is simple and clear. We can express its essence in a few words: In your inner core, behind the body, senses, prana, and mind, you are one with the universal Being. Your own Self is the Self of all existence. Discriminate between your inner nature and your outer manifestation, and you will find the entire universe residing within your own heart. There is only unity within and around you, above and below, which is your own deepest awareness. To realize that, simply withdraw from your personal thoughts into the witnessing seer.

Compared to the directness and simplicity of the Yoga of Knowledge – particularly such as Ramana Maharshi taught it – Vedic mantras seem unnecessarily obscure, difficult to understand, and of little relevance. Vedic deities and the complexities of the Vedic ritual seem like a detour, not a direct path to Self-realization. Particularly for those born in the West, it would seem that the Yoga of Knowledge by itself should be enough, and the Vedic teachings would only likely confuse people further.

Yet this view that the *Vedas* are irrelevant for enlightenment today is an overreaction that occurs from a lack of understanding the level from which the Vedic mantras arise. There are many Vedic mantras that can help us in the pursuit of Self-realization and can add a richness, depth and new dimension to our meditation. The Vedic approach is more symbolic and sound- based than rational, but this can compliment the limitations of intellectual approaches.

For those in whom the Vedic mantras are alive and awake, the Vedic language seems ideal for expressing the highest spiritual truths, realizations, and creative powers – which are beyond ordinary speech and mind, and cannot be reduced to any literal set of meanings. Sometimes the language of philosophical texts can seem too mental, obscuring the great mystery beyond speech and mind, in too precise a verbiage. The highest truth transcends reason and all dualities, and appears as paradox and mystery.

Yet appreciating the Vedic mantric knowledge does not require that one loses regard for the direct teachings of the Yoga of Knowledge. On the contrary, it enhances the Yoga of Knowledge, showing how to approach it with the mantric language of the soul. The Gayatri Mantra is good example of a Vedic mantra that can stimulate our aspiration towards the highest truth.

Ramana Maharshi's Vedic and Tantric Mantras through Ganapati Muni

Kavyakantha Ganapati Muni, disciple of Bhagavan Ramana Maharshi, has taught several important Vedic and Tantric mantras for developing Ramana's realization within us in the form of Lord Skanda, the son of Shiva, with whom Ramana is identified.[244] I am including the Sanskrit of the three mantras below, as their sound quality is important for their usage.

Ramana Maharshi's Root Mantra

Oṁ Vacadbhuve namaḥ

This is an important new mantra from Ganapati Muni designed to awaken the consciousness of Ramana within us. It honors Skanda-Ramana as the supreme Guru who arises from the power of speech (vacadbhūḥ). It refers to Agni or Fire as the inner speech, the inner guru, the supreme state of the word (Para Vak), which is Pranava or Oṁ, and the process of Self-inquiry that energizes it. Its six syllables represent the six heads of Skanda. Repeating this mantra awakens Skanda-Ramana as the inner guru through the silence of the heart.

Ramana Maharshi's Tantric Mantra

Śa ra va ṇa bhava

This is the primary mantra used to worship Lord Skanda, also called Subrahmanya, Kartikeyya and Muruga, commonly repeated in India today, not only for the highest Self-realization but for all the goals of life. The mantra is most important for its root sounds, but does have an outer meaning as "Arise in the forest of reeds." This refers to Skanda's birth amidst the reed grasses in the story of his birth. Reed grasses or Shara can be identified with Oṁ that is the arrow (shara, an arrow made from reeds), or with Soma (Shara is a type of reed grass that yields Soma in the *Vedas*). Skanda is born of the union of Shiva (Sa) and Uma, which gives rise to the highest light, and which is the most powerful weapon to destroy the ignorance within us. Repeating this mantra energizes Lord Skanda within us.

Ramana Maharshi's Vedic Mantra

Vṛṣā jajāna vṛṣṇam raṇāya tam u cin nārī naryam sasūva, pra yaḥ senānīr adha nṛbhyo astīnaḥ satvā gaveṣaṇaḥ sa dhṛṣṇuḥ

> *The bull has generated the bull. Him the great mother has given birth to as a noble son. He is the powerful, leader of the army, in the world below for noble soul, he is the leader, the warrior, in the search for the cows, who is daring.*[245]
>
> *Maitravaruni Vasishtha, Rigveda VII.20.5*

This verse from Vasistha in the *Rigveda* is highlighted by Ganapati Muni, showing how later deities like Skanda can be found prefigured in earlier texts. Skanda is well known as *Senani* or the "leader of the army," as he is the head of the army of the Gods. Shiva as the bull (spiritual power) has generated Skanda as his son or manifestation in the outer world. Shakti as *Nari* or the noble woman has given him birth as his mother. Skanda is the head of the army for the awakened souls. The search for the cows (gaveṣana) is the inquiry into the Self, the search for the primal light of the soul or reality, symbolized by the Cow of Light. Repeating this mantra energizes the Vedic practice of mantric Self-inquiry.

Non-Duality in the *Vedas*

"Veda" means "knowledge." This indicates that the Yoga of Knowledge should be the ultimate application of the Vedic mantras. Shankaracharya wrote his important commentaries on the three prime Vedantic texts of the *Upanishads, Bhagavad Gita*, and *Brahma Sutras*, in which he promoted an Advaitic or non-dualistic view of the Vedic teachings. However, he did not take that interpretation back into Vedic texts, much less to the *Rigveda*. This has caused both scholars and yogis to regard earlier Vedic texts as ritualistic in value, with the great Yoga of knowledge emerging only with the *Upanishads*.[246]

Early on in my Vedic research, I felt it was possible to take an Advaitic interpretation back to the mantras of the *Rigveda*. This was the view of Ganapati Muni, Sri Aurobindo, and several others. Most Vedic scholars regard the *Vedas* as the Book of Works, Karma or ritual, and the *Upanishads* as the Book of Knowledge. Ganapati and Aurobindo regard knowledge and ritual as two ways of applying the Vedic mantras, starting with the first mantras of the *Rigveda*.

Non-duality can be found as a prime interpretation in the earliest Vedic mantras. As this mantric Vedic non-dualism is not presented in a strictly logical language like later Vedanta, it retains a certain plasticity and variety of expression. The teachings of later Vedanta are present in the *Rigveda*, reflecting the Vedic language where each of the Vedic deities has its "Atmic" aspect or "application toward Self-knowledge."

Modes of Expressing Self-Realization

The great majority of Vedic hymns are formed in the mode of devotion, which is the 'thou-mode' or *tvam-bhāva* form of expression, addressing the Divine as thou (tvam). Very few Vedic hymns reflect the 'I-mode' or *aham-bhāva*, addressing the Divine as I or the Self. Yet those hymns that do have a special importance in the later Upanishadic literature, like Vamadeva's statement quoted by the *Brihadaranyaka Upanishad* that "I was Manu and the Sun."[247]

However, the *tvam-bhāva* or thou mode can express non-duality by way of glorification, as the verse below that honors Agni as the Divine light of consciousness that pervades all of nature.

> *Thou O Agni, shining bright through the days, from the waters, from the rocks, from the forests, from the plants, thou lord of souls of all souls, are ever born pure.*
>
> *Gritsamada Shaunaka, Rigveda II.1.1*

In addition, the Self can be indicated indirectly through deity forms and their activities, a third person expression (he or that). As the realization of the cosmic reality, it can be expressed through general or abstract terms like truth or the Vast Truth (Ṛtam Bṛhat). Self-realization can be indicated by a discovery of that which is hidden (guha), or by simple indicatives like that (tat). Self-realization can be taught through symbols, as in the case of the Sun in the Vedas, which serves as a metaphor for the Divine Self. The *Vedas* as usual prefer such indirect modes of expression.

The search for Self-realization can be expressed in pluralistic terms, such as becoming one with all. Below is such an expression of becoming unbounded in the Godhead and becoming both heaven and earth.

> *Adityas (Sun Gods), may we be unbounded, full in the Godhead and in the mortal realm, O pervasive powers. Winning, Mitra-Varuna, may we win you, becoming, heaven and earth, may we become you.* [248]
>
> *Maitravaruni Vasishtha, Rigveda VII.52.1*

All the Vedic Godheads, besides their ordinary functions, have a special status in the higher knowledge and can indicate different approaches to the Purusha or Supreme Self. Most notably, Indra, the foremost of the Vedic deities, commonly represents Self-realization. One must cultivate the Indra consciousness of transcendence in order to reach the higher Self. We see this in the case of Vamadeva, where he unfolds the power of Indra by degrees in various hymns to Indra, before bringing out the great statement of "I was Manu and the Sun," in which he identifies with the Sun as the Divine light.

The deeper Vedic Yoga is an unfoldment of Self-realization. Agni represents the inextinguishable and immortal fire of Self-awareness. The Sun or Surya indicates the supreme light of consciousness. Indra represents the Self that is the master of all. Soma represents the overflowing bliss of the highest Self. We need not take this lack of direct statements of Self-realization in the *Rigveda* as a lack of the higher Self knowledge. We must always remember that the *Vedas* prefer indirect to direct forms of expression. The Vedic language weaves abstract ideas and concrete images together and does not always separate them.

Self-realization is not an achievement of the lower self or ego, but requires the surrender and dissolution of the lower Self. That is why the practice of Bhakti Yoga or the Yoga of Devotion usually precedes and provides the foundation for Jnana Yoga or the Yoga of Knowledge. The mind and body need to be first purified in order to access the higher paths. This is the traditional approach of the Advaita Vedanta where the student must first be made ready in order to receive the higher knowledge. Without a suitable vessel in the form of a sattvic body and mind, the knowledge of the supremacy of the Self can be used to glorify the ego or the intellect. The *Vedas* deal with all aspects of Yoga along with the Yoga of Knowledge and weaves them together.

Purusha and Atman

The *Upanishads* emphasize the Purusha or cosmic person, and the Atman or the higher Self, as the Supreme Reality or Brahman. This appears to many people as different from the Vedic Gods like Agni and Soma, which seem mundane in their implications as nature deities. But actually it is not the case. The Vedic deities themselves are forms of the Purusha. The *Upanishads* emphasize the Purusha in the Sun, and also speak of the Purusha in the Moon, the Purusha in the Fire, the Purusha in Lightning, and the Purusha in the Waters.

> *The Purusha that appears in the Sun, he am I, indeed he I am.*
>
> *The Purusha that appears in the Moon, he am I, indeed he I am.*
>
> *The Purusha that appears in the Lightning, he am I, indeed he I am.*[249]
> *Chandogya Upanishad IV.11-13*

These light forms reflect the prime Vedic deities. The Purusha is the light of which all the Vedic deities are manifestations. The Sun is the illuminative aspect of consciousness or the Purusha. Fire is the immanent aspect of consciousness or the Purusha. The Moon is the bliss aspect of consciousness or the Purusha. Lightning or Wind is the energetic aspect of consciousness or the Purusha. Water is the reflective aspect of consciousness or the Purusha. All Vedic deities are aspects of the Purusha and each can indicate the Purusha as a whole!

Of the Vedic deities, Indra most prominently represents the supreme Self and the Seer. The Sun or Surya most prominently represents the light of awareness. Vayu most prominently represents the formless Spirit. Soma is the Self as bliss or ananda. Agni is the Self as the indwelling consciousness.

Self-inquiry and Agni, the Inner Speech

The *Rigveda* contains several hymns that pose questions, which reflect a kind of "mantric inquiry" into higher reality. Some of these questions are posed to the Gods as to their existence or the reasons behind their action. Others are about our relationship with the Gods.

Self-inquiry consists of following back our thoughts to the spiritual heart, a return to the core of our being – particularly to the small space or secret cavity of the spiritual heart that contains the entire universe. We find this practice of Self-inquiry central to the Yoga of Knowledge from the *Upanishads* to Ramana Maharshi in recent times. This process of search back into the heart is portrayed in many Vedic hymns, particularly those to Agni as the flame of awareness in the heart.

Now one may ask the question: "Is not Self-inquiry a movement into silence? How can speech relate to that state to enter where we usually have to first silence speech and the outgoing mind?" In response, the Vedic speech indicated by Agni is not ordinary speech, but the arising of the Divine Word within us. It is the voice of our inner souls, not the chatter of the mind. That voice of our souls is inherently a search for Divinity and Self-realization. Only in the silence of the outer speech can the inner speech, the spiritual fire of Agni, arise. This inner Agni voice is a natural movement of Self-inquiry. It is the awakening of the mantra or the Divine Word within us, which is ultimately the "Divine I am."

Agni can be a deity of Self-inquiry and Jnana Yoga, not just simply an indicator of Mantra Yoga, as is his more common role. Self-inquiry should be a mantric inquiry — the highest application of our power of speech, which includes the ability to question.

In the state of Self-realization, Agni, or the individual soul, becomes the Sun or the Supreme Soul. There are certain aspects of Agni that are most involved in this process of Self-inquiry. *Guha* is the form of Agni that dwells in the secret cave of the heart where the Self is realized. *Kumara* is the child form of Agni that represents our spiritual rebirth as a realized soul. *Vaishvanara* is the cosmic form of Agni identified with the Sun, but also indicates the liberated soul. Agni's Vaishvanara form reflects the process of Self-inquiry.

This inner search (anveshana) is metaphorically styled in the *Vedas* as a search for the cows (gaveshana) hidden in the cave, where they have been stolen by the powers of darkness. This occurs relative to the hymns of Indra, but also at times in the hymns to Agni and other deities. The Vedic cow or *Go* is a symbol of light, knowledge, and the soul. It is not to be literally regarded as a mere cow. The cave is the cavern of the heart.

Of the Agni hymns in the *Rigveda* relative to Self-inquiry, those of Parashara Shakti, grandson of the Rishi Vasishtha, are most notable, as Ganapati Muni has emphasized.[250]

> *Like a thief with a cow hiding it in secrecy, yogically developing our surrender (namo yujanaḥ), and carrying our surrender within, together the wise have searched for him by steps, and all the holy ones have approached you, O Agni.*[251]
>
> *The Gods have moved according to the observances of truth, be their horizon, like heaven the earth. The waters increase him with wonder as a beautiful child, well born in the womb, in the origin of Truth.*[252]
>
> *Parashara Shaktya, Rigveda I.65.1-2.*

As Ramana states, surrender and inquiry go together. Inquiry is a progressive surrender within. Surrender is a progressive search or inquiry within. The wise search out the different forms or steps of Agni, or light, back to the light of consciousness in the heart. The womb or the "garbha" that is the origin of truth is the womb of the heart, which is the golden womb (Hiranyagarbha), the heart of Yoga.

> *Holding in his hand all soul powers, he places the Gods in hiding and sits in secrecy. The sages who control their intelligence find him there, when they praise the mantras formed by the heart.*[253]
>
> *As the unborn he upholds heaven and earth. He has propped up heaven with the mantras of truth. Protect the beloved steps of the cow (perception). Agni enter with secrecy into the secret place, the universal life.*[254]
>
> *Those who perceive him dwelling in the secret cave, he dwells at the stream of truth; those who release the bonds, worshipping the truth, then Agni declares the vastnesses to them.*[255]
>
> *Parashara Shaktya, Rigveda I.67.2-4*

The sage Parashara is perhaps the most esoteric of the Vedic seers. His hymns to Agni are among the greatest Vedic treasures and compare well with any mystical poetic literature. By control of the intelligence, one gains the mantras of truth formed by the heart, such as *Oṁ* or *So'ham* (He am I). These reveal the reality of the Self. This teaching shows the combination of Dhi Yoga, Bhakti or Namas Yoga, and Mantra Yoga, meditation upon the Supreme Word within the heart.

There is a verse of Parashara's grandfather Vasistha that sums up the inner inquiry process. It has been highlighted by Ganapati Muni.

> *I yoke the chariot with two stallions that seeks the light (yuje ratham gaveṣanam). My mantras have reached him who welcomes them. He has spread apart heaven and earth by his greatness. Indra has destroyed unequalled obstructers.*[256]
>
> *Maitravaruni Vasishtha, Rigveda VII.23.3.*

Let us attempt to decode this esoteric Vedic statement. The chariot that is yoked is the Yoga practice or sadhana. It is a "gaveshana," which not only means a seeking of the light but an inquiry into truth, specifically a search for the Self within the heart. Indra's two horses are the dual powers of breath and mind. The Rishi expresses his realization of Indra as the pure Self or pure I within the heart. That Indra has broken open the two dualistic worlds. He has destroyed the unequalled Vritras, dragons or obstructive power of the Ignorance, revealing the One Truth of the Supreme Brahman.

Rigvedic Statements of Self-realization

Dhi relates to wisdom, insight, and discrimination. Dhi Yoga is inherently a Yoga of knowledge. Dhi Yoga serves to align the Buddhi, or intelligence of the soul (Jiva), with Cit, or the consciousness of Paramatman, and the being of Para Brahman. Self-realization is the natural culmination of the Vedic Yoga.

There are many statements of the Self-realization in the *Rigveda*, though most are veiled in a symbolic language. The great Vedic Rishis in their hymns reveal their deeper perception, experience and consciousness in different ways. Below we provide some examples.

Vamadeva

Vamadeva is probably the most famous of the Vedic Rishis quoted in the *Upanishads*. Two of the four main *Mahavakyas* or 'Great Statements' of Advaita Vedanta as found in the *Upanishads* also quote from Vamadeva's Vedic verses.

> *I was Manu and the Sun. I am the Rishi Kakshivan, the sage. I humbled Kutsa, son of Arjuna. I am the Seer Ushanas, behold me!* [257]
>
> *Vamadeva Gautama, Rigveda IV.26.1*

Manu here refers not just the historical original human being, but also to the cosmic person who dwells in the Sun. This statement of Vamadeva is related to the Mahavakya *Aham Brahmāsmi* or 'I am Brahman' in the *Brihadaranyaka Upanishad.* Vamadeva in this hymn also identifies himself with other great Vedic Rishis like Kakshivan and Kutsa. Like Krishna, he identifies himself with the Seer Ushanas. Here Vamadeva is speaking as Indra, and this is among his hymns to Indra. It is the "I am" as Indra, or the Supreme I am, that is making these statements, not Vamadeva at a mere personal level. Indra can also be identified with the Sun as the supreme light.

> *While still within the womb I investigated and learned the births of all the Gods. A hundred metal cities held me down, then I flew away with the speed of a falcon.*[258]
>
> *Vamadeva Gautama, Rigveda IV.27.1*

The womb (garbha) here is symbolic of the womb or sacred space within the heart, not the human womb. In that small space within the heart occurs the birth of all the outer Gods of the pranas and senses, and of the inner Gods or the experiences of Self-realization. It is where our inner inquiry or investigation should proceed. Here Vamadeva is referring to the birth of Indra, and the hymn occurs among his hymns to Indra, the birth of the consciousness of the Self.

This verse of Vamadeva is quoted in the *Aitareya Upanishad* as indicating the Selfrealization of one who learned the answer to the great question, "What is the Self?" (*ko'yam ātma*?) It relates to the Mahavakya or great Vedantic saying *Prajñānam Brahma* or "Intelligence is Brahman."[259] Through the soul's power of intelligence the Divine becomes conscious within us.

Vishvamitra

> *I am Agni, from birth the knower of all things born (agnir asmi janmanā jātavedāḥ). Ghee is my eye. The immortal nectar is in my mouth. The three natured ray, the measurer of the region, I am the undecaying heat, the offering, the Name.*
>
> *With three purifications he purified the ray, by the heart knowledge the thought according to the light. He fashioned the supreme treasure by his Self-nature. Then he saw all around heaven and earth.*
>
> *Gathina Vishvamitra, Rigveda III.26.7-8*

Here the seer Vishvamitra expresses his unity with Agni, the Divine flame of awareness in the heart. This flame of the heart, which is our soul, provides us with knowledge of our past lives and also the keys to the births of all creatures. Through Agni he is able to see all around heaven and earth, and become immortal. It is this realization of Agni that is the basis of Vishvamitra's vision of the Gayatri Mantra.

Dirghatamas

The hymn of Dirghatamas, *Rigveda I.164*, is one of the most esoteric both for astronomical knowledge and for deeper yogic wisdom. Several of its verses are commonly quoted in later Vedic and Upanishadic literature. Dirghatamas raises the fundamental questions that occur in the *Upanishads*.

> *Who has seen that which was born first, which without bones bears that which has bones. The soul of the world, the blood, the Atman, which knower should I go to in order to answer these questions? Ignorant I ask not knowing by my mind, what are the secret stations of the Divine powers?*[260]
>
> *Dirghatamas Auchatya, Rigveda I.164.4-5*

Later in this same hymn he expresses the answer to his questions, from his own inner perception. He has realized the inner spirit or guardian, the inner controller behind all the energies in the universe, animate, and inanimate, the Self within.

> *I have seen the guardian who does not falter, moving by the near and far paths. He wearing the converging and diverging forces ever revolves within these worlds.* [261]
>
> *Dirghatamas Auchatya, Rigveda I.164.31*

Vatsa Kanva

Vatsa describes his Self-realization in a simple and direct manner as being reborn like the Sun. Solar rebirth is another symbol for Self-realization, with the arising of the supreme light of awareness within us, like the Sun.

> *From my father I received the wisdom of truth (medhām ṛtasya), I was born even as the Sun.*[262]
>
> *Vatsa Kanva, Rigveda VIII.6.7*

Shrutivid Atreya

This is another declaration of the perception of the Supreme light of consciousness through the Sun, as the unification of all diversity.

> *By the truth, they hold that hidden eternal truth of yours, O Mitra and Varuna, where they release the horses of the Sun. Where the thousand stand together, I have perceived That One (Tad Ekam), the best of the beautiful forms of the Gods.*[263]
>
> *Shrutivid Atreya, Rigveda VI.62.1*

Releasing the horses of the Sun means going beyond the pranas, mind, and senses that are the horses or powers of the soul. That One is the Supreme Unity of all, not simply one among many. Here the reference is to the Sun as the light of the Self. Mitra and Varuna are the two main powers of the solar truth as compassion and judgment that lead us to the solar Self.

Dharuna Angirasas

> *To the ordainer, the seer-poet, who is to be known, bear your word to the original glorious power, Agni, who sits in ghee, who is almighty, most auspicious, the holder of the riches, the pillar of pervasive power.*
>
> *By the truth they held the foundation truth, in the power of Sacrifice, in the supreme ether. Holding the Dharma of heaven, worshipful sages, by the births attained the Unborn.*[264]
>
> *Dharuna Angirasa, Rigveda V.15.1-2*

This statement of Self-realization is indirect and in the plural sense indicating what the Rishis as great Yogis understood. Agni as the inner Self is the pillar of all existence. The sages merge into that foundation truth or higher Dharma, which is rooted in the supreme ether or highest state of consciousness. This Yajna or sacrifice in the supreme ether is referring to the yogic practice of meditation, offering the mind into the supreme consciousness. Through developing the births of the Gods or the higher truth powers within themselves, the sages attain the unborn reality of Brahman, Being-Consciousness-Bliss.

Virupa Angirasa

Mortals have a relationship of kinship, unity, and identity with the Gods. They can become immortal like the Gods. There are several terms for this kinship, one of which is 'yuj', the same root from which the term Yoga arises, and suggests a deeper unity, not simply a general association.

Virupa speaks of Agni and says, "If you were I and I were you my wishes would be fulfilled." This reflects his actual experience, mirrored in his very profound and esoteric hymns. Agni represents the inner Self-awareness that is ever awake within us at the core of our hearts. He also shines at the summit of the worlds in the highest heaven that is the highest realm of consciousness in our awareness. To realize that inner supreme light, we must remain ever awake, united to our inner awareness at the core of our being.

If, Agni, I were you and if you were me, then your blessings here would be true. As a sage at the session, as an ever awake enlightened one, O Agni, you shine in heaven.[265]

Virupa Angirasa, Rigveda VIII.44.23, 29

Part IV
Vedic Yoga and the Vedic Deities

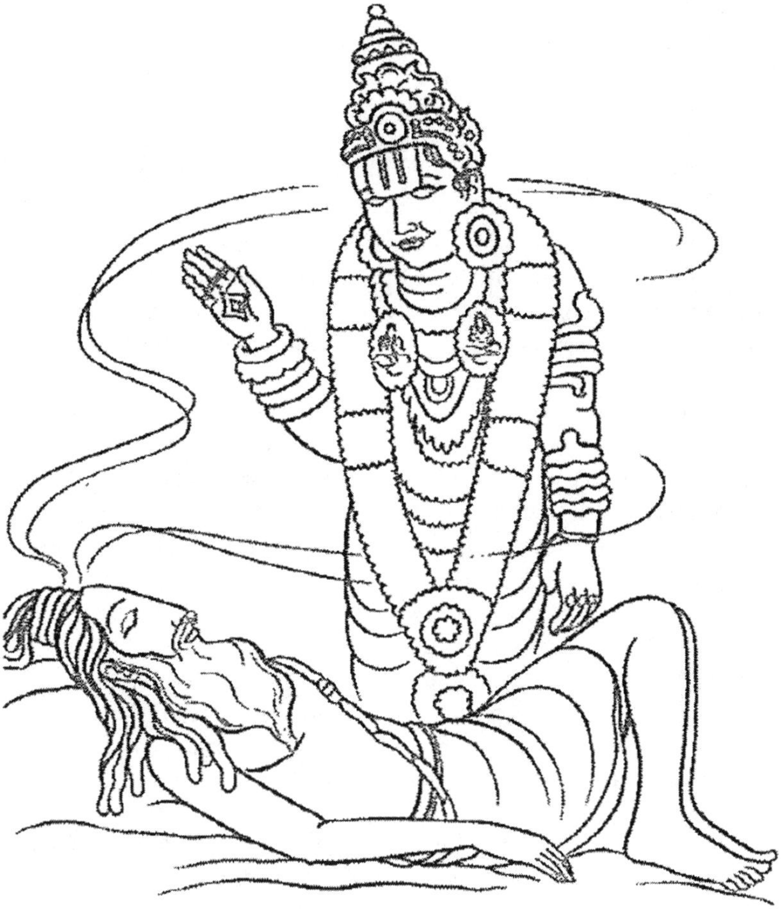

The Play of Agni and Soma: The Great Vedic Cosmic Duality

We live in a vast universe filled with powerful polarities, dichotomies, and dualities that reinforce the mysterious and dynamic nature of reality. Various systems of thought have formulated these cosmic dualities in different ways. The *Vedas* have their own special and insightful approach.

The Vedic view of the universe is of two fundamental principles of *Agni* and *Soma* that comprehend the main dualities of life which, though different in manifestation, are ultimately one. The entire Vedic Yoga is based upon the underlying polarity and mutual transformability of Agni and Soma. These two terms, like Yin and Yang, are untranslatable. The simplest way is to look upon Agni and Soma is as Fire and Water but this is just the first step of a greater set of correspondences.

Agni exists on various levels as light, not only manifest but also latent or working behind the scenes. It is the fire that can be enkindled at various altars or grounds of experience. These are called *chits* in Sanskrit, which means "layers." Chit also means "consciousness" that is the ultimate level or layer behind all that exists. Agni refers to various forces of light and energy that manifest on different levels of matter, life, and mind but are all ultimately interrelated.

Soma similarly exists on all levels of existence as the water, fluid, nourishment or delight hidden in all things. Soma develops in drops and flows in a stream or current, or pools in various receptacles. Each form of Agni requires its corresponding form of Soma as the fuel for it to burn. Agni is like the force, whereas Soma is the field out of which it manifests. Soma holds the substance of matter, life, and mind.

Whereas Agni or fire has to be churned out by friction, Soma as nectar or juice has to be pressed out by pressing stones (symbolic of various actions of pressure or concentration). Neither force is entirely evident, particularly in this physical world, though they have many derivative forms. We ourselves are a kind of fire, or power of light and intelligence, which exists in the field of body and mind as its Soma.

The Rishis work to awaken Agni and Soma within us as the great powers of Yoga, with an ascending current of fire or aspiration and a descending current of nectar or grace. Once manifested, the Rishis work to develop their powers further as the keys to the inner worlds, taking us to higher levels of Agni and Soma or perception and reception. The Vedic Yajna or ritual centers on developing Agni and Soma as cosmic powers. This requires the application of various forces of an electrical, magnetic, luminous or thermogenic nature as powers of higher awareness.

At the highest level of our nature, Agni and Soma are respectively the consciousnessforce (cit-śakti) and bliss (ānanda) aspects of the Supreme Self. At the lower level of the physical body, they are represented by the digestive fire or the eater of food (Agni), and the food that is eaten (Soma). Yet consciousness itself can also be called the eater or absorber, with the entire universe as its food or what it absorbs, so that these two levels are not entirely separate. This is made clear in *Taittiriya Upanishad* that outlines the five koshas or sheaths from food, breath, mind, intelligence, and bliss. It then concludes by calling all five sheaths as food and equates them with Ananda or bliss.

> *I am food. I eat the eater of food. I have consumed the entire universe; my light is like the Sun world.*[266]
> *Taittiriya Upanishad III.10.*

In the outer cosmic order, Agni and Soma are heaven and earth, the realms of light and nourishment. On the physical globe itself, Agni and Soma exist as the land and the waters. In the vegetable kingdom, Agni is the chlorophyll and Soma is the sap (rasa) in plants. In the atmosphere, Agni is wind and lightning, while Soma is the clouds and rain. In heaven or the sky itself, Agni and Soma are the Sun and the Moon.

Note the following correspondences below but do not take them rigidly. There is an Agni in each form of Soma and a Soma in each form of Agni. This great duality is ultimately a manifestation of the great mystery, with each merging into the other, and cannot be made rigid:

Agni/Soma Correspondences

Agni	Soma	Agni	Soma
Fire	Water	Spirit	Matter
Seer	Seen	Soul	Body
Time	Space	Male	Female
Present	Past	Heaven	Earth
Sun	Moon	Day	Night
New Moon	Full Moon	Summer	Winter
Mountain	Lake	Hot	Cold
Dry	Wet	Harsh	Soft
Pungent	Sweet	Ascending	Descending
Right	Left	Intellect	Emotions

Principles of Agni-Soma Interaction

The Vedic Yoga involves energizing and balancing Agni and Soma on all levels. This requires understanding the principles through which Agni and Soma work in their various manifestations.

Principle 1: Agni and Soma both exist on all seven levels of existence and each aspect of our nature.

Every level has its type of digestive fire and its type of food, its type of light and heat, and its type of water or reflective substance.

Level	**Agni**	**Soma**
1. Physical	Digestive fire	Food
2. Vital	Breath fire	Air
3. Mental	Emotional fire	Sensory impressions
4. Intelligence	Fire of intelligence	Ideas
5. Bliss	Fire of love	Experience
6. Consciousness	Fire of consciousness	All that can be perceived
7. Being	Fire of truth	All existence

Principle 2: Relative to the same seven layers, they can be divided into pairs as Agni and Soma.

Agni	**Soma**
Vital (Prana)	Physical (Anna)
Intelligence (Buddhi, Vijnana)	Mind (Sensory mind, Manas)
Consciousness (Chit)	Bliss (Ananda)

Being (Sat), the seventh principle is common to all the others. In the Vedic context, prana and Anna can refer to other dualities like intelligence as Agni and mind as Soma, or consciousness as Agni and bliss as Soma.

Principle 3: Agni as the eater is the subtler principle, of which Soma as the eaten is the corresponding grosser principle.

For each of these seven cosmic principles that which is more outward becomes its body, food, or Soma, and that which is more inward becomes its self, spirit, eater, or Agni. In this regard, the following dualities arise:

Agni - Eater	**Soma – Food/ Eaten**
Prana - breath	Anna - food

Mind	Prana
Intelligence	Mind
Bliss	Intelligence
Consciousness	Bliss
Being	Consciousness

- Prana or our life-energy is the eater of the food that we take in through the mouth.
- The sensory mind is the eater of the food that we take in through the breath or prana.
- The discriminating intelligence is the eater of the food that we take in through the mind and senses.
- Our bliss or love is the eater of the food that we take in through our discriminating intelligence.
- Our higher consciousness is the eater of the food that we take in through the love or bliss we gain in life.
- Our inner being is the eater of the food that we take in through our consciousness.

Principle 4: Interpenetration of Agni and Soma

Agni and Soma interpenetrate, work through and support one another in various ways. Agni as the heat that causes plants to grow allows the Soma or juice in the plants to develop and the fruits of the plant to mature. The Sun by its light causes the Moon to wax and wane. Yet the Sun also draws up the waters and helps bring down the rain.

Agni as the fire that cooks our food allows the Soma, or the taste of the food, to come out. Agni in the body causes appetite, while Soma (saliva) gives relish to the food. Pranagni causes our vital fluids (plasma and blood), which are Soma, to circulate and carry food to the different tissues. The mental Agni gives acuity to the senses through which they can better extract the colors and flavors, the essences of Somas of sensory experience. The fire of intelligence allows our ideas to mature so that they can be nourishing to our souls. The fire of bliss allows our experiences to mature so that everything yields us the eternal delight. The fire of consciousness allows us to extract the essence of delight from all that we perceive. The fire of truth allows us to extract the essence of the eternal, immutable being from all that appears to us.

Principle 5: Interchangeability of Agni and Soma

Agni and Soma as two interrelated polarities are like the two sides of the same coin, and each can turn into the other. Agni can become Soma, and Soma can become Agni. What is Agni on one level can become Soma on another level and visa versa.

Agni is at times lauded as Soma, and Soma is at times lauded as Agni. They are two aspects of the same reality. Soma is only real when it is burning with Agni. Agni is only real when it is fed by Soma. Agni is required to prepare the Soma. Soma is required to nourish and control the Agni. Agni or heat as it rises creates clouds, from which the rain comes.

The Kundalini Agni as it rises up the spine cools down. The Soma nectar as it descends down the spine becomes hotter. At a certain state of awareness, the Yogi can experience a light like a million Suns, in brightness and like a million Moons, in coolness and delight at the same time. Another example of Agni and Soma as becoming interchangeable is that dry ice can burn us, and excess heat around can eventually burn us out and render us cold.

Principle 6: Mutuality of Agni and Soma

Agni depends upon Soma for its manifestation and Soma depends upon Agni for its manifestation. Only when fully united with Soma can Agni burn the brightest. Only when united with Agni can Soma be its purest.

Soma is the fuel for Agni, indicating that only when Agni embraces the fullest and highest Soma can its own greatest manifestation occur. Chidananda or consciousness-bliss is the highest Agni and Soma, which unites as pure being. In Yoga we must learn the integral development of Agni and Soma. Perhaps the most important approach is to draw the Agni or Kundalini fire up from the lower chakras for purification, while drawing the Soma or Amrit down from the higher chakras for invigoration.

The play of Agni and Soma is the play of transformation that is the essence of life and the motivation for all spiritual growth. We need to let these powers awaken within us and follow their inspiration. Agni and Soma will take us through and beyond all duality.

THE SECRET OF THE COSMIC WATERS

Water connotes life, happiness, and delight, the very flow of existence. Water is not just an outer element but reflects internal realities of Soma, bliss, and samadhi. Along with Agni or fire, water plays an important role in Vedic thought. It occurs primarily relative to Soma, which is a watery deity. Yet there are many other water, river, ocean, and rain-based deities including Indra, Varuna, and Parjanya.

In addition, the Waters, *Apas*, as Goddesses, form an important part of Vedic symbolism, with several hymns to them, many verses, and numerous references. Woman is the essence of water, as the male is the essence of fire. She carries the special powers and sensitivities of water, its capacity to flow and to carry electrical force (lightning or Shakti).

The Goddesses (Devis) relate to the qualities of water. The rivers are great Goddesses, particularly those like Ganga that flow from high mountains like the Himalayas. They convey the rasa or essence of the mountains with them. Vedic Sarasvati is the great river of knowledge that provides wisdom and artistry in her flow. She is the prime river of Vedic culture and of the entire universe.

> *Filling the earth and the wide region of the atmosphere, may Sarasvati protect us from bondage. Who has three stations and seven levels, increasing the peoples of the five births, in every encounter, she should be invoked.*
> *Bharadvaja Barhaspatya, Rigveda VI.61.11-12*

Such waters have an inner reality as pervading the universe and manifesting on different levels. The Vedic rivers are often said to be seven, perhaps symbolizing the currents of the seven worlds or seven chakras.

Spiritual life or sadhana in the *Vedas* is symbolized as a journey on the waters, crossing a great river, or a crossing the ocean. The *Vedas* reflect a maritime vision of the cosmos, viewing the universe as a series of oceans or waters in various layers. Vedic thought recognizes the existence not only of earthly waters, but also of atmospheric and heavenly waters. Even the realm of pure consciousness in Vedanta is sometimes called the "ocean of consciousness," which reflects the Vedic view.

Water in this broader sense refers to the vibratory or wave like nature of reality, which includes space and air, not just to the material element of water. All the worlds are waters or vibratory mediums of expression. The Sanskrit term for waters, "Apas," is a plural term that literally means "the waves," and reflects the vibratory nature of the cosmic existence. The *Upanishads* connect Apas with Satya or the Waters with the supreme truth, reflecting this understanding.[267]

Out of the waves arises the lotus of inner light through which the Divine being takes birth in the manifest worlds. Both Prakriti, or nature, and Purusha, or the cosmic person, have a certain resonance or watery like quality, reflected in the power of bliss. Water is the main element behind life, and can symbolize nature as a whole. Life arises from the sea, which in the *Vedas* is the ocean of the heart that is the ocean of prana and ultimately the ocean of bliss that is immortal life.

> *The entire universe dwells within your nature, in the ocean, in the heart, in the power of life. That which is borne in the face of the confluence of the waters, may we attain your wave of bliss.*[268]
>
> *Vamadeva Gautama, Rigveda IV.58.11*

Without water, embodied life is not possible. This truth is evident in our own bodies, which consist of a special form of living water or plasma protected within the boundaries of our skin, energized by prana and Agni, the main vital energies of the life-force and the vital fire. Yet as the basis for life, water can represent all the five elements, which are all waves or mediums of expression for the indwelling soul.

The Vedic universe as a series of oceans resembles the waters of the firmament in Biblical, Babylonian, and other ancient systems. There is a universal continuum from the earthly to the heavenly waters to the waters beyond the worlds, and from the outer material waters to the inner floods of pure awareness. The form worlds are but islands in these all-encompassing waters. Mother nature is a personification of the cosmic waters. Our embodied life is but a special protected drop of the cosmic waters.

The Oceanic Universe

The inner eye reveals the universe as a series of oceans placed one on top of the other, with descending streams linking them together. The waters of the higher planes are clear and vibrant, yet as the waters enter into the lower worlds they become murky and stagnant, with the contact to their higher source gradually lost. This is our position in the human world and its dense spiritual ignorance like a marshy sea.

The waters cascade down from the higher planes like waterfalls. These waterfalls are Shakti or Parvati (mountain streams), the power that descends from above. They carry an electrical force that sets everything in motion, which is the *Vidyut* or *Tadit*, the prime electrical energy of Tantric thought.

Lord Shiva, as a mountain God, allows the heavenly river or heavenly Ganga to descend down upon his head. Without Shiva's head to hold them and break their fall, these waters would break the earth. Shiva here is symbolic of the crown chakra and the stillness power of meditation that can absorb the cosmic waters.

In the *Vedas*, the waters are often a synonym for space or ether. An important Vedic chant is the *Apam Pushpam* or "Flower of the waters" chant.[269] It describes the Sun (Aditya), Moon (Chandrama), Fire (Agni), and other primary natural forces as flowers in the waters, including time itself symbolized by the year (samvatsara). This means that the light powers of nature are nothing but vibrational designs, flowers if you will, formed in the waters of space. We are all vortexes of energy in the waters of space, which are the waters of consciousness. We are individualized patterns of the field of the waters and how it expresses itself in various ways.

This watery vibratory quality of space allows it to condense or crystallize into various forms or energetic structures, some living like our own body, some inanimate like the Sun. Yet these particularized forms are nothing but focal points of vibrations in the universal field. They are not separate entities and must return to the water or waves from which they arose.

Our minds work through the same vibratory processes. The waters of pure consciousness get condensed through waves of our thoughts, but must eventually return back to the ocean of awareness. The mind or manas principle is compared to the Moon, which has a reflected light and a watery nature.

Water in Vedic thought originates in space, not on earth. Ether contains the seeds of all the other elements within it. Water is inherent in the vibratory and reflective quality of space and its heavenly currents. The Sun draws in the heavenly waters and projects them downward along with its rays. They are transmitted to the Moon, which serves to reflect the subtle essence of water back to the earth, where the waters form clouds in the atmosphere, gather energy, and then condense and fall to the ground as rain to nourish and sustain life. The Jiva or reincarnating soul follows these watery currents to take birth in a new body.

Of course we are not talking modern science here but yogic science, which is mantric and poetic. Yet one can still experience this cycle of the waters inside oneself. One can connect with the descending flow of Divine grace, which is the spiritual side of the heavenly waters. When the inner waters are flowing, then we can understand the meaning of all life and go beyond all taint and limitation.

Water and Light

Water has a capacity to reflect light, which we see in the blue ocean or lake. Even a drop of water like a crystal can reflect a vast spectrum of light. The rainbow is made up of light reflected through water. Gems have a kind of metallic watery quality in their transparency.

Water and light (Apas and Jyoti) are the two main factors of cosmic existence and the two primary essences or "rasas" in the universe. The Gayatri Mantra as taught in the *Upanishads* ends with the closing mantras, "Water and Light as the immortal essence."[270] Actually water is light in its reflected form. Light reflecting upon itself creates water. Water becomes a mirror for the light, but a flowing mirror. Light touches itself through water, while water knows itself as light. Clear water is like the vibratory field of light. Light and Water in the *Vedas* represent an important aspect of the Agni-Soma or fire-water equation.

This essence of water becomes the *chitta* or reflective consciousness in the heart, in which the Self can be realized like a light shining in a pure mirror. Water allows us to see. At a physical level, it is the clear fluid in the eyes that enables visual perception to occur, which can reflect light back to us. What is purified by water allows the light to shine through it. Light is itself perhaps the purest form of water or clear medium of expression.

The unity of light and water is a profound Vedic insight. Water first of all refers to the nutritive power inherent in light. The watery or oily quality inherent in light allows light, as in the case of sunlight, to create and nourish life. After all, it is sunlight that draws up the waters from the earth by evaporation and releases them back in the form of rain. It is light that allows things to grow and ripen. Water and light are ultimately one in life that depends upon both. Light also has a quality of delight or bliss, which is a kind of watery energy. This bliss unity of water and light was called *madhu* or "honey" at a deeper level.

The Waters as the Inner Worlds

In Vedic thought, the inner or spiritual worlds are symbolized by the waters or the ocean. The inner worlds are like waters. They require our immersion within ourselves and letting go of our outer sense-based consciousness. Meditation means moving into the waters of consciousness beneath the surface mind, and is often symbolized as a diving deep within.[271] The waters are a symbol for the inner world of consciousness.

When we merge into meditation, it is like going under water, letting go of our ordinary senses, letting go of the prana itself, and going beyond the breath. Diving deep into the sea indicates withdrawal from the senses and entering into the deeper consciousness, the yogic state of "pratyahara." We must drown ourselves in the inner sea in order to find the One. We must go from the outer waters to the inner waters. We must return to the core ocean of the heart.

The calmness of meditation is like the water in a still or placid mountain lake. It is not an artificial or rigid stillness, but a gentle self-contained movement, like a lake with gentle waves. To be like water is a great teaching. It allows one to adapt to everything and to find energy everywhere. Water teaches us how to surrender, which is the essence of Bhakti Yoga, and how through surrender to move, change, and transform without personal effort or struggle.

The "fire in the waters" is a symbol of the light of the soul hidden in the deeper waters of the subconscious mind. The spiritual fire that we need to enkindle is the fire of the inner waters, which is the fire of bliss, not simply fire as a material force. The Vedic fire in its highest state as *Vaishvanara* or the cosmic person dwells in the waters, as the light that pervades the cosmic ocean. This was later honored as Vishnu and Narayana in Hindu thought.

Agni, the cosmic fire, is connected with the cosmic waters and the God mind in the *Rigveda*. It is the God mind and the God vision that dwells in the waters of the inner worlds, which are the waters of cosmic space. In that is the Supreme Name of the Divine consciousness.

> *From heaven, Agni was born first, then second from us as the Knower of all Births, third in the waters by the God mind, perpetually enkindled he is lauded by those of deep minds.*[272]
>
> *Agni, we know your threefold three aspects, we know the domain in which you are carried in many forms. We know the Supreme Name that is hidden. We know the fountain from which you have arisen.*[273]
>
> *In the ocean, in the waters, by the God mind, the God eye enkindles you at the udder of heaven. Standing in the third region, in the lap of the waters, the great buffalo has grown.*[274]
>
> *Vatsapri Bhalandana, Rigveda X.45.1-3.*

Yogic practice consists of accessing the waters of consciousness, which means opening the inner currents and channels, the nadis of the subtle body, to the flood of grace. Enabling our inner waters to flow is indicative of the awakening of the subtle body, which has more a watery and electrical nature than the dense earthly physical body. The electricity that flows through our inner waters is the higher prana of immortal life.

Another metaphor for Yoga practice is like tracing a stream back to its source in the higher mountains or higher oceans. Here the stream is the current of our own thought and prana. The source of the waters is the Divine bliss and love within us. This ascending the waters means tracing the current of our thoughts back to their origin in the spiritual heart.

One of the main Vedic metaphors found in Vedic hymns is of the great God Indra (the power of lightning-perception), who slays the dragon that lays at the foot of the mountain holding the waters and preventing them from flowing. The dragon, or Vritra, represents the limiting, veiling, and obstructive power of the ignorance.[275] His defeat releases the seven rivers to flow into the sea. This is symbolic of opening the seven chakras and their nadis or channels, an experience well known to the Vedic Rishis.

The dragon (Ahi-vritra) represents the concealment power of the ego, which dwells at the base of the spine keeping the Kundalini asleep or dormant. Indra is the lightning energy of meditative insight that dissolves the ego, the seer power of the witnessing Self. This allows the higher waters to stream through all the channels of the mind and body, breaking down all obstacles and clearing away all karmic impurities.

Water and Prana

Water as it flows or moves also carries energy or prana. Prana is the electrical force created by the currents of the waters. Our own life prana is sustained by the circulation of our blood and bodily fluids. Prana is the force that allows these fluids to move and sets them in motion. To sustain a proper prana, we need the right fluid base in the body in order to hold it. Yet to have proper water or dynamic liquidity, we need the moving power of prana in order to sustain its flow.

The higher great prana exists and moves in the waters of cosmic space, only a small portion of which ever becomes embodied in living creatures. To create space within ourselves is to create prana as well. Prana requires the inner waters to grow and to flow. Prana is the lightning of the waters.

In Vedic thought, the atmosphere (antaṛkṣa, or intermediate realm of space between heaven and earth) is the main realm of the waters, the source of the rains that create and sustain the earthly waters. In this regard, there are three worlds of the earth, waters and heaven (light or fire). The atmosphere is also the sphere of the Atman, which is the inner prana. In other formulations there are the waters beyond heaven, up to the waters of the Absolute or Supreme Brahman.

Water allows life or prana to be embodied. The soul enters into the body and into the world through the element of water. There is an interesting Upanishadic statement:

> *In the shoreless waters, in the center of the world, on the ridge of heaven, greater than the great, through the inner radiance having entered into all forms of light, the Lord of Creation stirs within the seed.*

> *Which the seers weave within the ocean, which is the creation in the Supreme Word. From this is born the Mother of the world, who through water produces creatures on the earth.*[276]
> *Mahanarayana Upanishad 1*

Ritual Bathing and Baptism

Ritual bathing is an important part of Vedic practices and of religious rituals worldwide. It is a facet of Dharmic living, including bathing in sacred rivers. *Snana*, which refers to all types of bathing from water to mantra, is one of the main principles of Yoga practice found in the *Yogi Yajnavalkya*, the main traditional yogic text after the *Yoga Sutras*.[277]

Vedic water rituals are complementary to Vedic fire offerings, and water is offered to the sacred fire at certain points of the ritual, or also to the Sun. Water cleanses away all impurities if we allow it to flow freely through us. This means that we must become like water in order to be pure. Meditation itself is a kind of inner bathing process in which we bathe the mind in the waters of contemplation.

The idea of a spiritual rebirth or baptism reflects our immersion in the stream of the heavenly waters, which constitutes our second or spiritual birth. This inner current of waters is also the waters of the sound current or Oṁ. Outer rituals are external means to stimulate that internal flow. We all need immersion in these inner currents for our spiritual rebirth. The waters are the womb of Shakti through which the Divine Mother can bring about our inner transformation, our inner arising as the Divine child.

Water and the Chakras

The water element relates to the water chakra, the Svadhishthana, just above the root chakra or Muladhara, like a pool of water on the earth. At this site we can experience the creative and formative power of water, which provides nourishment and stability to the physical body, and forms the basis for procreation. Yet water exists in different forms in the other chakras. The waters of the heart are the waters of consciousness and of prana. The waters of the head and crown chakra are the ambrosial waters, the nectar or ananda. Each chakra has its own water as it has its own fire or light.

One must learn to drink these inner waters from the chalices of the chakras, which the *Vedas* compare to various cups for drinking Soma. This procedure is often done at the third eye where the stream of Shakti flows down from the higher planes of the thousand petal lotus of the head. At that point one can breathe in the inner waters to satiate the thirst of the soul for immortal life. Yet from the third eye, the waters are taken deep into the heart.

The higher waters are Soma, the bliss, Ananda or nectar of immortality, or the streams of honey-wine. These pervade all space, light, and consciousness. Such waters bring about the rejuvenation of body and mind. They carry the essence, the rasa, the delight hidden in everything.

Water brings joy. Many of our recreational activities are performed through water, on the water or by the water. Certain special waters or beverages bring about intoxication. The Yogi imbibes the inner waters that intoxicate the Spirit and bring the soul to ecstasy. He learns to play on the cosmic waters, in which he can never die. The lotuses of the chakras bloom in these Soma streams that flow through the central channel of the Sushumna.

Water and Sound

Sound is the vibration of the heavenly waters of space. This vibration of space is the origin of sound at a cosmic level. All mantras are the songs of the inner waters resounding in the space of pure consciousness. As the great Rishi Vasistha states in the *Rigveda*:

> *They know the origins of heaven and earth, the waters listen as they flow.*[278]
> *Maitravaruni Vasishtha, Rigveda VII.34.2*

Learn to hear the secret of the waters, which is the Nada, the unstruck sound from the core of your being. The heavenly waters chant Oṁ in their waves, while the electrical current within them forms the sound Iṁ. From these two all other letters or mantras arise. These sounds of the waters, or vibrations of space, are the basis of all sounds, verbal or non-verbal. Everything is hidden in the sound of the waters, which are both without and within. We are all the children of the waters and need to return to their universal flow.

Agni Yoga: Vedic Fire Yoga

Human culture in its prehistorical origins developed from the discovery of fire, which brought the power of light directly into the human world. Ancient humanity developed many forms of fire as the cooking fire, the counsel fire, the hunting fire, and the sacred fire. Yet fire as a material element was only the first of the many fires that our species discovered. The inner fires are more important and the ancient seers had a greater knowledge of them than does our culture today. The Rishis were able to use the sacred fire as a doorway into the worlds of the Gods or the celestial lights – and to the light of universal consciousness itself.

Agni as the sacred fire is the key to the Vedic Yoga, just as he is the basis of the Vedic ritual or Yajna. Yoga arose as the inner aspect of the fire ritual, the offerings of speech, mind, and prana into our inner fire of Self-awareness. The Vedic Yoga is a cultivation of Agni in its various spiritual forms, and its complementary forces of Soma, Vayu, and Surya, or Moon, Wind, and Sun. Agni is a prime factor in all later Yoga teachings, including Hatha, Siddha and Tantric Yogas that emphasize the Kundalini Fire or root form of Agni. Yoga culminates in the fire of meditation that burns up all of our karmas, taking us beyond the process of ignorance and rebirth. Traditional Shaivite Yogis of the Himalayas today are known by the sacred fires that they keep perpetually burning.

The author's book *Yoga and the Sacred Fire* discusses all aspects of Agni, starting with the *Rigveda* and can be consulted for more detail.[279] In this chapter, we will emphasize the Vedic Agni relative to its relationship with the other great powers of Yoga. Ganapati Muni related Agni to four primary forms; 1) the earthly or material Fire (Pārthiva), 2) Speech as a faculty that is also his electrical form (Vāk, Vaidyuta), 3) the sacrificial Fire or Yajna (both inner and outer, yogic and material), 4) and the Soul (Jīva, both bound and liberated).[280]

The fire on the earth is the beginning of a set of profound cosmic correspondences. As Ganapati Muni states:

> *The earth has a soul and is not unconscious. Just as our body is the abode of our souls, so the earth is the body of a greater Soul. That great Soul of the earth is the Divine nature of Agni. He is the hearer of our hymns to the Fire.*[281]

The Agni that the Rishis acknowledge is the soul of the earth, which has its own central fire. Yet the entire universe is the greater body of the Universal Soul or cosmic Fire.

Agni or the Vedic sacred fire represents the Divine consciousness-force or Chit-shakti, a spark of which descends into matter and becomes the individual soul or Jivatman. Agni as the Divine child builds up the worlds from within by his will, wisdom, and aspiration, with the soul evolving through many births, ascending through the kingdoms of nature. He is responsible for all transformations, for all development of substances and creatures in the universe, which he creates as various layers or levels, taking on new forms, turning old creations into new fuel in order to evolve life further.

Agni or fire symbolizes the individual soul hidden in the body, like the fire hidden in wood. All yogic practices involve awakening our soul's aspiration to immortality within us, which means developing our inner Agni. Our inner soul, hidden like a secret flame deep within our hearts, abides inextinguishable throughout all our states of consciousness of waking, dream, and deep sleep. It endures as the witness through our every birth and death, through all our many sojourns in the various worlds and planes of existence of the Divine's vast manifestation. Meditation consists of merging into the cosmic fire and universal light, life, and love.

Agni's most important aspect for Yoga is probably his role as the central fire in the heart, the very core of our being. This Agni or flame of the spiritual heart is like the pilot light that lights and sustains all the other fires of body and mind. These fires merge in the flame of the heart in deep sleep and at death, as well as in the state of samadhi.

Agni as the individual soul or Self dwells in the lotus of the heart, which is an eight-petal lotus representing the eight directions of space (four cardinal and four intermediate directions). In our ordinary state, the petals of this lotus are turned downward and the fire of Agni gets directed to the navel region as the digestive fire, and remains primarily a personal and biological force. As we grow in awareness, the heart lotus gradually opens and turns upward, unfolding all the higher potentials within us as the light of awareness.

From this central heart fire, three interrelated currents arise as breath, speech, and thought.[282] These three sustain our mind, emotions, and spirit. Of these three, the fire of intelligence (Dhi or buddhi) in the mind is the most important for our awareness. Three fires similarly descend as digestion, elimination, and reproduction. These three sustain the physical body and our instincts. Of these three lower fires, the digestive fire or "Jatharagni" in the navel is most important and is the central power in the physical body.

The *Rigveda* reflects the image of the fire sacrifice as a universal metaphor, representing the underlying process of all existence as the transformation of the light. This yogic fire sacrifice shows that all our thoughts and actions are offerings to our soul in order to help it grow and evolve in consciousness, as it moves back through the world of nature to the Godhead or Brahman. Agni is the mystery of our birth and death and the doorway to the infinite and the eternal.

Agni is the Divine child, seed or embryo, the spiritual consciousness that enters into creation and builds it up from within. Agni contains the essence, the source, and the matrix of who we are and all that we can become. All the forces of nature are the mothers of this Divine child that nothing can limit or overcome. His supreme Mother is the Divine Shakti herself, the Great Goddess.

Our Soul Fire Journey as Agni

Let us take a quick look at the journey of this Divine flame of Agni because it is the journey of our own souls. The soul is like a flame that moves through the kingdoms of nature both creating and participating in them. It is fire that develops their particular substances and structures, and becomes the beings or life-forms that inhabit them. Yet Agni is not only fire, but also color, heat, and light. In addition, Agni is life, perception, mind, and consciousness, which are the inner factors of light.

Each one of us is a flame and a form of Agni, which is the light that illumines our body, senses, breath, mind, and consciousness. We are "fire beings," not simply as portions of a material fire but as manifestations of a spiritual and universal fire (symbolized by the God Shiva or Rudra). All that we see around us as fire, light, color, heat, energy, or motion is the great God Agni. As a manifestation of Agni, we contain all these powers within ourselves.

Agni takes many forms on earth. In fact everything on earth is a form of Agni. All forms of matter are forms of Agni. Within all material forms some process of fire or combustion is continually going on, sustaining it. There is a fire within the earth and within the waters, a fire within the rocks, a fire within the plants, a fire within animals, and a fire within human beings. Each of these levels of life is a different birth or manifestation of the cosmic Fire.

Agni arises from the Divine Mother, who is space (Aditi), as part of the cosmic breath called *Matarishva*.[283] It takes shape as the stars and then through the rays of the Sun descends to the earth through the waters of the atmosphere, which get charged with its electricity as it becomes the lightning force or *Vidyut shakti*. It then falls to the ground and becomes the waters of the ocean and streams, which become pranically charged and can gradually develop life and intelligence.

Yet at the same time that the cosmic Agni descends from the periphery of space, another form of Agni arises from the center of the earth. It produces the earth from within and abides in its core as the mineral or volcanic fire. When these earthly and watery forms from below and above of Agni meet, life is born and plants take shape (the Agni of photosynthesis). After the plant kingdom has evolved, a new fire arises as the animal fire, the fire in the belly or Jatharagni, which transforms plants as food into animal tissue. However, the ultimate essence of the plants and the highest animal form is the human being, which through the digestive fire develops the higher fire of intelligence and discrimination that is capable of knowing the Divine.

Agni represents our soul or psychic being,[284] the inextinguishable flame of awareness that follows us through every birth and death and through all our states of waking, dream, and deep sleep. As such, he is called *Jatavedas* or the "knower of all births." Where does this flame of our soul come from? It is a portion of the solar fire that has descended into the earth, which in turn the Sun receives from the light of consciousness (Chit-tejas) behind time and space, and from the lords of universal life and karma (the Bhrigu and Angirasa Rishis). Our soul's flame is a spark of the original cosmic Agni.

The development of this spiritual fire is the real purpose of our lives, which should be a Yajna, a sacrifice or conscious worship. This cultivation of the flame of awareness is embodied in the practice of the Vedic ritual, which is connected to the universal powers of time, space, energy, matter, and mind. Ghee or clarified butter symbolizes the pure or sattvic mind in which the flame of awareness can burn cleanly. Ghee or ghrita is Agni's source, main food, and prime abode in which he lives.[285] Ghee is the essence of food, which has an oily quality and represents our nerve and brain tissue, which has an oily quality.

Agni is the Divine child that is born within us the child of heaven, the son of the waters, the son of strength. He dwells in the cavern or secret place of the heart. As he comes forth in his full glory he becomes the liberated soul or Mukta-Purusha, one with the supreme Self or Paramatman, the Divine Fire incarnate.

The Soul in Yoga

Yoga's main concern is a higher human evolution—the manifestation of the soul or Agni in its full glory, to turn the human person into a universal being. The fire of Yoga is meant to change our crude human nature into something genuinely spiritual, to replace our egoic mindset with a pure awareness beyond desire. The Agni or flame within us naturally seeks to return to his Divine solar home. Our soul's fire carries the Divine will within us to return to God. We must bring that spiritual fire out of the earth of our body and mind in order to illumine our lives and reconnect us with the greater universe of consciousness.

All the different practices of Yoga serve to develop Agni on different levels. Asana practice purifies, and balances the digestive fire (Jatharagni). Pranayama purifies, balances, and energizes the pranic or breath fire (Pranagni). Pratyahara, or internalization, purifies and internalizes the fire of the sense and motor organs (Indriya-agni), particularly the eye and speech, which are the main forms of Agni in the sense and motor organs. Dharana, or concentration, focuses and heightens the fire of the mind (Manasa-agni). Dhyana, or meditation, increases the fire of wisdom (Buddhi-Agni). Samadhi, or absorption, merges us into the Divine fire to transform our consciousness at a soul level (Jiva-Agni).

So too, the different paths of Yoga cultivate different forms of fire. Jnana Yoga or the Yoga of knowledge burns our samskaras and karmas in the fire of knowledge (Jnana-agni). Bhakti Yoga or the Yoga of devotion burns our lower passions in the fire of Divine Love (Prema-agni). Karma Yoga burns our egoistic impurities in the fire of sevice (Seva-agni). Raja Yoga, the integral Yoga, burns our conditioned habits in the fire of samadhi. Hatha Yoga, the Yoga of psychophysical practices, uses Yoga postures and pranayama to purify the body and mind.

We must learn to sublimate our inner life fire from an animal to a Divine level. This is not to suppress it or try to put it out but to take it to a higher level of manifestation. It requires the fire of austerity and simplicity (tapas), recasting the base metal of our lower humanity into the pure gold of the enlightened nature. This is the alchemical yogic fire. In this process, a new form of the Divine fire, the Kundalini force, which is a higher aspect of the Pranic fire, arises from the base of the spine and carries our consciousness upwards out the top of the head, and into the higher consciousness beyond all time and space.

Agni, like Kundalini, is a power of fire, prana, and speech. Both are connected to the earth and to the earth altar in the body (the Muladhara or root chakra). Kundalini is comprised of the letters of the Sanskrit alphabet that reflect the powers of cosmic sound and the Divine word. The Vedic fire sacrifice symbolizes the rising of the Kundalini from the earth or root chakra to heaven or the crown chakra, followed by the descent of Divine grace or Soma from heaven by the falling rain. Kundalini is the inner Agni, and awakening it is the essence of the Vedic worship of Agni.

The Universal Soul

Through the process of Yoga, the individual soul can expand into the universal soul, which is its inherent potential, and the real goal of our journey through the kingdoms of nature. In Vedic thought, the individual soul is called "Agni Jatavedas," the knower of all births. As the Rishi Vishvamitra states:

Oh Agni, these your eternal births for you the ancient we proclaim anew. For the great bull these sessions are made. Hidden in all births is the knower of all births.[286]

Hidden in every birth is the Knower of All Births, by the Vishvamitras he is enkindled inextinguishable. May we abide in his good thoughts and in his auspicious good mindedness.[287]

Gathina Vishvamitra, Rigveda III.1.20-21

We must learn to awaken at the level of the soul and the spiritual heart, as beings of consciousness seeking immortality through many bodies and many births. We must arise to our Divine mission of Self-realization, not just for our individual needs, but also for the evolution of life and consciousness in the world of nature. Agni is not just the ignorant soul, which is its inferior status, but the indwelling Divine presence within us, our inner guide, guru, and Divine connection.

He is the seer, among those who have not developed the seer vision. Wise in consciousness, Agni is the immortal placed in mortals. May Agni with this strength protect us from difficulty. May we ever abide in your happy right mindedness.[288]

Maitravaruni Vasishtha, Rigveda VII.4.4

This Divine fire is born within all creatures as the soul and core sense of Self. Through the practice of Yoga, our inner fire expands into the universal and becomes Vaishvanara, meaning the fire as the universal soul person. In the process Agni unfolds all the Gods or Divine powers (the Vasus, Rudras, and Adityas) and takes us through all the worlds or realms of consciousness from the earth to the highest formless heavens (the Rochanas). Notably, Agni unfolds the Lords of Dharma as the great Gods, Varuna, and Mitra, who symbolize the truth principles of purity and compassion. Agni merges with the descending Vayu or electrical/lightning force of Indra (truth perception), which destroys all ignorance and brings the soul into the infinite.

The eternal light is placed within us for the vision, the swiftest mind among the moving senses. All the Divine powers of common mind and common perception follow perfectly that single will.[289]

Wide moves my ears and wide my eyes facing this light that is placed within the heart. Wide moves my mind in a deep understanding. What can I say, indeed what can I think?[290]

All the Gods surrendered to you in awe, O Fire, as you endured throughout the Darkness. May the universal soul (Vaishvanara) protect us with his grace. May the immortal one protect us with his grace.[291]

Bharadvaja Barhaspatya, Rigveda VI.9.5-7

Whatever we see on earth is a form of Agni. All human beings are forms of Agni. The Sun, Moon, and stars in the sky above are also forms of Agni. The highest form of Agni is the Brahmagni (Agni of Brahman or the Absolute), the Agni of pure being (sat). This is Shiva, the fire that creates, preserves, destroys, and transcends the entire universe.

May we abide in the favor of the universal Fire, for he is the ruler resplendent over all the worlds. Manifesting from us he perceives the entire universe. The universal Fire expands himself through the Sun.[292]

Present in heaven, Agni is present on earth. Present here he has entered into all the plants. The universal Fire by his sudden power is present everywhere. May he protect us by day and by night.[293]

Kutsa Angirasa, Rigveda I.98.1-2

Names and Forms of Agni

Agni has many names in Vedic thought, a few of the most important of which are listed below.

- *Agni* – the inner guide, guru, soul or transforming power
- *Jātavedas* – the knower of all births, the one who is aware at his birth
- *Vaiśvānara* – the universal person, or cosmic soul
- *Kumāra* – the child or youthful principles
- *Guha* – that which is hidden, the secret essence, the light in the cave of the heart
- *Aṅgiras* – the primordial seer power, the hidden fire as in the coals
- *Sahasputra* – the son of strength or the one born immediately or by power
- *Hota* - invoker
- *Purohita* – chief priest
- *Ṛtvik* – seasonal priest
- *Ṛṣi* – the seer or the sage
- *Kavikratu* –He has the will of the seer

- *Vipra* – the illumined one.
- *Pāvaka* – the purifier
- *Apām napat* – the son of the waters

Agni is the head of the earth deities called the eight Vasus or indwelling powers. As the priest of the sacred ritual, he has many names and functions. He can be identified with all the Vedic priests and their outer and inner correspondences. Agni has several related Goddess forms, particularly relative to different aspects of the Vedic ritual including *Ilā, Bhāratī,* and *Sarasvatī.*[294]

Agni does not disappear from later Hindu thought but is found in fiery deities like Rudra, Bhairava, and particularly Skanda, the younger son of Shiva, who is his later incarnation (also called Kartikkeya, Subrahmanya, and Muruga). The *Mahabharata* contains a long section explaining how Agni takes birth again as Skanda.[295] Fiery Hindu Goddesses like Bhairavi, Uma, Durga, and Chandi reflect a symbolism of Agni.

Agni Dhi, the Meditative Insight of the Sacred Fire

Dhi is not only light, but also heat and transforming power. The awakening of this inner intelligence ripens, cooks, and transforms our nature. Dhi is also Agni or fire. While the Sun stands more for comprehension and awareness, fire is more a power of wakefulness, concentration, and discrimination.

Agni is the soul (Jiva) in its most conscious power of intelligence (Dhi). He represents the immanent divinity and its ability to ascend upwards to the heavens or higher lokas. He is our inner guide. The basis of the Vedic Yoga is to awaken and follow that Agni in its Godward journey.

> *Agni is conscious with intelligence (dhiyā sa cetati), the original ray of the sacrifice, to achieve his goal.*[296]
>
> *Gathina Vishvamitra, Rigveda III.11.3*

Agni is our inner guide on our spiritual practice which is our yogic self-offering to the indwelling Divine Light.

> *May Agni knowingly lead us to the treasure that is enjoyed by the Gods, which all the immortals made by intelligence (dhiyā yad viśve amṛtā akṛṇvan), and our Father Heaven and creator raining the Truth.*[297]
>
> *Vamadeva Gautama, Rigveda IV.1.10*

Agni takes us to the highest immortality, which is the ultimate fulfillment of Yoga. For that he is the God, the guru, the Rishi, and our own inner guide.

> *Thou, O Agni, were the first Angirasa Rishi, the God of Gods, you became our auspicious friend.*[298]
>
> *Thou Agni grant the mortal the highest immortality and glory every day, who thirsts for both the Divine and human births; you give blessings and delight to that illumined soul.*[299]
>
> *Hiranyastupa Angirasa, Rigveda I.31.1, 7*

Agni is not just the fire in this world but the original light of consciousness carrying and transcending all the worlds. His is the Divine Son that carries both the Father and the Mother, the Shiva and Shakti principles.

> *He is Being and Non-being in the supreme ether, in the birth of the discerning Father and the lap of the Infinite Mother, Agni comes to us as the first born of truth, he is the Bull and the Milch Cow in the original Life.*[300]
>
> *Trita Aptya, Rigveda X.5.7*

This Divine fire brings about the development of all our higher yogic potentials, unfolding the thousand petal lotus of the head.

> *Thou Agni from the lotus, the Rishi Atharva enkindled, from the head of every sage.*[301]
>
> *Bharadvaja Barhaspatya, Rigveda VI.16.13*

Soma Yoga: Vedic Bliss Yoga

Our lives are based upon the pursuit of happiness in one form or another, which implies the avoidance of sorrow. The yogic path consists of a pursuit of the highest bliss and immortality, with a complete and final end to all suffering. As such, Yoga is the highest and most intelligent use of our energies and aspiration that we all can share at our deepest level.

The Vedic hymns culminate in a vast epiphany of delight – the experience of Soma – which is not simply an outer intoxication, but the joy of experiencing the entire universe, with all of its beauty, love, and wisdom, as our true nature that can never be lost. That Divine inebriation is the goal of art and mysticism worldwide, yet the ancient Vedic Rishis succeeded in tapping into it thousands of years ago in a way that is as comprehensive and enduring as anything that humanity could develop since.

The *Vedas* teach us how to find our ultimate peace and well-being within our hearts and remove all afflictions from our consciousness. This Vedic pursuit of happiness is symbolized by Soma, the immortal nectar of Divine Bliss at the core of our being that pervades the entire universe. Only through that bliss or Ananda can we go beyond all sorrow and malaise. This inner Vedic search directs us to our eternal joy, not simply to outer sensory enjoyments that all must eventually end in disappointment.

This same inner Soma that affords us immortality in consciousness can also rejuvenate body and mind, and forms the ultimate medicine or healing balm. Vedic Soma encompasses all forms of healing, art, and spirituality, beautifully blended together in a great symphony of transformation. In the current chapter, we will examine the Vedic Soma or Bliss Yoga. The author's book on Soma deals with the subject of Soma in great detail, along with its Ayurvedic and yogic implications.[302]

Whatever we seek happiness from in life becomes our bliss or our Soma, as it were. Our sought after goal may be wealth, prosperity, sensory delights, food, sexuality, beauty, love, art, or religion. It may extend into intoxicants, drugs or addictions at an outer level, or higher states of consciousness within. These are all potential forms of Soma on various levels, which is the essence of delight that we seek in all objects and actions. Yet Soma does not dwell in any outer form or action, which are merely temporary containers for it. We project our inner Soma into outer objects, only to lose it, if we are not connected to the Soma inside ourselves. Our own consciousness is the ultimate source of Ananda, and external enjoyments are but its reflection or its mere shadow.

Yoga looks to a lasting internal happiness and bliss that is not dependent upon any external factors, which always bring in an element of uncertainty. This inner happiness is defined as the yogic state of mergence or absorption, *samadhi*, in which we become one with all that we perceive. Samadhi is the yogic form of Soma. *Soma Yoga* relates to the development of the state of samadhi, particularly as arising from inspiration, love, and delight. This Soma-Samadhi is the pinnacle of all yogic striving and the eighth of the eight limbs of classical Yoga that encompasses all the other limbs. Soma is the fruit of the Vedic Yajna or worship and the Soma book is said to be it highest of all the books of the *Rigveda*. Soma is the great king, connecting to whom we can gain power over all things, including over our own minds, not through intimidation but through sheer delight.

Soma represents the immortal nectar that is the life of the Gods, and the basis of all manifestation in the universe. We want to live only because we experience a delight in being alive. Only that immortal nectar of Soma, however, can feed and energize the immortal aspect of our own nature, through which even our mortal enjoyments proceed. The entire universe arises from that bliss, abides in it, and must return to it, and we are part of it at every moment. The Vedic Yoga is about our return to bliss, which is the return to samadhi, our own inner Self-awareness and Self-realization.

All Vedic deities drink the Soma and gain strength by its power. This is a metaphor for the Divine wisdom, energies and faculties that are born of abidance in the state of samadhi or absorption into the inner consciousness. The Vedic deities are manifestations of samadhi, particularly the deeper samadhis of the silent mind, what are called Nirvikalpa Samadhi (thought free), and Sahaja (natural) Samadhi in later yogic thought.

Forms of Soma in the Universe

Soma has many forms in the universe that is itself a manifestation of Soma as the prime creative power. Soma relates to whatever provides nourishment, moisture, sustenance, cohesion, or delight—and such potentials are in everything.

There are many forms of Soma on our planet earth through the waters, plants, and animals, and the fertility of the earth itself that is centered in the ground. Water forms of Soma are the ocean, rivers, lakes, and ground water. Plant forms include trees, flowers, herbs, and grasses, particularly those plants that have significant juices or fruits. Animals reflect their Soma through their playing and their mating rituals.

The main atmospheric form of Soma is the rains that nourish life on earth. The clouds, the mist and the fog, the atmospheric forms of moisture are types of Soma. The air itself has its pranic or nourishing aspects, particular air arising from water sources like the ocean, lakes, meandering rivers, or mountain streams. The main heavenly form of Soma is the Moon that gives delight to all and inspires poets and mystics, ruling over the tides of the ocean and the fertility cycles in animals. In addition are the solar waters, the waters of space, and space itself, the ocean of heaven that are subtle forms of Soma.

There are many biological forms of Soma that represent the harmony of life and body. These include the sap in plants and the blood in animals. Most bodily tissues are forms of Soma including plasma, blood, nerve, and reproductive tissues that are watery in nature. The food and beverages that we rely upon are additional forms of Soma. There are special Soma foods like fruit, milk, ghee, sugar, and honey. There are special Soma-increasing herbs that open the mind and heart, and promote rejuvenation and longevity, such as the *rasayanas* or rejuvenative agents of Ayurvedic medicine.

Soma exists in the body as the tongue and the sense of taste. It is the basis of Kapha, or the biological water humor that supports the body, and of Ojas, the ultimate energy reserve of the body that upholds the immune system. Vedic Soma is compared with honey (madhu), ghee (ghrita), and milk (go). It can be prepared or cooked in milk (gośrita), yogurt (dadhyāśrita), grain (yavaśrita), or plant juices (rasaśrita). Vedic Soma is not a single plant but the healing essence of all the plants. Ultimately, Vedic Soma is the nectar of our own inner plant, the nervous system, subtle body and its chakra centers.

My knowledge of Ayurveda has helped me understand the role of Soma in the *Rigveda*. Ayurveda provides a link between the Vedic Yoga with the Tantric Yoga that similarly revolves around Agni, Soma, Vayu, and Surya, the light forces of Fire, Moon, Lightning, and Sun, including the Vedic view of the chakras or energy centers of the subtle body. Ganapati Muni explains them simply and directly, "The Moon in the head, the Sun in the heart, Lighting in the Eyes, and Fire in the seat of Kundalini."[303]

Soma is the basis of the mind, particularly in its reflective, contemplative, receptive, and emotional aspects. Soma as a plant symbolizes the subtle body, the chakra system, which springs from the center of the Moon or the lotus, the crown chakra of the head. Soma develops through concentration, which extracts it, from which it flows in drops. This is the meditative mind that produces the drops or *bindus* of higher awareness. The flow of Soma is the flow of the mind in samadhi.

Soma is the power that holds and sustains the entire universe, like the great Shiva linga:

> *The pillar of heaven, firm and extended wide, the full filament moves around us on every side. He honors both heaven and earth that he encompasses. With a common energy, the seer-poet holds these connected worlds together.*[304]
>
> *Kakshivan Dairghatamasa, Rigveda IX.74.2*

Names of Soma and Its Related Deities

Soma as a cosmic power has many names and forms in Vedic thought. These reflect the process of preparing the Soma, which serves as a metaphor for the distillation of the bliss in all aspects of our lives.

- *Soma* – that which swells, particularly expanding with moisture, implying growth and happiness.
- *Indu* – meaning the drop, as Soma develops and grows in drops like water drops and raindrops, or inner drops of nectar.
- *Pavamāna* or Self-purifying. If we let our Soma flow like letting water flow, it naturally purifies itself. This means that through letting go of enjoyment our enjoyment will increase.
- *Dhārā* – the stream, a steady flow of moisture, delight, and concentration.
- *Samudra* – the ocean or the gathering place of all powers, which are one in delight.
- *Rājā* – Soma is the king because it is the highest and most powerful principle.
- *Ṛtam* – Soma is the law and truth behind the universe.
- *Madhu* – honey wine or bliss
- *Mada* – ecstasy, including that of going beyond the mind.
- *Matsara* – intoxication

Soma has joint forms and functions with many other Vedic deities, Soma is their food, their life-blood, and energizing power. Most important of these are Varuna as the Lord of the cosmic ocean; Indra as the main drinker of the Soma, sometimes along with Vayu and the Maruts as powers of air; Agni as the power that prepares the Soma; and Surya or the Sun as the immortal nectar of light. Soma is closely connected to the Goddesses, especially water and river Goddesses, and has a number of related Goddess forms, particularly the Divine sisters who aid in its development.

The priestesses have sung, the powerful Mothers of truth, adorning Soma, the child of heaven. Wealth from four oceans and from every side, Flow, Soma, a thousandfold![305]

Trita Aptya, Rigveda IX.33.5

Soma continues in later Hindu thought, where the term becomes primarily a name for Shiva, particularly Shiva together with his wife Uma, with Soma indicating *Sa* or he (Shiva) plus *Uma* (Shakti). Soma relates to Chandra or the Moon God in various forms, and with the many forms of the Goddess that are associated with the Moon. Soma is reflected in benefic forms of the Goddess associated with beauty, bliss, water, abundance, and fertility. This includes Gauri, Lakshmi, Kamala, and Sundari. Even Krishna has his Soma, which is the ecstasy of devotion. Shiva wears the crescent Moon on his head, in forms like *Chandra Shekhara*, as do many forms of Shakti.

Soma Dhi and Soma Yoga

The main Soma offering of the yogic inner sacrifice is that of the mind or manas, to which Soma corresponds at a psychological level. This consists of offering our intentions, motivations, desires, and pursuit of enjoyment to the Divine within. The turning of the mind within, not out of suffering, but out of a deeper Divine love and joy, is the basis of the Soma Dhi Yoga, the Soma Yoga of the intelligent mind. This inner Soma mind offering means offering the soul to the Godhead. Extracting the Soma bliss or Ananda from the mind is one of the most important Yoga practices and constitutes the essence of meditation. It means offering the Anandamaya kosha or "bliss sheath," the inmost of the five sheaths, to the Divinity. That is why Soma in the *Rigveda* is said to be the highest offering.[306]

Held by seven insights (sapta dhītibhir hito), unharmful he has directed the rivers, which have grown a single eye.

Asita and Devala Kashyapa, Rigveda IX.9.4[307]

The seven insights are perhaps the enlightened forms of the five sense organs plus mind and intelligence, or the seven chakras that these relate to. These through the power of Soma or Divine Bliss, the river or nadis of the subtle body, grow a single eye or unitary perception of truth.

Welcomed by the thought, held by the intelligence (dhiyā hitaḥ), Soma moves in the beyond, the poet by the flow of the seer.

Ayasya Angirasa, Rigveda IX.44.2[308]

The flow of Soma or Soma Dhara is the concentration of the calm or peaceful mind. This is not simply the Yoga practice of dharana but that of *samyama*, the combination of dharana, dhyana and samadhi, which is the basis of both the Siddhis or powers of Yoga, and Self realization or Kaivalya.[309] It grants vast creative powers.

> *Soma by the original thought (pratnena manmanā), Divine from the divine powers, flows pressed out in a stream.*
> *Medhyatithi Kanva, Rigveda IX.42.2*[310]

Soma is pressed out as the flow of nectar through the streams of mind and prana that spread from the individual to the universal. The original thought is that of the pure I or the Self, the "I am all."

> *Together with a discerning mind (dakṣeṇa manasā), the poet is born, the seed of truth, hidden beyond the twins.*
> *Vatsapri Bhalandana, Rigveda IX.68.5*[311]

Soma reflects the discriminating mind of the seers, which dwells beyond the twins or beyond the realm of duality. This faculty of discernment is called Daksha in Vedic thought and compliments Kratu or the power of right judgment.

> *The tongue of truth pours the beloved honey-wine, the speaker, the lord inviolable of this insight (patir dhiyo). As the son, he holds the secret Name of the parents, in the third luminous realm of heaven.*
> *Kavi Bhargava, Rigveda IX.75.2*

The honey-wine that Soma produces is the bliss or ananda. This is the basis of the Soma Dhi, which is to perceive and meditate upon the beauty and delight inherent in all things. Soma relates to the highest heaven, which is also our true nature in the spiritual heart. As the Divine child of immortality, he carries both our parents as heaven and earth.

> *Where there is bliss (ānanda) and delight, happiness and joy, where there is the attainment of all desires, there make me immortal, flow on Soma, flow for Indra.*[312]
> *Kashyapa Maricha, Rigveda IX.113.11*

Soma as the nectar of bliss flows for Indra, the Self as the perceiver of all. Soma flows in drops, which are the intoxications of the concentrated mind. This power of bliss is the creator of all things, the Divine delight from which the universe first arose and sustains it anew at every second.

Soma flows the father of thoughts, the father of heaven and the father of earth, the father of Agni, the father of the Sun, the father of Indra, Soma flows through the purification filter singing.

The Rishi mind, the maker of the Rishis, who wins the world of light, who has a thousand guidances, the leader of the poets.

Ushanas Kavya, Rigveda IX.96.5[313]

Soma as bliss or Ananda is the origin or father of all higher thoughts and of the entire universe. Soma is the supreme Rishi, as it is the bliss of Ananda that is the main inspiration for the Rishi vision and Rishi power, which has the capacity to create entire worlds and cultures. It is that Soma or mystic wine that inspires poets everywhere.

Flow for the winning of great power over all the seer wisdoms. You, Soma extend the original ocean for the Gods, as ecstasy.

Flow, Soma, around the earthly realm and through heaven by the dharma. You, clear in vision, the seers direct by their thoughts and by their insights.[314]

The Seven Rishis, Rigveda IX.107.24

Soma reflects a cosmic symbolism that indicates the state of samadhi or supreme bliss that allows us to perceive the entire universe within our own consciousness. He holds all seer-wisdoms or powers of higher perception.

The king of all flows in the vision of the Sun-world. The ruler of the Rishis has entered into the insight of truth. He is cleansed by the filter of the Sun, the Father of knowledge, of unequalled seer-power.[315]

Kavi Bhargava, Rigveda IX.76.4

Soma is the king of all, the father of all wisdom, the supreme seer-poet, who has the vision of the entire realm of light. The *Vedas* are meant to provide us that Soma of the Divine Word, which is the power of Divine Love behind all manifestation. Soma is the grace of the Rishis, which is the grace of our own higher Self.

THE ANCIENT SOLAR YOGA

What if the most powerful force for energizing all Yoga practices were as obvious and visible as the Sun? The fact is, that it is. The Sun, properly understood is not merely an outer but an inner energy source, reflecting the supreme light of Yoga both in our own hearts and in the world of nature around us.

The Sun is the most powerful influence in nature, responsible for the light through which all life on earth functions, and sustaining the force of gravity through which the earth revolves. The Sun is the ruler of our solar system and all that occurs within it. Yet though we all may welcome the sunlight every day, we seldom consider the spiritual reality of the Sun or honor the sacred presence and higher spirit behind it. We take the sunlight for granted or value it for providing us better health or an alternative energy source!

However, if we look at traditional cultures from throughout world, we discover a strong awareness of the Sun as a spiritual force, and a secret doorway to a higher reality. We note extensive religious, yogic, astrological, and shamanic traditions that revere the Sun in various ways and seek to understand the wisdom and grace behind its outer form, intuiting through the Sun the supreme force behind all existence. The Vedic Yoga is a "Yoga of light," which is also a "Solar Yoga" or "Yoga of the Sun." Vedic Dharma is probably our most well-preserved ancient system of the original religion of light and the Sun.

The Sun is the visible representation of the deity, the veritable face of the Gods. The Sun is the great symbol of the Self, spirit or Divine presence in the world (Atman).

> *The bright face of the Gods has arisen, the eye of Mitra, Varuna, and Agni. He has filled heaven, earth, and the atmosphere, the Sun, the Self (Atman) of all that is stable and moving.* [316]
>
> *Kutsa Angirasa, Rigveda I.115.1*

The Sun is no mere luminous material globe, but the source of life, intelligence, love, and consciousness – light in the inner sense. We are all rays of the central Sun of consciousness that illumines the entire world. Throughout the ancient world, continuing in some areas down to present day, we find a worship of the Sun as part of a greater religion or spiritual path of light, enlightenment, and Self-realization. This "solar religion" or "solar Dharma" occurs along with an honoring of the sacred Fire, the mystic Moon, and other aspects of light – as part of a worship of nature as a whole and of the cosmic mind behind it.

The Sun is the One God, the Light of lights, the God of gods of the ancient world. This religion of the Sun pervaded the ancient world. It predominated among the Egyptians, Persians, Hindus, and Scythians, to name but a few, extending to the Aztecs, Mayas, Incas, and Pueblo Indians of the New World. Ancient Pre-Christian European traditions of the Greeks, Romans, Celts, Germans, and Slavs, contain strong solar symbolisms. Monotheistic approaches like Judaism, Christianity, and Islam contain a symbolism of light. There is a strong solar symbolism in Zoroastrianism, Buddhism, and Shinto, and many other traditions. Such spiritual teachings of light link the human being to the Sun and regard us as "children of the Sun," forms of light on earth taking birth to fulfill the solar will towards greater life and consciousness. We could say that the natural religion of our species is the religion of the Sun. Yoga is first taught to humanity by the Sun God in various forms as Vivasvan, Hiranyagarbha, or Savita. The ancient solar religion of humanity reflects its original Yoga tradition.

While scholars downplay the spiritual implications of ancient solar cults, as we begin to understand native traditions, it is becoming clear that there is a mystic meaning behind the ancient worship of light. Earlier humanity was probably more spiritual than our current humanity, owing to its ability to connect with the inner Divine light behind the great illuminating power of the Sun. This ancient path of light beckons us both from the future as well as the past, as the ecological age dawning today requires that we once more honor the sacred and Divine presence in nature, especially in the Sun.

The Vedic Religion of the Sun and Light

The *Vedas* are based upon a solar symbolism as a religion of light and of the Sun. The Sun is the supreme deity of the *Vedas*, the Divine power in heaven, which functions in the atmosphere as Lightning, and on earth as Fire, which are the three main manifestations of light in our visible world. The Vedic ritual involves making offerings to a sacred fire in order to connect with the beneficent powers of the solar deity. The *Vedas* teach that we are children of the Sun born on earth to carry forward the Divine light of truth.

The Vedic Yoga involves resurrecting the Sun out of darkness, which means returning to the Sun of our own true Self that is hidden in the darkness of the material world and the ego-mind. Each one of us is a Sun, a universal light of consciousness, but that solar aspect of our being must be regained through the process of Yoga Sadhana, which is a cultivation of the light within us.

Chanting mantras in the sunlight, particularly along with standing in water and offering the mantras to the solar deity, is one of the most powerful Mantra Yoga practices. It works particularly well with solar mantras like Oṁ, Hrīṁ, or the

Gayatri Mantra. Sound is also light and we can use the Sun to energize all mantras. Hrīm is the most important of the bija mantras said to carry the power of the Sun. But the solar energy is the root of all mantras. The Vedic mantras are said to dwell in the rays of the Sun. They number 432,000, which is 360 X 1200, reflecting a solar mathematics of the zodiac.[317]

The Gayatri Mantra

The Gayatri Mantra to Savita, a powerful form of the Sun God, is the most important of all Vedic mantras, and one of the most commonly used mantras in Yoga practices. The Gayatri Mantra is an important tool for drawing the spiritual energy of the Sun into our minds, hearts and bodies, serving like a solar panel drawing in energy for our inner life.

> *We meditate upon the supreme light of the Divine transforming Sun (Savita) that he may stimulate our intelligence.* [318]
>
> *Gathina Vishvamitra, Rigveda III.62.10*

Savita represents the Divine light of awareness hidden within us that Yoga serves to activate in order to bring about the evolution of our consciousness beyond time and mortality. Here we see the seeds of Yoga explained in terms of a solar symbolism.

There are many Gayatri based hymns in the *Vedas*, as Gayatri also refers to one of the three main Vedic meters in which more than a hundred hymns are composed. There are two other Gayatris to the Sun God in the *Rigveda* that are beautiful and powerful, which I have commonly used. This second Gayatri Mantra of Vishvamitra occurs in the *Rigveda* as the very verse immediately before the more famous Gayatri Mantra. It lauds the Sun as *Pushan*, the power of perception, which serves to nourish us from within.

> *Who discerns and sees together all the worlds, may that nourishing Sun (Pushan) be our protector.*[319]
>
> *Gathina Vishvamitra, Rigveda III.62.9*

The next Gayatri brings in Aditi, the Divine Mother and a seeking of bliss and happiness. Aditi is the great World Mother and all the Sun Gods called Adityas are regarded as her children.

> *Sinless before the infinite Mother (Aditi), in the impulse of the Divine Solar father (Savita), may we meditate upon all things as beautiful.*[320]
>
> *Shyavashva Atreya, Rigveda V.82.6*

Vedic rituals, like *Agnihotra*, are performed at sunrise, noon, and sunset, the main points of solar transformation during the day. The deity of the Gayatri Mantra, Savita, represents the transformational power inherent in the Sun, not only to change night into day, but also to take us beyond the darkness of the ego into the infinite light of the higher Self. Savita is the deity of Yoga and meditation, who sets the yogic process in motion within us as a manifestation of the Divine Will. Yet we should remember that this Gayatri is only one of many Vedic verses to the Sun that can be used in a similar manner.

The Purusha or Higher Self as the Being in the Sun

Yoga and the *Vedas* are linked together by the common conception of the *Purusha* or *Atman*, the Supreme or Universal Self, which is the goal of classical Yoga and the main subject of the Upanishadic teachings. The Purusha or Atman is identified with the Sun both in Vedic and Yogic thought. The idea of union with the Sun occurs in several Vedic verses, to quote a few examples below.

> *I have known that Supreme Person, of the luster of the Sun beyond darkness. Only knowing him can one go beyond death. There is no other path for transformation.* [321]
>
> *Shukla Yajurveda XXXI.18, Shvetashvatara Upanishad III.8*

While the solar Purusha is mentioned specifically in the *Yajurveda*, in the *Rigveda* it is lauded indirectly through the Vedic Sun Gods.

> *Arising from the surrounding darkness, seeing the higher light, we have reached the Godhead, the Divine Sun, the supreme light.* [322]
>
> *Praskanva Kanva, Rigveda I.50.10*

> *From my father, I have received the wisdom of truth. I was born even as the Sun.* [323]
>
> *Vatsa Kanva, Rigveda VIII.6.10*

The great Upanishadic prayer is to merge into the Solar Self. The famous *Isha Upanishad* ends with a chant to merge in the solar Self, which also contains the oldest reference to the *So'ham* mantra. In fact, the great Hamsa or Swan of yogic thought is originally a Vedic Sunbird.

> *Sun, O nourisher, single seer, controller, power of the Lord of creation, remove your rays and gather up your heat that I may see your most auspicious form. The Purusha (Person) that is within the Sun beyond, He am I!* [324]
>
> *Isha Upanishad 16*

The *Upanishads* tell us that the Sun chants Oṁ as it moves in the sky. The Sun is not only the source of light, but also that of sound and mantra. Mantra Yoga is rooted in the worship of the Sun as in the inner light.

> *Thus indeed that which is the upward chant (udgītha), that is the primal sound (praṇava). That which is the primal sound that is the upward chant. That which is the Sun beyond is the upward chant. He is primal sound. He chants Oṁ as he moves.* [325]
>
> *Chandogya Upanishad I.5.1*

The Sun and the Branches of Yoga

Relative to the Yoga of Knowledge, the inner Self or Atman is symbolized as the Sun, ever shining in the hearts of all. After introducing the famous mantra "I am Brahman" (aham Brahmāsmi) or "I am God," the *Upanishads*[326] quote a verse from the Rishi Vamadeva in the *Rigveda* that states, "I was Manu and the Sun."[327] Relative to the Yoga of Devotion or *Bhakti Yoga*, the first and main images used in worship were that of the deity in the Sun disc, *Surya-Narayana*. This is the background of the ancient Vaikhanasa tradition of India, which is still followed in the famous temple of Tirupati in South India, the largest and wealthiest shrine in the country.

A solar symbolism enters into the great trinity of Hindu deities. *Brahma*, the Creator, has a solar aspect. *Vishnu*, the preserver, is worshipped as the Sun, particularly as *Surya-Narayana*, the Sun as the cosmic person who enters into the hearts of all beings. *Shiva*, the transformer, is honored as the supreme deity behind the Sun, particularly as *Rudra*, who represents the highest light and color of the Sun. Brahma, Vishnu, and Shiva are identified with the three aspects of solar energy as creating, sustaining, and transforming the universe.

The Solar Yoga and Solar Yogis

Krishna in the *Bhagavad Gita* states that he taught the original Yoga first to *Vivasvan*, the Sun God, who passed it on to Manu, the primal human sage, who is called the son of the Sun. [328] Krishna is traditionally regarded as the *Yogavatara* or "incarnation of Yoga," a status that is not afforded to any other human personage. This statement of Krishna refers to the Vedic teaching that we as human beings are descendants of the Sun.

Manu, the son of the Sun, is the first king, law giver and great Yogi in this particular world-age. From him originate both the great solar and lunar dynasties of kings, with Rama and Buddha hailing from the solar side, and Krishna and Arjuna from the lunar side. This statement of Krishna is similar to that of Vamadeva quoted earlier from the *Rigveda* stating he was Manu and the Sun. Krishna here relates to the royal sages or Rajarshis. There were other priestly sages or Brahmarshis associated to the Sun. Rama is also connected to the Sun.

The traditional founder of *Yoga Darshana* or the "Yoga system of philosophy" – which the *Yoga Sutras* of Patanjali represents – is said to be *Hiranyagarbha*, which means the "Golden Embryo," and is identified with the Sun. Kapila, the founder of the Samkhya system, is similarly identified with the Sun. In the *Mahabharata*, Krishna states: "As my form, carrying the knowledge, eternal and dwelling in the Sun, the teachers of Samkhya, who have discerned what is important, call me Kapila. As the brilliant Hiranyagarbha, who is lauded in the verses of the *Vedas*, ever worshipped by Yoga, so I am also remembered in the world."[329]

Yajnavalkya is an important figure in both Vedanta and Yoga. He is the most famous of the Upanishadic sages, to whom most of the *Brihadaranayaka*, the longest of the ten main classical *Upanishads* is ascribed. He is said to have received his Vedic mantras directly from the Sun God as Aditya. The *Yogi Yajnavalkya*, an ancient Yoga text, reflects a strong solar symbolism. It has extensive teachings on Oṁ and the Gayatri Mantra. It states, "The Sun, the Self of the world, is the prana placed in the heart."[330]

The Sun and Prana

Relative to the practice of Yoga, the Sun as Prana is a key to many pranayama practices. In the *Upanishads*, the Sun is identified with Prana:

> *The Self bears himself in two ways, as Prana and as the Sun. Such are his two paths, outer and inner, which revolve by day and by night. The Sun is the outer Self and Prana is the inner Self. The movements of the inner Self (Prana) are measured by those of the outer Self (the Sun).*[331]
>
> *Maitrayani Upanishad VI.1-3*

Our prana is our inner Sun that marks our inner days and nights that follow a similar course as the outer days and nights.

This Upanishadic idea reflects older Vedic views. Yajnavalkya's *Shatapatha Brahmana*[332] states that we have 10,800 breaths by day and night. This equals 720 breaths every 48 minutes (1/30 of a day), which he identifies with the general number of days and nights in a year. It amounts to one breath every four seconds. Our term of 21,600 breaths lasts for a life of 100 years. This means that we can make our lives longer by breathing longer and make our lives shorter by breathing more quickly.

In the yogic view of the subtle body, the right or solar (Pingala) nadi governs fire, heat, and activity at a physiological level. The Sun is present physically as the solar plexus fire in Hatha Yoga, and as the Atman in Raja Yoga. The key to pranayama is to draw in the prana of both the inner and the outer Suns.

The Sun and Meditation

One of the simplest and most important meditation techniques is to meditate upon the Supreme Self or Divine presence as the Sun within the heart, of which the mind and brain is but an outer reflection like the Moon.

Relative to modern Yoga masters from India, Sri Aurobindo taught an integral Yoga of Self transformation through the Supramental light and Shakti, which he lauds under the symbolism of the Sun. Ramana Maharshi, the greatest of the sages or Jnana Yogis, speaks of the heart and the Self as the inner Sun.

In Tantric Yoga as in the *Upanishads*, the Sun at a deeper level, is identified with the heart. The spiritual fire force of Shakti in the root chakra and the lunar or water force (Soma) of Shiva in the crown chakra unite in order to create it. Agni is the red point, drop or sphere (bindu), and Soma is the white bindu, which unite to create the Sun as the golden bindu.

Forms of the Solar Divinity

The Sun God, which is the god of light, has many forms throughout the universe. All forms of light are forms of the Sun, including all the stars and planets or lights in the sky. In our own body, the solar light has created the head, the brain, and the light of our intelligence, particularly the eyes, and our powers of perception and discrimination. The Sun sustains prana. The Sun is the heart. The Sun is the soul within the heart.

The Sun has heavenly or sky forms as the Sun and the planets that shine by its reflected light. The stars themselves are distant Suns. The Sun is regarded in Vedic thought as the gold or golden light of heaven. Yet there are also earth forms of the Sun or solar energy. There is the sunlight reflected on the ground and rocks or absorbed by the waters. There is the sunlight absorbed by plants, which allows their sap to rise. There is the sunlight absorbed by animals, the solar warmth that allows them to move. We human beings strive to take in the sunlight or to be in the sunlight. This is an unconscious honoring of the solar deity.

The solar force is symbolized by certain animals, notably the horse, and birds like the eagle and falcon. The Sun is the foundation of Dharma or cosmic law, portrayed in Vedic thought by the wheel of Dharma or the *svastika*. The Sun is the light of law and truth. The Sun has many forms in the individual as prana, the eye, perception, intelligence, discrimination and awareness, but above all as the inner Self or Atman. It is the light of the Sun that is the field of light and energy, the subtle body, behind our physical encasement.

Names of the Sun God

The Sun God has the largest number of names of any of the Vedic deities. These reflect different aspects or powers of light, transformation, or Dharma for which the Sun is the prime motivating power.

- *Sūrya* – the one who sets everything in motion; the most common name for the Sun.
- *Savita* – the power of inspiration, motivation, and higher evolution, Yoga and meditation.
- *Āditya* – the unbounded light and primal intelligence.
- *Mitra* – the Divine friend and lord of compassion .
- *Varuṇa* – the Divine lord, giver of wideness.
- *Āryaman* – the Divine companion, friend, and helper is the third after Mitra and Varuna, and together rule the three higher heavens or rochanas beyond the ordinary three realms of earth, atmosphere, and heaven.
- *Bhaga* – the blissful lord, Bhagavan.
- *Puṣan* – the nourisher, the seer, the guide of the soul beyond death and darkness.
- *Viṣṇu* – the pervader, ruler of the highest heaven.
- *Tvaṣṭaṛ* – the maker of forms, associated with the great Goddesses.
- *Hiraṇyagarbha* – the golden seed or fetus; the causal body.
- *Indra* – Indra as the Supreme Lord is often a name for the Sun or higher light, though more commonly he relates to the atmosphere.
- *Vivasvān* – the radiant one, associated with the dawn.
- *Prajāpati* – the lord of creatures, more common in later Vedic texts.

Surya Dhi and Surya Yoga

Surya Dhi is the illuminating power of our higher intelligence that reveals all things like the Sun. Surya Yoga is the culmination of the Dhi Yoga, the union with our higher Self that, like the Sun, is pure light.

Seers of the vast illumined seers yoke their intelligences and their mind. The one knower of the ways of wisdom ordains the invocation. Great is the glory of the Divine creative Sun. [333]

Shyavashva Atreya, Rigveda V.81.1, Shvetashvatara Upanishad II.4, Shukla Yajurveda XI.4

Here, yoking is done of the mind, manas, and Dhi, powers of intelligence by the Divine Sun or Atman as Savita. This Vedic Yoga of controlling the mind and buddhi is well evidenced here.

That Lord the ruler of the stable and moving world, who stimulates our intelligence (dhiyam jinvan), we invoke for grace. So that nourishing Sun will give growth to our knowledge, our protector and inviolable guardian for well-being. [334]

Gotama Rahugana, Rigveda I.89.5

This Sun God is the One Creator and Lord of all the worlds, the Sun of suns, the God of Gods, the Light of lights. The *Veda* invokes him in various forms, here as the provider of nourishment, Pushan, to stimulate our intelligence and guard over the unfolding of the treasures of the spiritual life. Yet there are various forms of Dhi Yoga connected with the other Vedic forms of the Sun God. There are seven or twelve Sun Gods or Adityas as representing the seven rays of the Sun or the twelve months of the year.

The Sun Gods uphold the stable and moving world. They are the guardians of all the universe. With a profound intelligence (dīrghā dhiyo), guarding their celestial powers, the carriers of truth, they note our debts.[335]

Gritsamada Shaunaka, Rigveda II.27.4

The very rising of the Sun every day indicates our own deeper light, purity and Self-realization as the Rishi Vasishtha lauds:

When rising today, you declare the truth to Mitra and Varuna that we are sinless, may we abide in the unbounded Godhead, O Aryaman, your beloved singers![336]

Maitravaruni Vasishtha, Rigveda VII.60.1

Vedic Shaivism

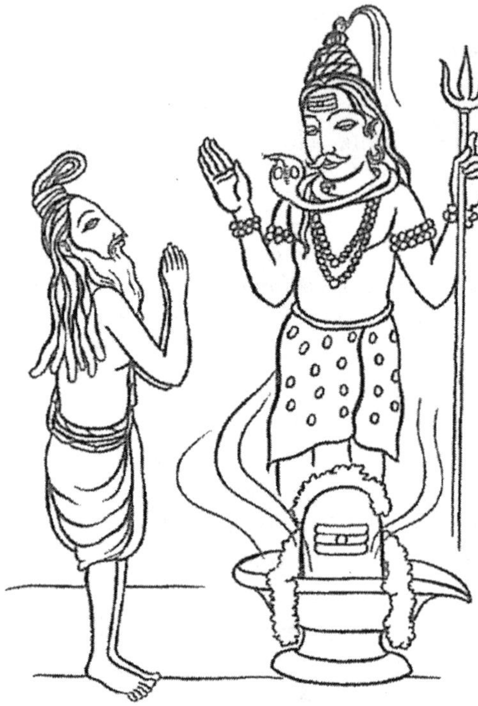

Shiva as the Supreme Reality of Being-Consciousness-Bliss (Sacchidananda) represents the great Unknown beyond the senses, speech, and mind. This formless reality cannot be reduced to any particular historical depiction, description, or nomenclature. Shiva in Sanskrit is not a name but a description of that which is auspicious, indicating something beyond words. One needs a deeper vision to understand the Supreme Reality that both contains and transcends all things, and is beyond speech and mind. The vision of the Supreme Shiva takes us beyond all dualities and contradictions, and remains forever a matter of paradox and mystery that cannot be reduced to any linear time-space coordinates such as characterizes physical reality. Even quantum physics, with its ability to deconstruct time and space realities, is just beginning to approach or to emulate the language of Shiva.

There are scholars who claim that Shiva is a pre-Vedic or non-Aryan deity, and who would not connect Shiva's origins with Vedic teachings or practices. They point out that the name "Shiva" for a deity as occurs in Shaivite texts is not found in any obvious way in Vedic texts. Such statements are made, even though Shaivism is an integral part of the Vedic teaching throughout India and has been historically for many centuries, or for as long as the literature can be found.

We must not forget that mantric texts like the *Vedas* cannot be understood through a superficial vision, by semantics, or through mere word comparisons. It is the deeper or mystic meaning that matters, not simply the outer name and form that is always subject to variations. The deeper yogic teaching remains dynamic and changes with time in outer expression. We need to understand this power of transformation behind the teaching, not simply the visible forms it may leave behind as it manifests through the movement of time.

Shiva as Oṁ and Primal Sound, the Deity of Sanskrit

Let us examine the connections of Shiva with the *Vedas*. Shiva's drum is said to be the origin of the Sanskrit alphabet, starting with great Sanskrit grammarians like Panini. Shiva is the prime deity of the Sanskrit language, which relates him to the Vedic language that is the oldest form of Sanskrit. Shiva is said to be *Omkara*, the sacred syllable Oṁ, which is called the essence of the *Vedas* in texts from the *Upanishads* back to the *Yajurveda*. The *Rigveda* similarly states that its comprehension rests upon the imperishable syllable (akshara) of the chant in the supreme ether, which indicates a similar mantric foundation for it.[337]

As *Pranava* or primal sound, Shiva's expression is the *Vedas*, which arises from Oṁ. To try to separate Shiva from the *Vedas* is to try to separate Oṁ or the Sanskrit language from the *Vedas*. Shiva is the great lord of mantra, and the *Vedas* are the oldest Sanskrit expression of mantra. The *Vedas* are the expression of Shiva as mantra, which means that Shiva in his totality is the *Vedas*.

Shiva and Rudra

Shiva as *Rudra*, which means "the maker of sound," is an important deity in the *Rigveda*, who is approached with great reverence as an awesome power. There are not very many hymns in the *Rigveda* specifically addressed to Rudra, but his roles and those of his children and companions (which include Indra, Agni, and Soma) are significant. Rudra is the father of the *Rudras* or *Maruts*, the Vedic storm Gods, who are led by Indra who is *Marutvan*, and who between them have many hymns of their own in the *Rigveda*. The twin horsemen or Ashvins are also called *Rudras* and have a number of hymns of their own. Rudra can be regarded as the great father of all the Vedic Gods.

Rudra and the Maruts reflect both the wandering Yogis and the power of pranayama. The *Vedas* speak of the *munis* or silent sages or *keshis* (who have matted hair), who control the breath (*vāta rāśana*) as connected to Rudra,[338] and as associated with other Rishi groups.[339]

The munis who control the breath wear unclean clothes. They move by the course of the wind, which the Gods have developed. Ecstatic by our muni-power, we ascend the winds, our body is all that you mortals see.[340]

Munaya Vatarashana, Rigveda X.136.2-3

The Maruts are also lauded as having human forms as sages and are not simply deities or personifications of natural forces like lightning and the storm.

Who have spotted horses, Maruts, whose mother is Prishni, who move with beauty and are visitors to the sessions of knowledge. Men who have the tongues of fire and the eyes of the Sun. May all the Gods come to us with their grace.[341]

Gotama Rahugana, Rigveda I.89.7

The *Rigveda Tryambakam* or *Mahamrityunjaya* mantra to Rudra remains the main verse used to worship Shiva today and is the most commonly used Vedic verse chanted after the Gayatri Mantra.

We worship the three-eyed one, who has a pleasant fragrance and who gives nourishment. Like a cucumber from its stalk, may he release us from death but not from immortality.[342]

Maitravaruni Vasistha, Rigveda VII.59.12

Rudra becomes the predominant deity worshipped in the *Yajurveda* or the later Vedic period. Most notable is the famous Rudram chant of the *Krishna Yajurveda*, which remains the most important long chants use in Shiva worship throughout India today as it has been for centuries, and is the first text in which the famous "*Namaḥ Śivāya*" mantra appears.[343] In this *Yajurveda* text one can find most of the names of Shiva that are worshipped in later times like Rudra, Shiva, Shankara, Shambhu, Bhava, Sharva, Pashupati, Kapardi, and Nilagriva.

Shiva as Rudra has a prominence earlier in the Vedic texts than either Vishnu or Brahma, the other two deities in the Hindu trinity, which similarly to Shiva gradually come into prominence in the late Vedic era. Rudra is also honored in a number of names and forms in the *Atharvaveda*, including Bhava, Sharva, and Manyu.[344]

Shiva as the All Vedic Deity

Shiva appears as the essence and integration of all the main Vedic deities, which represent his diverse manifestations. Shiva is said to be *Agni-Somatmakam* or "composed of both Agni and Soma," the fire and nectar that are the main factors of the Vedic mantras and their inner and outer rituals. Agni, or harsh forms of

Shiva, include Rudra and Bhairava; Soma, or soft forms, include Shiva, Shankara, and Shambhu.

Shiva is *Tryambakam* or "he who has three eyes," which eyes are Sun (Surya), Moon (Chandra or Soma), and Fire (Agni). These three eyes of Shiva reflect the three main deities of the *Vedas* as Agni, Surya, and Soma (Fire, Sun, and Moon). Vedic Indra is the Vayu or Vidyut (lightning form), which can be added to these three as the fourth and their underlying power. Shiva represents all four primary Vedic light forms as Agni, Soma, Indra/Vayu, and Surya – Fire, Moon, Lightning, and Sun, which are the four lights of Shiva or the four forms of Shiva's light.

Shiva is strongly connected to the Vedic Deity Soma, which remains a name of Shiva in later times. Soma and Rudra form a pair in Vedic thought. Both are related to the healing process that in later times is associated with Shiva. Rudra is the foremost of doctors in the *Rigveda*[345] and Soma is the magical elixir of immortality.

> *Soma and Rudra grant to our bodies all medicines. Release and remove whatever bondage or sin committed that is in our bodies.*[346]
> *Bharadvaja Barhaspatya, Rigveda VI.74.3*

Shiva is similarly closely connected to Agni and with all aspects of fire. Agni is called Rudra in the *Rigveda*. Rudra, which means red, is associated with the color of the fire. The fierce nature of Rudra correlates with the dangerous energy of fire.

> *Your king of the sacred ritual, Rudra, the invoker, for the truth sacrifice for heaven and earth, Agni, before the thunder of the ignorance, in golden form for grace, bring into manifestation.*[347]
> *Vamadeva Gautama, Rigveda IV.3.1.*

The eight names of Shiva in the famous *Shiva Mahimna Stotra 28* – perhaps the most important hymn to Shiva in classical Sanskrit literature – are Bhava, Sharva, Rudra, Ugra, Mahadeva, Pashupati, Bhima, and Ishana, which are largely Vedic. In the *Shatapatha Brahmana* for building up the fire altar, nine forms and nine names of Agni are mentioned. These include Rudra, Sharva, Pashupati, Ugra, Ashani, Bhava, Mahadeva, Ishana, and Kumara. Seven of these names are identical with seven of the eight names of Shiva in the Shiva *Mahimna Stotra*, another name, Kumara, is a name of Shiva's son Skanda who is identified with Agni.[348]

Shaivite yogis and ascetics – such as continue to exist in the Himalayas today – are devoted to fire and maintain their own undying fires, which they worship along with Vedic mantras. They collect and anoint their heads and bodies with the *bhasma* or sacred ash from the fire, with which Shaivite ascetics are identified. This fire form of Shiva worship reflects Vedic fire worship and appears as its continuation.

Shiva as Agni is one of his most important manifestations. The Agni worship of the *Vedas* and the Shaivite Agni worship are part of the same sacred fire tradition.

The Sun is the great deity of the *Vedas*, which have many forms of the Sun God. Sometimes as Rudra he identified with the destructive and transformative aspect of solar energy; but often he is identified with the Sun overall. Shiva is said to be pure light (Prakasha) in later Tantric philosophy, whose outer manifestation is the Sun, which symbolizes the light of the spiritual heart.

Shiva is a deity of prana and ayus, the life-force, which is ultimately the energy of consciousness. He relates to Vayu or the cosmic wind, spirit, and breath. This association of Shiva with prana connects him to Yoga traditions of Prana Yoga and pranayama. Most Yogic pranayama-based teachings are largely Shaivite in origin, like the Hatha Yoga tradition that goes back to Adi Nath, Lord Shiva.

The Unity of Indra and Shiva

Of the four main Vedic deities and their connections with Shiva, Shiva has the most in common with Indra. Vedic Indra and Puranic Shiva share many of the same names and functions, making them almost inseparable. In the *Mahabharata* one of the first names of Shiva is *Shakra* or Indra.[349] The following information is based on the work of Kavyakantha Ganapati Muni.[350]

Indra as a Sanskrit term means the "Lord" or "ruler" as does "Ishvara," an important name for Shiva. In Vedic hymns the term Indra is used as general term for Lord, just as Ishvara is used in Puranic hymns. Both Indra and Shiva are lauded as the Supreme Deity and the ruler of all the other Gods. Puranic Shiva is the great God, *Mahadeva*. Vedic Indra is the king of the Gods, *Devaraj*.

Shiva is the destroyer among the trinity of Puranic deities, along with Brahma, the Creator, and Vishnu, the Preserver. Indra in the *Vedas* is a destructive God, a destroyer of obstructions. "Vritra," the enemy of Indra, literally means "obstruction." Indra is the "destroyer of cities," *Purandara*. Shiva is the "destroyer of the three cities," *Tripurahara*, which he actually accomplishes for the benefit of Indra in the Puranic stories.

Indra and Shiva both have a consort named power (Shakti in the case of Shiva, Shachi in the case of Indra), who herself is a fierce Goddess. Indra's consort Indrani is in fact the Goddess of the army in the Vedic tradition. The martial role of Shiva's consort as Durga or Chandi, the destroyer of all enemies and opposition, and the leader of the Divine army, is well known. Indra and Shiva are both renowned as destroyers of demons and have terrible or wrathful forms. Indra in the *Vedas* is frequently called *Ugra, Ghora*, and *Bhima*, meaning fierce, terrible, and frightful, which are common epithets for Shiva in later times.

Shiva is said to be a non-Vedic God because he fights with Vedic Gods like *Bhaga* and *Pushan*, and destroys the sacrifice of *Daksha*, who is the son of Brahma or *Prajapati*, from which he is excluded. Yet this Puranic myth is not entirely new. A similar story occurs in the *Brahmanas* as Rudra slaying Prajapati or Brahma with his arrow,[351] which story is echoed in some hymns of the *Rigveda*.

Indra kills the son of *Tvashta* in the *Rigveda*,[352] who symbolizes the sacrifice. Tvashta is identified with Prajapati or Brahma in Vedic and Puranic thought. After slaying the son of Tvashta, Tvashta tries to exclude Indra from the drinking of the Soma, much like Shiva's being excluded from getting any share of the sacrifice. Indra elsewhere destroys his own father (who is Tvashta) and fights against the Gods.[353] Ultimately all the Gods abandon Indra and he has to slay the dragon (Vritra) alone. By *Brahmana* and Puranic accounts, Vritra is a Brahmin and Indra commits the great sin of slaying a Brahmin by slaying Vritra, for which he must seek atonement.

Indra, like Shiva, is a fierce God who transcends good and evil, going against social customs and doing what is forbidden. Indra does things like eats meat and drinks wine (sometimes in enormous quantities), and goes into various states of intoxication and ecstasy. Indra is born as an outcast and in some hymns in the *Vedas* he grants favor to outcasts. Shiva similarly is a deity of ecstasy (Soma) and transcends all social customs.

Indra, like Shiva, is called the dancer[354] and is associated with music and song. The letters of the Sanskrit alphabet come forth from Shiva's drum. Indra in the *Vedas* is called the bull of the chants, and all songs go to him like "rivers to the sea."[355] Shiva is identified in Tantric thought with the vowels of the alphabet. Indra in the *Chandogya Upanishad* is identified with the vowels among the letters of the alphabet.[356] Shiva is identified with the mantra Oṁ. Indra in the *Vedas* and *Upanishads* is also identified with the Oṁ.

Shiva is a mountain God, similarly Indra is a God of the mountains.[357] Shiva allows the heavenly Ganga to descend on his head. Indra's main action is destroying the clouds (mountains, glaciers) to allow the rivers to flow from the mountains into the sea. Both deities are interwoven with the myth of the descent of the heavenly waters. As Shiva is identified with the Ganga, Indra is identified with the Sarasvati River, and Sarasvati in the *Vedas* is lauded as Indra.[358]

Shiva is worshipped by the linga or standing stone. Indra, Soma and other Vedic Gods are worshipped by a pillar (stambha, skambha). The pillar and the linga are the same, symbols of the cosmic masculine force. Both Shiva and Indra represent the cosmic masculine force. Shiva's vehicle is a bull. Indra in the *Vedas* is frequently called a bull (*vṛṣa, vṛṣabha*). Shiva's bull is also identified with the rain cloud. Indra as the bull is lauded in the Vedas as the bringer of rain. The bull is also a symbol of the cosmic masculine force. Oṁ, which is identified with both Indra and Shiva, is identified with a bull.

Shiva is identified with the Vedic deity Rudra, and most of the sacred chants to Shiva, like the Rudram from the *Yajurveda*, are Vedic chants to Rudra. Vedic Rudra is lauded in the *Vedas* in hymns to Indra.

> *That power of Rudra appears in the primal abodes, where those wise in consciousness hold their minds to it.*[359]
> *Narada Kanva, Rigveda VIII.13.20*

Both Indra and Rudra are deities of the middle region or the atmosphere (Antariksha). Indra is the wielder of the thunderbolt, just as is Rudra. The Vedic sons of Rudra are called the Maruts. The Maruts are the companions of Indra, who is their leader. Shiva travels with his host of Bhutas or ghosts. The Maruts are also spirits or Bhutas and in the *Vedas* they travel with Indra. Indra is the main deity of the Vedic Rishis. Shiva is the main deity of the yogis. The yogis are usually Rishis and Rishis are usually yogis. In fact, the Maruts, the sons of Rudra and the companions of Indra, are sometimes lauded as Brahmins, Rishis, or Yogis.

Rudra-Shiva is propitiated to overcome death: the same is the case with Indra in the *Vedas*. There are Vedic prayers to protect us not only from the wrath of Rudra, but also from the wrath of Indra. Both Rudra and Indra are propitiated to grant us fearlessness and for defeat of our enemies.

The early *Upanishads*[360] identify Indra with Paramatman, the Supreme Self, just as the later *Upanishads* identify Shiva with Paramatman. Indra is called prana or the life-force in the *Upanishads*.[361] Shiva is also identified with prana. The Maruts, the sons of Rudra-Shiva and the companions of Indra, are identified with the pranas.

Shiva is a God of time, Kala. Indra is also a deity of time and eternity, and rules the year in Vedic thought. Both Indra's and Shiva's roles of destroying Prajapati or his son relate to eternity (absolute time) destroying time or the year (relative time) represented by Prajapati and the sacrifice.

The members of Shiva's family have Vedic equivalents, which is a topic in itself that will be mentioned only briefly. Skanda, the son of Shiva, is born of Agni or fire and is clearly identified with Agni.[362] Agni in the *Vedas* is called Kumara and Guha, which are later names of Skanda. Ganesha, the other son of Shiva, is commonly lauded by a chant to Brahmanaspati from the *Rigveda* (*Ganāṇām tvā gaṇapatim*).[363] Brahmanaspati and Brihaspati are considered to be the same deity in the *Vedas*.

The conclusion that we must draw is that Indra and Shiva are essentially the same deity, according to a shift of language. The two are so close in function that they must have arisen from a common source as part of a common tradition. This does not mean that Indra and Shiva are identical. According to Ganapati Muni, Indra refers more to the light aspect of the atmospheric force or the lightning and the power of perception. Shiva is more the sound aspect or thunder, and more specifically indicates the power of the Divine Word Oṁ. The symbolisms of Indra and Shiva can also be different at times. Indra is equated with horse and chariot symbolism, while Shiva is portrayed as a hunter, though they both share the symbolism of a bull.

Vedic deities like Indra, Agni, Soma, and Rudra are as freely identified with each other just as are Puranic deities like Shiva, Vishnu, and Devi (the Goddess). The Hindu approach has always allowed devotees to regard their chosen form of the Divine for worship as the supreme – whether Shiva, Vishnu, Devi, or other deity forms. Yet at the same time it insists that devotees of one form allow devotees of another form to have the same freedom of view.

Shaivite Dharma

When we study or chant the *Vedas*, we should try to connect to their essence (*rasa*) or central meaning (*sāra*), found in their sound vibration (*svara*). This is not merely a material or human sound but a vibration of consciousness. Look for the presence of Shiva in that. As the *Upanishads* eloquently state:

> *He who is lauded as the essence of sound (svara) in the Vedas, and is established in the Vedanta, who is beyond mergence in primal nature, he is Maheshvara (Shiva).*[364]
>
> *Mahanarayana Upanishad, Dahara Vidya*

Shiva does not represent the outer form of the Vedic terms but their inner essence of sound, meaning, energy, presence and power, which is *svara*. This ultimately takes us back to primal sound or Pranava and to Oṁ. The Upanishadic statement here reminds us of the *Yoga Sutras* that identifies Ishvara with Oṁ. It suggests the older Vedic Yoga that was based upon the power of sound, which in the later Vedantic Yoga became more philosophical in language.

Shaivism reflects the eternal tradition of Yoga, which is the practice of the Vedic Rishis. Many great Vedic Rishis were also proponents of the Shaivite Yoga, not as a literal worshipping of Shiva in his Puranic form, but as understanding that same primal reality of consciousness, vibration, sound, and light. The Rishi Yoga and the Shaivite Yoga are not different. The Rishi is one who knows how to work with all the light and sound forms of Agni, Soma, Surya, and Indra, and on all levels from the body to the highest awareness, which are all the forms and manifestations of the supreme Shiva.

Vedic Rishis that are important in Shaivite dharma include Vasishtha, from whom the Tryambakam Mantra arises,[365] his son Parashara, whose Rigvedic hymns are among the most mystic in the text, Vamadeva, which is also a name of Shiva in later times, Vishvamitra, who is a personification of Agni, and Agastya, who connects the northern and southern Shaivite traditions. Vasishtha and his followers like Rudra-Shiva are called *Kaparda* or who wear their hair in a special matted lock at the top of the head.[366] The Indus Valley seals contain several depictions of the three-headed, lord of the wild animals, in siddhasana, a prototype for Rudra-Shiva.

The *Kena Upanishad* prominently mentions Uma Haimavati, Shiva's consort.[367] Shvetashvatara, of the name of the *Upanishad* ascribed to him, taught the Vedic-Shaivite Dharma, weaving in Vedic deities of Agni, Soma, Vayu, and Surya into his explanations of Yoga and Vedanta.[368]

The older Shaivite teachings, such as found in the *Mahabharata*, are called the *Pashupata Dharma* from Shiva's name as Pashupati, the Lord of the wild animals, which is his main Vedic name after Rudra. Pashupati on a deeper level means Shiva as the lord (pati) of souls (pashu), or the seer as the lord (pati) of perception or the seen (pashu). This in turn connects to the Rudra and Marut traditions of the *Vedas*.

In the *Mahabharata*, Upamanyu who praises Shiva and the sage Tandi, who taught the *Thousand Names of Shiva (Śiva Sahasranāma)*,[369] shows that all the main aspects of Shiva and Shaivite Dharma were well known at the time of that text. The great Yogi Lakulish from Kayavarohan in Gujarat revived the Shaivite Dharma in the late ancient period, at least two thousand years ago. The great Nath Yogis, most famous of which is Gorakhnath, did so again around a thousand years ago, with important disciples and followers in Kashmir, Maharashtra, Nepal, and Bengal. The great Shankara not only revived the Vedantic teaching some fifteen hundred years ago, but also promoted all aspects of Shaiva and Shakta Yoga, and recognized Hatha Yoga as well.

Medieval Tantric Hinduism is dominated by the role of Shiva, but echoes a Vedic symbolism. Shaivite and Vedic Dharma rests upon a cultivation of the sacred fire of awareness or Agni, a development of the cosmic prana or immortal life-force or Indra, a flow of the nectar of bliss or Soma, and the dawning of the supreme light or Surya, the inner Sun of the heart. Later Shaivite Tantric Yoga centers on drawing the Agni or Kundalini Fire up from the earth altar of the Muladhara to the Soma vessel of the thousand petal lotus of the head, reflect the inner aspect of the ancient Vedic Yajna. There is a continuity of Shaivite Dharma from the Vedic Rishis to modern times.

The Universal Dharma

One basic and universal teaching can be found in India from early ancient times and characterizes the essence of the tradition. This Vedic presence of Shiva, however, does not mean that there are no other revelations of Shaivite Dharma apart from the *Vedas*, either before or after them. The higher teachings are always unlimited and even one great guru can produce many great volumes of teachings. But to understand the *Vedas*, we need to recognize the light and sound of Shiva behind them, not Shiva as a separate deity, but Shiva as the great unknown, absolute pure awareness.

Throughout the ancient world, and in most indigenous and pagan traditions today, we find a similar worship of the sacred fire (Agni), sacred plants, trees, forests, and groves (Somas), sacred grottos, streams, lakes, and waters (Somas), sacred animals (particularly wild animals), the worship of the Sun (Surya), Moon, stars, and constellations, and the worship of Wind God (Indra), lighting, and the thundercloud. They worship that supreme pervasive power or Shiva as the sacred mountain, sacred rock, standing stone, or pyramid, as they worship his feminine counterpart Shakti as the sacred valley, river, cave, ring stone, or altar. Shaivite and Vedic Dharmas reflect the same teaching that arises out of nature and the cosmic mind, and is present for all those who are willing to embrace the deeper spirit. Whether one calls that Shiva or uses another name, the same teaching can be known by its insights and its practices.

Vedic Vaishnavism

As a closing note relative to other primary Hindu deity forms, Lord Vishnu can be identified with the Sun Gods or Adityas of the *Vedas*, among which his name first arises in the Vedic hymns. Vaishnava Dharma, like Shaivism, forms an integral part of the Vedic or Sanatana Dharma. Vishnu is also associated with the Vaishvanara form of Agni as the spiritual light within the heart or Narayana. He is said to be *Upendra* or the "companion of Indra." The iconic worship of Vishnu arose through the image of the solar Purusha, such as from the Vedic Vaikhanasa tradition that is still followed at great Vaishnava centers like Tirupati in South India. This would be the subject of another extensive study, but I did want to propose the idea, so that the approach to Shiva here is not looked at in a sectarian light. The unity of Shiva and Vishnu should also be considered.

In addition, a sophisticated Vaishnava view of the *Vedas* was developed centuries ago by the famous Vaishnava teacher, Madhva or Madhvacharya, the founder of the Dvaita or dualistic view of Vedanta, who lived in the twelfth century. Madhva, also called Ananda Tirtha, produced a brilliant commentary on the *Rigveda* from a Vaishnava perspective, of which the first forty hymns of the *Rigveda* are still available. His worked can be consulted in this regard and is important for any deeper Vedic studies.

The Secret of Vayu: The Cosmic Spirit

The term "spiritual" goes back to the word "spirit," which refers to the wind. This association is not incidental but reflects many deeper connections. The spirit like the wind represents an unseen invisible force that motivates all things and imparts life to all visible forms, though itself has no form.

The idea of spirit is commonly associated with the breath, the wind that animates our own bodies and minds. The outer wind of nature is reflected in the inner wind or breath within us. We are like winds or spirits trapped in the confines of the body, evidenced by the breath that keeps us alive. Air is the supreme element behind life and consciousness, imparting movement to body and mind. The mind with its fast movements and connections is said to be like wind in nature or as hard as the wind to control.

Many spiritual traditions refer to the Divine as the "Great Spirit," in order to discriminate it from the mere power of the breath or lesser spirits, gods, or powers of the wind and air. The Great Spirit is the universal breath, the breath behind the breath or wind behind the wind, what one could perhaps call "the breath of God." This is one of the early definitions of Brahman, the Godhead or Absolute of Vedic thought. The *Upanishads* call the *Vedas* the very breath of Brahman or the cosmic Spirit.[370]

At a lower level, spirit as the vital force reflects vigor, strength, courage, and daring. For example, we speak of a horse that runs fast and is hard to tame as high-spirited. The Spirit provides us energy and motivation, impelling us to seek success, superiority, dominion and transcendence in various ways. The state of our spirit is perhaps more important than that of our body or mind. A strong spirit can overcome innumerable afflictions on both physical and psychological levels.

Prana in Vedic thought does not simply equate with the breath or vital force, which is its lower manifestation but, at a higher level, with the energy of consciousness. This supreme energy of consciousness is the power of immortal life that does not die with the death of the body. The great prana (Maha Prana) behind the universe is the same as the great or cosmic Spirit.

Vayu, the Cosmic Spirit

"Vayu" is one of the key concepts of Vedic thought and has great importance in the Vedic Yoga and Vedic sciences. Vayu has profound implications at a cosmic level and relative to our individual lives. If one understands Vayu, one understands everything, including time, space, and karma, life and death, and one's own deeper Self. Vayu in various names and forms is one of the key Vedic deities. All Vedic deities can be described as different forms or aspects of Vayu as the power of the Spirit.

Vayu is regarded as the element of air at a material level. This is a good place to begin a study of Vayu, but only the start of many correspondences. In Vedic thought, Vayu includes the concept of space or Akasha. Space in motion is air, while air at rest is ether. These are the two sides of Vayu, which is the unity of air and ether. Ether is the field in which air as a force operates. Yet as air is prana, space is also mind. Vayu can be both.

Modern science recognizes that the universe consists of a fabric of space filled with various channels, currents, or wormholes that are filled with dynamic energies undergoing innumerable subtle interchanges. This is a good picture of the cosmic Vayu, which consists of the energy currents within space, both potential and actual. One could say that potential energy is space, while activated space is air. The universe itself is Vayu in its ethereal vibration.

However, Vayu is more than the material or subtle elements. Vayu is the power through which everything comes into manifestation and into which everything eventually returns. Vayu is the cosmic principle of energy and space that pervades body, life, mind, and consciousness. The entire manifest universe arises from space and energy, which is Vayu at an outer level. At an inner level, Vayu stands for the formless principle of air and space, the invisible Spirit or Brahman behind the visible world of the earth, water, and fire elements, the realm of name and form. The famous *Shantipatha* or opening Peace Chant of the *Taittiriya Upanishad* declares this:

> *Namaste, Vayu, you are the directly perceivable Brahman. As the directly perceivable Brahman I will address you.*[371]
> *Taittiriya Upanishad I.1*

Vayu symbolizes the supreme Deity in Vedic thought, the Spirit that is formless in nature, yet full of power like the wind or air. Vayu as the creative or causal force is the power of Ishvara or the cosmic Lord. Yet Vayu as the receptacle of all power and the ground of all existence can symbolize the Supreme Brahman beyond all manifestation. Vayu can refer to the presence of being and consciousness that exists everywhere but cannot be seen anywhere.

Vayu is the *Kriya Shakti* or universal power of action, from which all other powers emerge. It is the causal power that guides and directs things from within. The entire universe is a manifestation of Vayu, which is the hand of God that shapes all things. The very nature of Brahman is like Vayu, which is beyond all limitations, appearances and divisions. So Vayu is more than action and ultimately relates to the formless, changeless reality that creates the entire universe without undergoing any modification itself.

Vayu sets everything in motion at a cosmic level, which is its play or dance. Vayu governs all cosmic forces, movements, and actions – the movement of the stars and galaxies, the gravitational network underlying the universe, electromagnetic forces, and the forces that govern subatomic particles. Everything exists in Vayu, which is the field of space as energized by air. Vayu is the field of our existence that is the basis of our expression. Fire, water, and earth are but different densifications of the energy of Vayu, different degrees of its many currents.

Vayu is the connecting principle that links everything together in various force fields. From it mind, speech, and intelligence arise, allowing communication and interchange on all levels. Vayu creates various channels, currents, nadis, or orifices in its movement. These can be found in every object in nature and in the bodies of all creatures. All the channels of the nervous, respiratory, and circulatory systems, including the Sushumna nadi, are aspects of Vayu.

Deities in the Sphere of Vayu

Deities in the sphere of Vayu predominate in the *Vedas* like Indra, the foremost of the Vedic Gods, as well as Rudra, Brihaspati, and the Maruts. Indra is often called Vayu and Vata, synonyms for air or prana. Indra rules all the other Vedic deities including Agni, Surya, and Soma, the principles of Fire, Sun, and Moon that can only operate under the guiding power of Vayu. What is said about Indra in this book can help us understand the nature of Vayu.

Vayu though by nature invisible is not devoid of light, it is the matrix of all forms of light. Vayu holds the power of lightning or *Vidyut shakti* that sets all other forms of light in motion, just as the atmospheric lightning can start fire on earth. As the power of lightning, Vayu relates most to Indra, the supreme Vedic deity who governs the power of perception and the higher prana.

In ancient yogic thought like the *Brihat Yogi Yajnavalkya Smriti* it is said that Ishvara is Vayu or air and the soul or Jiva is Agni or fire, which both dwell in the heart.[372] Yoga consists of expanding our individual fire to merge into the cosmic air. Vayu is Ishvara, God as the ruling will, causing everything to move.

Other Upanishadic ways of knowledge like the *Samvarga Vidya* of the *Chandogya Upanishad* identify Vayu and prana as Brahman and the supreme resort of all (samvarga), which absorbs all things in the end.[373] Such teachings are not identifying Brahman with the air element, but using the air element as a symbol for Brahman as the supreme formless energy, power, and presence. Vayu is said in the *Upanishads* to be the *Sutra*, the thread that links everything together.[374] It is the subtle or energy body that links all physical forms in a network of forces through the chakras that it creates in its movement.

Vayu in the human body is prana or life-energy, which circulates in the form of various winds. Vata is prana or the cosmic life energy that manifests from Akasha or cosmic space. Prana is Vayu as the guiding force of life and intelligence in the universe. Vayu holds the pranas of all living beings in its energy network that links them all together in the web of life. The soul is a portion of Vayu that has entered into the body with the help of fire or Agni.

Vayu holds the cosmic prana or life-force from which our individualized prana comes into manifestation. Vayu is the cosmic breath, which enters into the individual as the individual power of breath. We connect to Vayu and prana through the breathing process. Pranayama allows us to work with and develop our connection with the cosmic prana. The purpose of pranayama is not just to bring in more air or give us more control over the breathing process, but also to link us to the unlimited energy of the cosmic Vayu. This occurs when we unite the dualistic energies of prana and mind so that our awareness can enter into the unitary force of Vayu.

The great prana mantras of *Hamsa* and *So'ham* are the vibrations of prana, the natural sound of the breath that is the presence of Vayu resonating within us. Yet at a higher level, prana mirrors Sat or pure existence. *Hamsa* and *So'ham* are the sounds of *Aham* or the Divine Self. When the prana enters into the sushumna or central channel, the individual prana connects to the cosmic Vayu, which allows our awareness to ascend and expand into Brahman.

Vayu is the Shakti or cosmic power that electrifies everything and without which everything is inert. Vayu manifests from the power of the Purusha as the energy inherent in consciousness, which is the power of prana or life itself. The lightning force of Vayu both creates life in creatures and sustains all inanimate processes in the universe. All the Devis or forms of Shakti are connected to Vayu, particularly Kali who represents the Vidyut Shakti and the Yoga Shakti that takes us back to Brahman.

This primal lightning of Vayu is the source of sound, which is the energy vibrating in space, the thunder that arises from it. This primal sound is Pranava, the Divine Word or Oṁ, which sets in motion the underlying cosmic intelligence that structures the worlds. As the principle of sound or vibration, Vayu is called Rudra (Shiva), through which speech and language arise. Vayu as primal sound is Pranava or Oṁ, which is the sound of Shiva's drum.

Vayu at rest serves to create the ground of space. Vayu in motion creates the movement of time, which is the vibration of cosmic sound. The movement of time is the movement of cosmic prana. This power of time or *Kala*[375] is the main force of Vayu through which everything moves and changes. Time like Vayu is responsible for the birth, growth, decay, and death of all creatures, and for the beginning, middle, and end of all processes. Kala, or time, is in turn connected with karma or action, which is the effect of Vayu. Vayu carries and distributes all the karmas of living beings and the worlds or lokas in which they reside.

Vayu and Vata: Internal Winds

There are many internal forms of Vayu, just as there are those of Agni. There are pranic forms that work in the physical body and its tissues and organs, sustaining the life-process on an unconscious level from cellular respiration to the conduction of nerve impulses through the brain and spine.

Vayu gives rise to *Vata dosha*, the biological air-humor, which is the dominant force governing the movement and development of life-energy in the body. There is the primary form of Vayu as the life breath working through the lungs, energizing the brain through the sinuses, and nourishing the skin along the surface of the body. The five pranas also called five Vayus (prana, apana, samana, udana, and vyana) are prominent in the *Upanishads* and mentioned in the *Vedas*.

The five sense organs have electrical or Vayu energies receiving and transmitting sensory information to the mind. The main Vayu senses are hearing, which relates to space and touch that relates to air. Sound is the main communicative force behind all our sensory and mental movements. Touch is the main connective force behind all of our actions and interactions. The cosmic Vayu maintains the music of the spheres. Vayu itself, particularly in the form of the great God Shiva is the cosmic dancer. The five motor organs are specific forms of Vayu discharging pranic impulses through the mouth, arms and hands, legs and feet, reproductive and eliminatory organs. Most important for Vayu is the vocal organ, followed by the hands.

Vata is the biological principle of movement, energy, change in location, velocity and creation of equilibrium, which sustains the organic network of forces within our bodies and minds down to an autonomic level. Vata dosha when calm and balanced gives health, while when agitated or disturbed causes disease. Vata moves Pitta and Kapha doshas, the biological fire and water humors, just as air moves fire and water, creating the vibrations that sustain them, allowing digestion to occur and our tissues to be built up and energized.

Vata dosha is the main life-energy (pranic force) behind health and disease in body and mind. It is air or Vayu as a psycho-physical principle. The body as a material entity adds a factor of doshas, meaning entropy or decay, to Vayu as a cosmic force. Vayu must eventually seek to leave the body and return back to its formless nature, which means that everything that is born must die by the same power of breath that gives it life in the first place.

One must master first Vayu in order to master any of the forces in the universe, in the body or in the mind. All healing occurs through the power of Vayu and its Pranic manifestations. By connecting to the cosmic Vayu we can bring in the cosmic prana. That is the key to all higher healing. In Yoga, the higher prana or cosmic Vayu takes us to the realm of immortality by removing our attachment to the body and giving us back our freedom as formless awareness beyond birth and death.

Vayu creates all the wonderful synapses in the brain through which our human intelligence can function. Vayu is the key to the mind and how it works. Our emotional psychology is the atmosphere created by the Vayu within us and its storms. Through harmonizing Vayu all psychological problems can be resolved. Vayu is the very thread that holds our life together. Its currents connect all levels of our being, with not only energy but also intelligence.

Cosmic Forms of Vayu

In the earth or at a mineral level, Vayu is responsible for earth currents and energy movements of all types including plate tectonics, earthquakes, and the gases held beneath the ground. When this earth Vayu beneath the ground moves, all living beings quiver in fear. A portion of the cosmic Vayu is hidden in the earth as the magnetic and electrical forces running through the planet. Serpents and snakes are the Vayu creatures in the ground, which have their powerful poisons.

In the biosphere, Vayu is the life-wind that functions in the lower atmosphere and the life-currents that flow along the surface of the earth. This life-wind stimulates and cleanses the plants, and aids in their pollination. It helps in the weathering of the rocks to create the soil. It carries pollen, dust, and prana, and is the home of airy creatures like birds. This benefic life Vayu keeps our bodies and mind clean and energized by its purifying flow.

The life-wind is connected to the water-wind that flows along rivers, across lakes and moves along with the ocean, stirring its waves and stimulating its currents. It carries moisture and vitality. The atmosphere has its own creatures as birds and flying insects of various types.

Vayu is the dominant force of the atmosphere, just as Agni is on earth, and the Sun in heaven. There are many atmospheric forms of Vayu as air, clouds, or gases in motion. Everything we see in the atmosphere is a form of Vayu, including the wind that has no form. The weather is mainly a force of Vayu. That is why exposure to the elements and changes of seasons mainly serves to increase Vata dosha. Meteorology is a study of Vayu or a *Vayu Vidya*.

All of us regularly experience the power of the wind. Strong winds are generally unpleasant. Light breezes are usually pleasant. These are the touch of Vayu or the hand of God. Vayu as the dominant force in the atmosphere rules over the weather through the seasons. He has many forms as wind, clouds, lightning, rain, dust, and space

As the wind, Vayu blows from various directions, in differing velocities, at different temperatures, and with different degrees of moisture, bringing in various energies, including those of a spiritual nature. Vayu gathers the water particles in the atmosphere in the form of clouds, and causes them to rain and bring nourishment to the earth. Dust in the atmosphere represents the particles of earth held by Vayu. The wind is a carrier. The wind is a purifier. It keeps everything in motion. As the master force, the atmospheric Vayu can create powerful storms. Hurricanes, typhoons, tidal waves, and tornadoes are among its more powerful manifestations.

Vayu is responsible for directional influences, such as are described in *Vastu Shastra*, which is an important consideration for clinics, hospitals, and treatment rooms. The different directional influences are special types of Vayus, the winds from different directions.

Vayu at the level of the solar system is responsible for the movement and revolution of the planets. The Sun itself has its solar wind or solar Vayu, its electromagnetic forces that hold the solar system together. The stars are gaseous forms of fire, sustained and generated by the powerful cosmic Vayu. At the level of the galaxy, Vayu is responsible for the movement and revolution of the stars. The galaxies themselves are smoke clouds created by the cosmic Vayu. Vayu governs the creation and equilibrium of the universe as a whole, yet stands beyond the universe as well.

Another atmosphere exists between the stars in which an interstellar or cosmic Vayu operates. Various types of winds and electrical currents come forth from the stars, galaxies, quasars, and black holes. Gravity is another force of Vayu that links the heavenly bodies together. Even the galactic clouds have their lightning through which stars are born.

Control of Vayu

Our modern technology rests upon certain outer powers of Vayu like electricity, combustion engines, and jet propulsion. This technological power over Vayu allows us to run electrical equipment and accomplish actions with speed, power, and efficiency. The mass media itself is another power of Vayu with its currents of communication through the atmosphere driven by radio waves. Yet though modern humanity has a better control over the outer Vayu through technology, we have probably less control over our inner Vayu or mind and prana. This is because we are disturbed by the outer Vayu, which works through inorganic energies that can disturb or short circuit the human nervous system. The modern person through computers and the media is addicted to an outer form of Vayu that can distract us from connecting to the higher Vayu within.

Controlling Vayu is one of the most difficult of all things, but it is the basis of Yoga Sadhana. It proceeds through purifying and calming body, speech, senses, mind, and prana. There is a trick, however. Only Vayu can control Vayu. The human ego cannot control Vayu but remains under the rule of many different forms of Vayu. Only the cosmic Vayu can control our individual Vayu and the prana and mind that are ruled by it. This cosmic Vayu is rooted in the Atman, the inner Self. By rooting our awareness in the Atman, we connect to the cosmic Vayu and have the power to master all things.

The Atman stands at the center of all the currents and forces of Vayu, which are but its outer expressions. If we hold to that center, then all the powers of the universe must revolve around us. Nothing in the world will be able to disturb us, just as the axis of a wheel cannot be disturbed by the movement of its periphery. The Self is the Vayu behind Vayu, the source of all energy, power, and prana, hidden in the cavern of the heart. From the Self-in-heart radiates all energies and powers. The Self is the link between all beings and all worlds. Resting in our own being we can hold all power and accomplish all things without trying to do anything at all.

Vayu Names and Forms

Vayu's many names refer mainly to its energy and its power.

- *Vāyu* itself refers to expansion and vibration, particularly as the cosmic energy.
- *Vāta* refers to Vayu's nature as the cosmic life force.
- *Vidyut*, lightning or electrical energy.
- *Marut* indicates his lightning vibrations.
- *Rudra* as the power to create sound.

- *Niyutvan* indicates his ability to network and link together.
- *Bṛhaspati*, the lord of the Divine Word as the maker of sound and mantra.
- *Parjanya*, as the power of storm and rain.
- *Indra*, as the lord or ruling power.

Three of these names of Vayu are most important. Indra represents Vayu as a power of perception, the lightning of the force of consciousness and Self-realization. Rudra, the prototype of Shiva represents Vayu as primal sound, which is manifest through the Divine Word Oṁ. Vata is Vayu as the force of life in creatures that is the great healer. Vayu like Indra and the Maruts is an important deity for drinking or absorbing the Soma, the Spirit that absorbs our soul and life-experience back into itself. This is particularly true of the Vayu in the head or the crown chakra that absorbs the Soma there.

Vayu is represented by several groups of deities, the Maruts, that represent the powers of Vayu, the Rudras, which represent its sound forces, and the Indras, which represent its perceptive forces. In later Hindu symbolism Vayu is associated with Shiva and Bhairava, and with Goddesses like Kali and Bhairavi. Hanuman is the son of Vayu and a form of Shiva. We will discuss more about Vayu and *Vayu Yoga* in the next chapter on Indra.

While the first hymn of the *Rigveda* is to Agni, the second is to Vayu.

> *Come, O beautiful Spirit (Vayu). These Somas are prepared for you. Drink of these and hear our call.*[376]
> *Madhuchchhandas Vaishvamitra, Rigveda I.2.1*

Vayu as the cosmic spirit in the head, drinks the Soma of the crown chakra, taking the offering of the mind and soul represented by it. The Vedic Yoga is not just about realizing the Sun as the Divine light of the Self within, but also about releasing the Vayu, the Spirit encased in the body.

> *Increased by the power of surrender, the ancient Gods were free of fault. They for the Spirit (Vayu), for the human being in bondage, illuminated the Dawn by the Sun.*[377]
> *Maitravaruni Vasishtha, Rigveda VII.61.1*

Indra Yoga: The Yoga of the Supreme Self

Throughout the various religious traditions of the world there is a recognition of God, the Lord, the Ruler or the Creator – a Supreme Being or higher principle behind the manifest universe. Early ancient humanity was no different, but simply recognized that Supreme Lord in a greater variety of names and forms, reflecting a broader and perhaps more tolerant perception of the sacred, and one more inclusive of life and nature.

The Vedic tradition is firmly rooted in an awareness of the Supreme, not merely as the Creator of the universe, but also as the Absolute and higher Self beyond time and space. The foremost of the Vedic Gods is Indra, which literally means "the Lord." Indra represents that which is greatest, highest, most powerful and vast, as well as that which is most beneficent, compassionate, caring, and befriending – traits reflected in the many Vedic hymns dedicated to him.

Indra is the same ruling power as God, the Divine will, and wisdom, later honored as *Ishvara* in Vedantic philosophy. The two words Indra and Ishvara are synonyms, meaning "lord." Indra is the form in which the Vedic-seer poets visualized the Supreme. Indra is the power behind the Vedic chants, which are mainly hymns of praise directed to the supreme Lord and formations of the Divine Word or primal sound.

> *All the chants glorify Indra as bounteous as the sea, the chariot lord of all chariot lords, the ruler of all powers, the lord.* [378]
> *Rigveda I.11.1*

In later India, the name Indra came to refer to the lord of heaven only, a lesser deity, not the supreme deity, and to a being subject to desire, limitation, and ignorance. This Indra of the *Puranas* should not be confused with Indra of the *Vedas*. Vedic Indra is akin to Shiva as the supreme Lord of all. He sustains both heaven and earth and is not limited by time and space. His actions are rooted in the Soma, which is the supreme bliss. He generates the Divine Light of awareness. He not only creates the worlds but also enters into them as the inner Self of all creatures. This reflects the Vedic view that the individual soul is a manifestation of the Supreme Brahman.

> *Indra's actions are well done and manifold, all the Gods do not diminish his laws, who upholds earth and heaven, and possessing magic powers generates the Sun and the Dawn.* [379]

> *Inviolable is the truth of your greatness, when suddenly born, you drank the Soma. Indra, the heavens cannot limit your strength or your power, nor can the days, nor the months, nor the years.*[380]
>
> *When suddenly born, you drank the Soma for ecstasy in the supreme ether, then you entered into heaven and earth and became the original support of the seers.*[381]
>
> *Gathina Vishvamitra, Rigveda III.32.8*

Indra like Ishvara is God as the creator and the lord of all, with the entire universe under his power and reflecting his energy.

> *Let us now declare the greatness of his great actions, the truths of the truth. In the formless realm he upheld vast heaven, and he filled heaven and earth, and the atmosphere. He upheld and extended the earth. This is what Indra accomplished in the ecstasy of Soma.*[382]
>
> *Gritsamada Shaunaka, Rigveda II.15.1, 2*

We may find the Vedic symbolism of Indra difficult to understand as the supreme cosmic Lord. Indra's drinking of Soma symbolizes the state of bliss absorption behind all manifestation. The state of transcendence, such as Indra represents, takes us beyond all ordinary dualities and conventions. The language is magical, cataclysmic, transformational, paradoxical, and awesome.

God and the Absolute

Indra, like the Brahman in Vedantic thought, is not simply a theistic image. Indra as Brahman has two aspects as *saguna*, with qualities, and *nirguna*, without qualities. With qualities, at a cosmic level, Indra is *Ishvara*, the ruling power behind the creation, preservation and dissolution of the universe, much like God in theistic traditions or Saguna Brahman. Without qualities, at a cosmic level, Indra is the Supreme Self, Absolute, or Supreme Brahman, the formless Godhead beyond all manifestation, Nirguna Brahman.[383] In addition, at an individual level in the human being, Indra is Atman or the inner Self, which can become one with Ishvara, the cosmic Lord, or with the Supreme Brahman beyond all time and space. It is that Indra or Paramatman that enters into the individual soul.

> *Indra extends beyond heaven and earth. Half of him is equal to both the worlds.*
>
> *That is the truth (Satya), Indra there is no other God or mortal greater than you.*

You are the king of the creatures of the world. You generated together the Sun, heaven and the Dawn.[384]

Bharadvaja Barhaspatya, Rigveda VI.30.1,4,5

Only a portion of this Indra consciousness is manifest through heaven and earth; an equal portion dwells beyond all manifestation as the Absolute. The worship of the Divine as both the cosmic lord and as the Absolute behind the universe, as in later Vedantic thought, is present in a symbolic form as the worship of Indra, just as in later times it took the symbolic form of Shiva. Indra reflects the Vedic foundation for the philosophy of Advaita or non-dualist Vedanta. Indra as the Supreme Self is beyond all otherness. There is nothing other than him.

If, Indra, if we extended the earth tenfold and multiplied it by the days and by all creatures, then Maghavan your glorious power would still be with strength and energy transcending heaven.[385]

You in the Supreme region of space by your own Self-power, for grace, of powerful mind, you have made the world an image of your strength. You have pervaded with energy the waters, the Sun world, and move beyond heaven.[386]

You are the prototype of the earth. You are the lord of the vast with sublime and heroic strength. You have pervaded the atmosphere with greatness. That is the Truth. There is no other like you.[387]

Savya Angirasa, Rigveda I.52.11-13.

The *Upanishads* quote the *Rigveda* relative to Indra as the ruler of Maya, for explaining the Self (Atman) that is the ruler of Maya.

Indra is the counter form of all forms. That is his form for the counter vision. Indra by his Maya power moves in manifold forms. His horses are yoked a thousand.

Garga Bharadvaja, Rigveda VI.47.18, Brihadaranyaka Upanishad II.5.19

His horses are ten and many thousands, and unlimited. That is this Brahman that has nothing before or after, within or without, that Self is Brahman, the experience of all.[388]

Brihadaranyaka Upanishad II.5.19

Indra is perhaps the foremost of the Vedic deities involved with the yoking process that contains the basis of the idea of later Yoga as a coordination of our faculties and energies. His two horses, which are mind and prana, are yoked to his chariot.

Indra is the greatest of the charioteers. Here we can also understand Indra's role as the lord of the senses (Indriyas or powers of Indra).

Indra by his Maya power is the counter form of all forms. All forms are his form. Pure consciousness is the inner energy behind all manifestation. Indra's thousand horses are the many minds and pranas of living beings. He brings these under his yogic power. Indra is ultimately the supreme Self who controls the Maya of the world. His martial symbolism and his destruction of the serpent and dragon (the powers of ignorance), reflects his negation of the manifest realm into the unmanifest Supreme Brahman.

A verse to the Universal Gods in the *Rigveda* reflects this great non-dual truth of Indra:

> *You are the good guardian, not to be deceived, you of good judgment. Beyond all Maya, your name is truth (paro māyābhir ṛta āsa nāma te).*[389]
>
> *Avatsara Kashyapa, Rigveda V.44.2*

Indra as the Ruling Power or Master Force: the Supreme Self

Indra represents that which is highest and best in all beings. We can speak of whatever is predominant in its particular field as its ruler or its Indra. Whatever is the greatest, most powerful, or most successful is the Indra, the ruler or the lord in that context. Indra is the ruling power of the fire on earth, the wind in the atmosphere, and the Sun in heaven, which are the Indras of the three worlds. More specifically, Indra is the mountain on the earth and the thundercloud in the atmosphere that brings the rain. In society, Indra is the ruler or the king.

The term Indra also refers to the power of perception, which is our main guiding sense. At an individual level, the eye is the guide or Indra of the senses. Prana is the Indra or guide of the body as a whole. The mind is Indra and the senses are called Indriyas or powers of Indra. The Buddhi or Dhi is the guide or Indra of the mind. The Atman or Purusha, the inner Self, is the guide or the Indra of the being as a whole. Relative to the chakras, Indra is the third eye or the center of command.

Indra relates to the supreme principle of *Sat* and *Satya*, Being and Truth, the presence behind all things that leads us to transcendence.

> *Carrying your power, bear your hymns of affirmation to Indra as the Truth (Satya), if in truth he exists. "There is no Indra, some say to you. Who has seen him? Why should we praise him."*[390]

"I am here, O singer, perceive me here. I transcend all beings by greatness, the directions of truth increase me, as the one who breaks things open, I break open the worlds".[391]

Nema Bhargava, Rigveda VIII.89.3-4

The ultimate ruling power behind the mind, prana, and senses is the sense of Self or I. Indra represents this Divine Self or seer, the "I am" or *aham*. This "I" or *aham* is the basis of all our pranas. It is the supreme prana that is our own life.

The "I" is the basis of all sounds and words. Aham in Sanskrit reflects the alphabet whose first letter is a and last letter is *ha*. Indra is this Divine *aham*, the "I am that I am." It is for this reason that all the Vedic chants are said to enter into Indra as rivers into the sea. Indra is the Divine Self that is the essence of all mantras. Indra is the bija or seed mantra, akshara, which in the *Upanishads* is identified with Oṁ. In Vedic symbolism, Indra is the manifestation of the Divine Self or the realization of the Divine I am. Indra gives us the power of our own deepest Self, the confidence to move the entire universe and master all forces.

The supreme spiritual energy that is Indra is the prime evolutionary force in nature. It is the inner Self that impels all creatures to grow, expand, and develop in various ways. That self-sense is ever motivating us to accomplish something new and to develop new faculties within us. This is another reason that I have called Indra the Master force. It compels us to seek mastery, with the highest mastery being mastery over our own selves. Indra is the ruling power, the seeking of self-supremacy that rules the universe. Indra is the Self of all creatures that causes us to seek Self-expression and Self-realization. Indra thus contains all the Gods.

Great, O seers, is that blissful Name, that all the Gods exist in Indra. A friend with the beloved Ribhus, manifoldly called, fashion this insight for the realization.[392]

Gathina Vishvamitra, Rigveda III.54.17.

Indra as Prana and Vayu

Indra represents prana as not only the life-force and power of the atmosphere but the cosmic energy that pervades all space. Indra is the original, great or *Maha Prana* that is the lord of the mind and senses. This ultimate prana is the Purusha itself, the Prana Purusha often referred to in the *Upanishads*. Invoking Indra is literally calling down the Great Spirit and the original life force in which is immortality. Indra as the master force in the universe is the will and power of God as it were, guiding all creation from above. Once Agni or the soul has matured, Indra enters into him and he eventually comes forth as the Supreme Purusha, the cosmic Being.

Indra is most commonly associated with Vayu as the cosmic Spirit. Like Vayu, Indra is lauded as the deity ruling the atmosphere (Antariksha). Both Indra and Vayu represent the air and ether elements, and the power of the spirit. Most of what was explained under Vayu applies to Indra as well. The difference is that Indra relates more to the ruling power of the spirit, while Vayu reflect its pervasive presence. Another difference is that Indra relates to the perceptive power of the Spirit, while Vayu relates more to the energy of the breath. Indra and Vayu are lauded together relative to meditation and the ability to yogically control the mind:

> *They (the seers) meditating with a truthful mind (satyena manasā dīdhyānāḥ), move yogically controlled by their own will power. Indravayu, to the hero-carrying chariot of you the lords, delights attend.*[393]
> *Maitravaruni Vasishtha, Rigveda VII.90.5*

Main Names of Indra

Indra has many names in the *Vedas* of which the most important include these:

- *Indra* – the lord of perception, the seer, the supreme ruler
- *Maghavan* – the great giver of abundance
- *Śatakratu* – who has a hundredfold will power
- *Śacipati* – the lord of power or the Goddess energy
- *Vṛtrahan* – the destroyer of Vritra as obstructions, ignorance, the serpent
- *Harivan* – who has two gold horses, dual powers of prana and apana, inhalation and exhalation
- *Vajrī* or *Vajrabhṛt* – wielder of the vajra, thunderbolt, or power of enlightenment
- *Purandara* – destroyer of the city or citadel, the body as the seat of the ignorance
- *Vṛṣa* or *Vṛṣabha* – the cosmic bull or Purusha principle
- *Marutvan* – lord of the Maruts or subtle electrical energies

As the world ruler, Indra works behind all the other deities. Indra is often invoked as a dual deity with other deities. This is because he represents what is supreme in all the deities. There are many dual deities with Indra in the Vedic hymns as Indra-Agni, Indra-Soma, Indra-Surya, Indra-Vishnu, Indra-Varuna, Indra-Pushan, Indra-Brihaspati, Indra-Vayu, and Indra-Vata. Indra has his consort as Shachi, who indicates the power of Shakti. Even the Goddess Sarasvati is compared to Indra through her ruling power of speech and mantra.

Goddess Sarasvati we call when the wealth is placed, like Indra in the piercing of the obstructer.[394]
Bharadvaja Barhaspatya, Rigveda VI.61.5

Ganapati Muni recognizes four main powers of Indra. These are 1) space, which includes the space of consciousness; 2) time, which includes primordial sound and prana; 3) the Sun, which includes all forms of light; and 4) the electrical force or Shakti working within the worlds.[395] He regarded Indra as the Supreme Consciousness in the universe that is the basis of space, time, light, and energy.

Indra Dhi and Indra Yoga

The *Upanishads* provide three important keys to the reality of Indra at a yogic level.

- First, Indra is the seer. Among the Vedic deities he most represents the Purusha or cosmic person that is the witness of all. Indra is the cosmic spirit that enters into the body from the top of the head. This occurs in the *Aitareya Upanishad.*

"He saw that Purusha as Brahman, as 'I have seen that.' Thus his name was *Idandra* (the seer of that). Though his name was *Idandra*, he is called Indra, as the Gods prefer what is secret."[396]

- Second, Indra is the bull or guiding power of the chants or Vedic mantras. Indra represents primal sound, nada, mantra, and Pranava. This occurs in the *Taittiriya Upanishad.*

"Who is the bull of the chants and has all forms, who is born from the immortal chants, may that Indra deliver me with wisdom."[397]

- Third, Indra is prana and ayus, immortal life. Indra is the power of awakening prana through which Divine grace pours into us from above. This occurs in the *Kaushitaki Upanishad.*

"He (Indra) said, I am Prana, the Self of intelligence, as the immortal life, worship me."[398]

Indra is Ishvara, the original Lord of creation through his lightning force. Dhi Yoga occurs when the heart and mind are united by the power of wisdom. Dhi is the intelligence of the heart, which seeks the Lord.

To Indra by heart and mind, to the original lord, the wise purify their intelligence.[399]
Nodhas Gautama, Rigveda I.61.2

The following verse is from a hymn to Brihaspati, the lord of speech. He is connected with Indra, the lord of the mind and senses. The sacrifice of the illumined is the inner sacrifice of Yoga.

> *The wonderful lord of reality, the beloved of Indra: May I attain the victorious wisdom (sanim medhām). Without which the sacrifice of the illumined is not complete, he directs the Yoga of intelligence (sa dhīnām yogam invati).*
>
> *Medhatithi Kanva, Rigveda I.18.6-7*

Indra generates from the truth, the intelligence or insight (Dhi) that is yoked to the mind (*manoyujam*).

> *Indra, wielder of the thunder, you are your worshippers protector. From the truth I generate your insight yoked to the mind.*[400]
>
> *Narada Kanva, Rigveda VIII.13.26*

Indra as the awareness of the Self that manifests in human beings is the natural ruler of the mind.

> *Indra, who was born as the first ruler of the mind.*[401]
>
> *Gritsamada Shaunaka, Rigveda II.12.1*

Indra as the force of prana is closely connected with Vayu or the power of the wind. Both are lords of insight. Here Vayu is the power of the Spirit, not simply the air element.

> *Indra and Vayu, with the speed of the mind, sages call you for aid, you who have a thousand eyes and are the lords of insight (dhiyaspatī).*[402]
>
> *Medhatithi Kanva, Rigveda I.23.3*

Part V
The Way of the Rishi

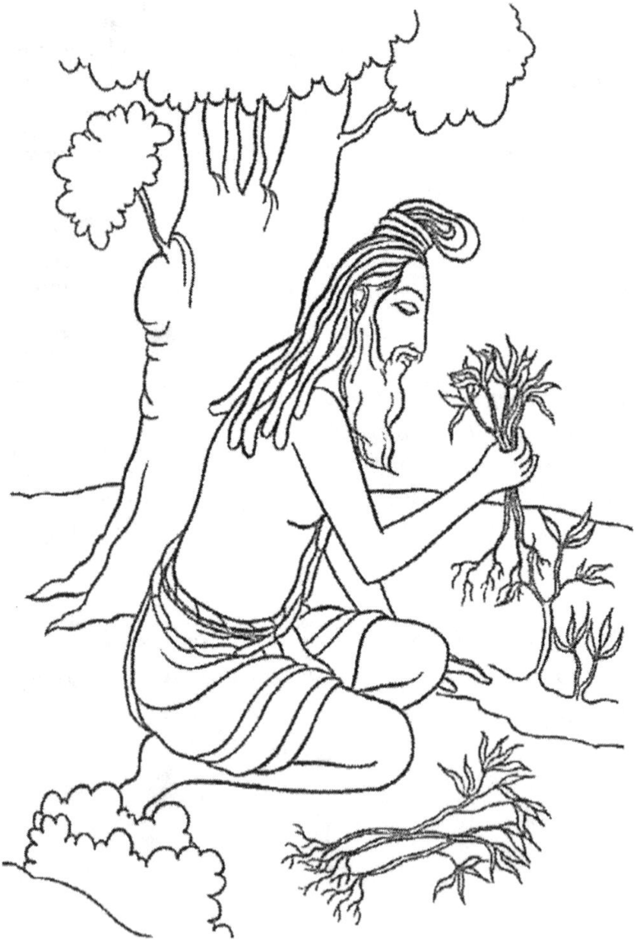

Pictures of Great Modern Rishis

In the following chapter are photographs of the great modern Vedic Rishis mentioned in the book: Kavyakantha Ganapati Muni, Brahmarshi Daivarata, Ramana Maharshi, K. Natesan, Sri Sadguru Sivananda Murty, Sri Aurobindo, Kapali Shastry and M.P. Pandit.

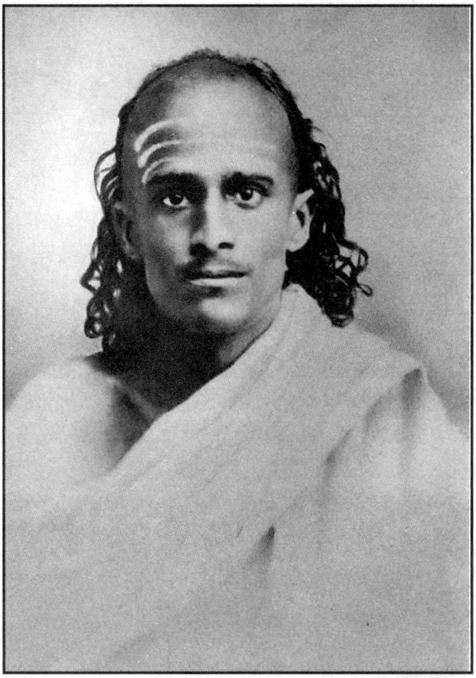

Kavyakantha Ganapati Muni, seer-poet of modern India, chief disciple of Bhagavan Ramana Maharshi, in his early years

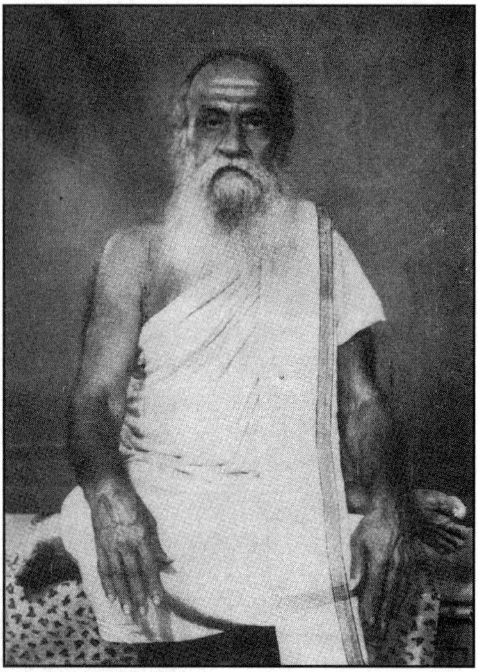

Brahmarshi Daivarata, chief disciple of Kavyakantha Ganapati Muni, guide to Maharishi Mahesh Yogi

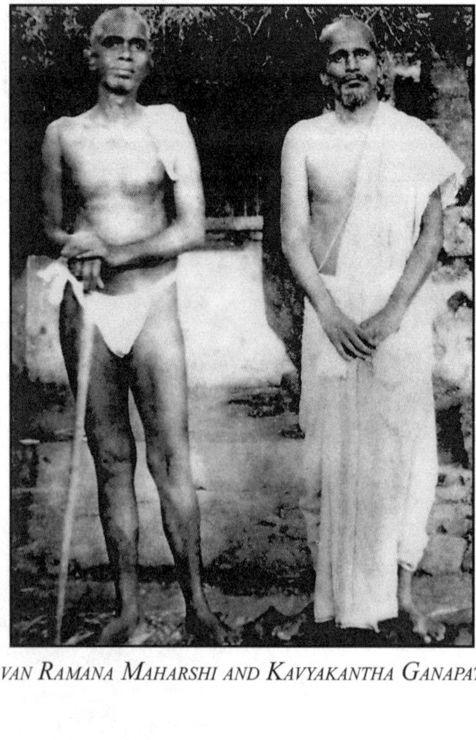

Bhagavan Ramana Maharshi and Kavyakantha Ganapati Muni

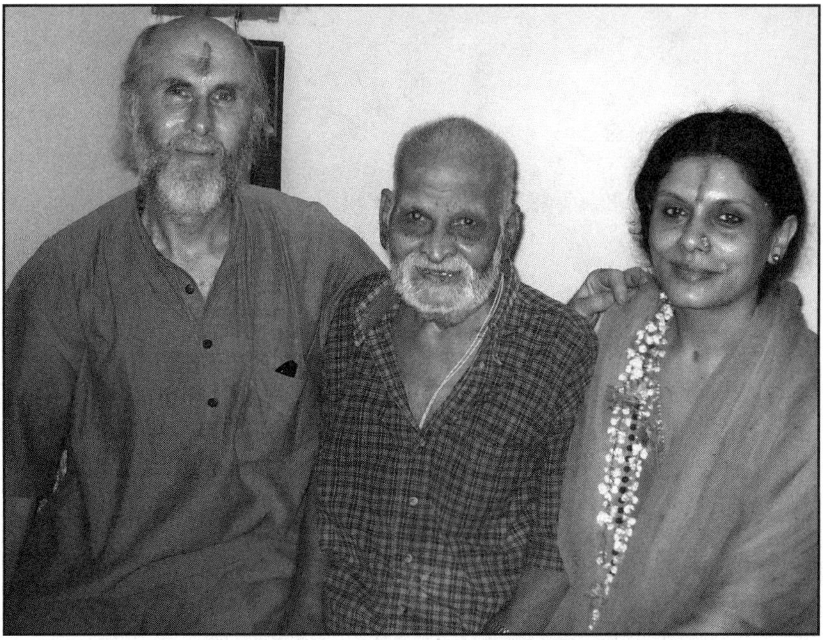

VAMADEVA, YOGINI SHAMBHAVI, AND K. NATESAN IN 2009, SHORTLY BEFORE HIS PASSING

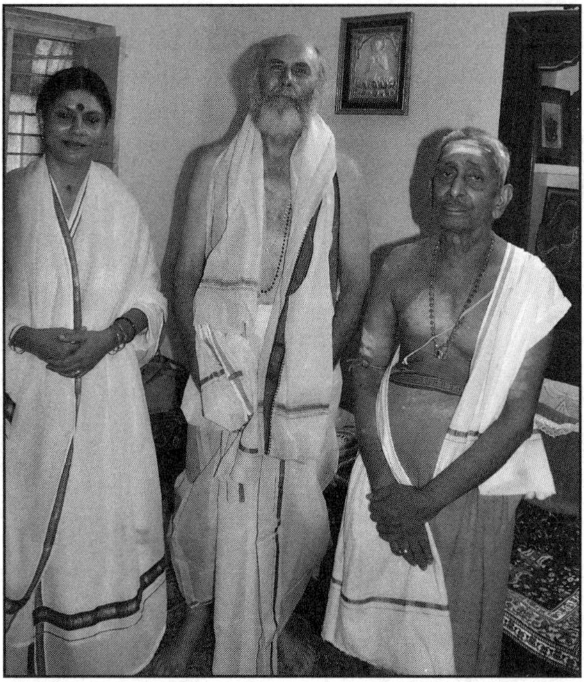

SRI SADGURU SIVANANDA MURTY, VAMADEVA SHASTRI AND YOGINI SHAMBHAVI

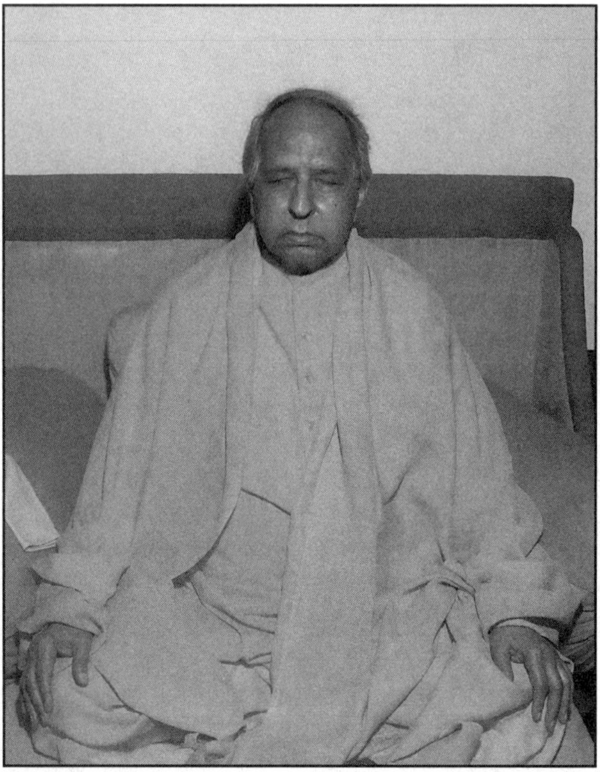

Swami Veda Bharati, seer of the Rigveda and the Yoga Sutras

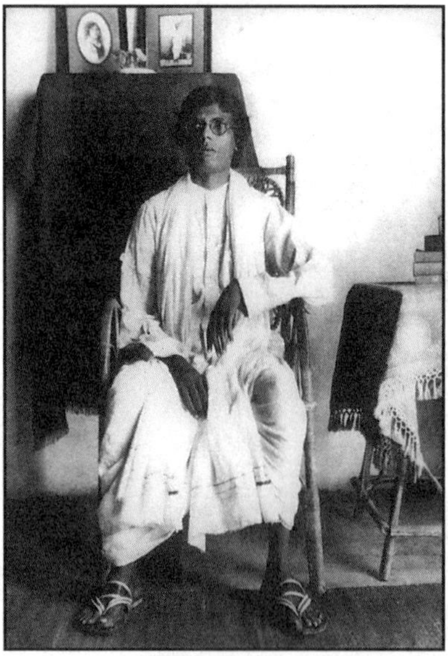

Kapali Shastry

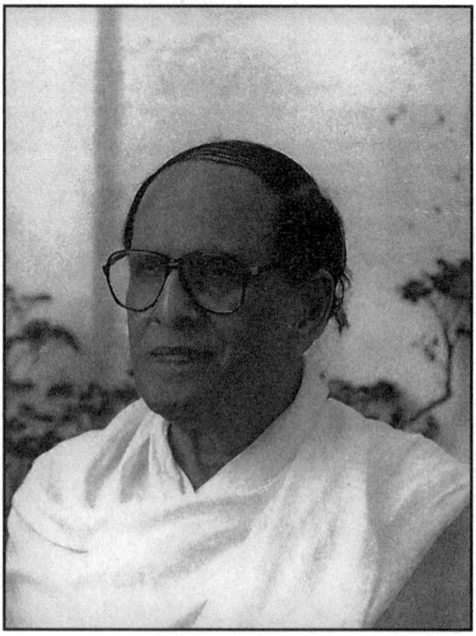

Sri M.P. Pandit

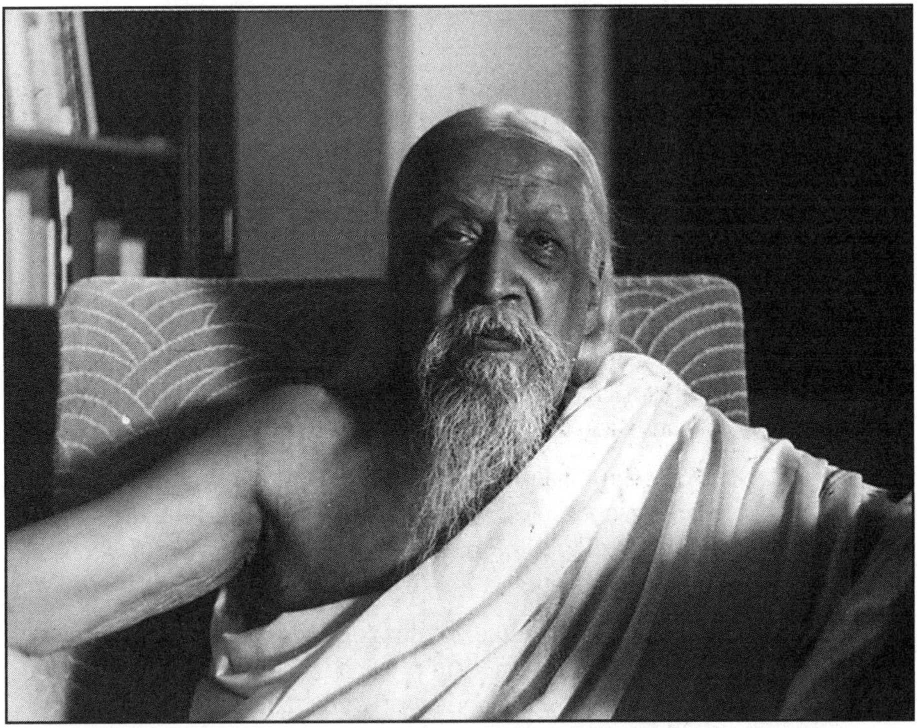

Sri Aurobindo

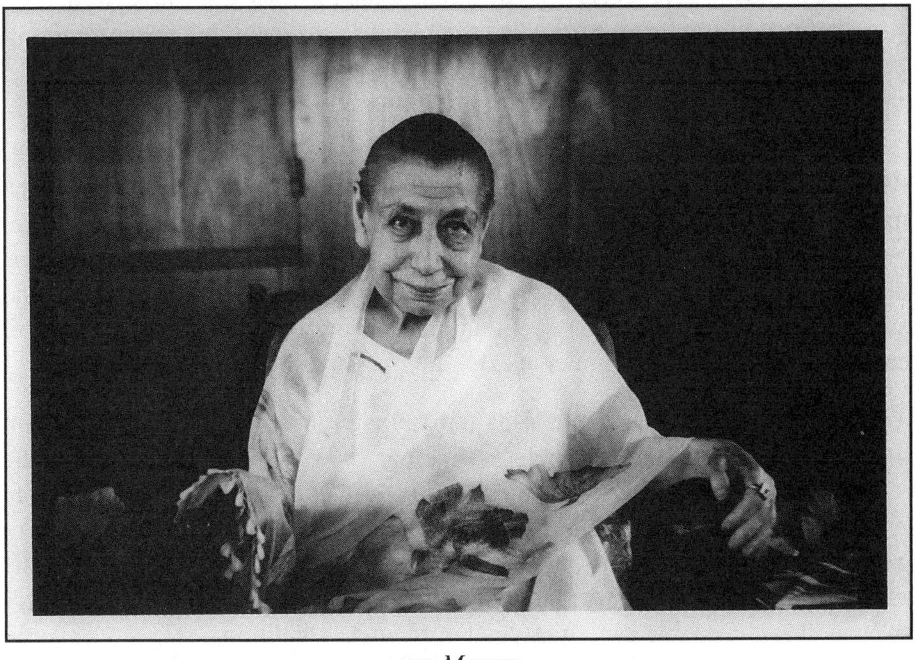

the Mother

Keys to the Vedic Rishi Yoga

The practice of the Vedic Yoga is part of a great art, labor, and sadhana extending through many lifetimes – the many births of the Vedic fire of the soul (Jivagni) by the power of the Rishis. The Vedic Yoga has numerous dimensions, manifestations, and energies that continually work to expand our awareness and break down our limiting concepts. To be able to realistically approach practicing the Vedic Yoga ourselves, we must consider certain key points:

- First, we must remember that the Vedic Yoga comes from a different world-age and reflects a different mentality and perception of self and world. It requires a change of mind and heart, a radical shift of our perception outwardly and inwardly for us to appreciate the Vedic language.
- Second, the Vedic approach is individualistic and requires adaptation of teachings and practices at a personal level. We need to understand our own unique nature and the balance of our energies, karmas, and capacities, along with their variations over time.
- Third, because the basis of the Vedic Yoga is mantric, it requires knowledge of Vedic Sanskrit, not simply at a technical level but at the level of inspiration. A mere memorization of certain chants along their right pronunciation and intonation may not be enough. One must know the meaning, essence, and application of the mantras at the level of the spiritual heart. A living knowledge of Vedic Sanskrit is indispensible to enter into the Vedic mind. While much of later Yoga and Vedanta can be understood in an English idiom, it is extremely difficult to do this with the Veda that is symbolic in nature.

Above all, developing the Vedic Yoga depends upon leading a Vedic life, which means having Vedic values and looking at the world in a Vedic light. This requires being connected to nature at the level of the heart and not having our minds dominated by the human world. We must be able to feel the land, waters, air, and sky, as well as the rocks, plants, and animals in our own blood, with our spirit encompassing all that we perceive extending beyond the horizons.

Yet if the summits of the Vedic Yoga remain daunting, Vedic teachings contain many dharmic approaches to help us live our lives rightly, through the Vedic sciences of Ayurveda, Vedic astrology, and Vastu. The truth is that the human mind, with its collective karmas, is quite limiting for everyone. It is difficult to become free of its distortions, even if we can avoid them most of the time. Vedic teachings contain many tools and insights to awaken the Yoga Shakti or power of Yoga that can enable us to transcend our human condition.

Rishi Yoga

The Rishi is one who has fully mastered the Vedic Yoga and become one with the Vedic deities in the experience of samadhi. Such a Rishi can create new Vedic teachings and new cultural forms for the upliftment of humanity, promoting a spiritual renaissance in the outer world.

The Rishi is a realized soul who carries the cosmic creative and evolutionary force that is the essence of life. For this reason, Rishis have been classified in Vedic and Puranic thought as a special order of beings, a level above the human. Through the Rishi Yoga one can enter into the cosmic order of the Rishis, and into Rishi Loka or realm of the Rishis, from which perpetual blessings, guidance, and creative powers perpetually flow into the earth consciousness. One can open the Rishi vision within and access the Rishi Prana that guides all pranas to a higher level of expression. The Rishi does not die and can take birth at will, or he may simply work through his subtle energy body, without needing to take on another physical form.

Becoming a Rishi resembles becoming a great Yogi in the Raja Yoga tradition or a Siddha. It requires tremendous work on body, heart, and mind, from the deepest subconscious levels to the highest consciousness. This entails a great deal of tapas and sadhana, including that performed outdoors in nature, not simply in front of a computer. It is a matter of total immersion in the practice without seeking any personal goal or result, not a short term practice or an expectation of instant enlightenment.

The Rishi Yoga requires the highest Self-knowledge just as in the Yoga of Knowledge, along with a well developed and articulate mind and a capacity for great silence. It also depends upon the most consummate Bhakti or devotion, particular to the Goddess who is the Shakti of all higher evolutionary transformations. It similarly requires a decisive and dynamic power of action and ritual as in Karma Yoga.

In addition to the skills and attainments of an integral Yoga, the Rishi Yoga requires that one must be an occultist who can read the secret forces of nature, whether those on the earth, in the atmosphere, or in the cosmic Space beyond. It benefits from an understanding of the energies of Ayurveda and the inner powers of healing. It similarly benefits from an understanding of Vedic astrology as to right timing and connecting to celestial influences.

One should be able to work with the forces of nature, something like the role of a shaman. One should be receptive to the secret powers of the plants and trees like an herbal healer. One should be able to communicate with the nature spirits in the mountains and in the valleys. One should know how to commune with animals and understand the consciousness and energy that they carry. One should be able to connect with the forces of the wind, clouds, and atmospheric energies and their subtle effects. One needs a sense of the cosmic light and intelligence in fire, lightning, Sun, and Moon.

One must be a poet who knows the secret messages of our deepest emotions and of the moods of nature. One must be a philosopher who knows the secrets of being, immanent and transcendent, both the creative and the absolute. One must be capable of envisioning new cultures and new civilizations through the power of the cosmic mind, which can integrate all human potentials outer and inner. Yet these powers and insights should be subordinated to a deeper Self-knowledge and a surrender to the Divine within. We can look to such examples as Sri Aurobindo and Kavyakantha Ganapati Muni for what an accomplished Vedic Yogi is likely to resemble in modern times.

The Vedic Rishi Yoga is not a matter of individual effort, though it may begin with personal striving. One benefits from becoming attuned to the "Rishi consciousness" or *Rishi Chaitanya*, through one of the traditional Rishi lines or Gotras. A Rishi life means living with the *Vedas*, studying, and chanting them regularly as part of a regular practice of ritual, mantra and meditation, with the Vedic deities awake and vibrant both within and around us. One needs to study the Vedic teachings in depth, not merely reading texts but comprehending the structure of Vedic mantric knowledge in the cosmic mind.

All souls are evolving toward becoming world-creating seers and Rishis, which is the full development of our inner nature and its creative Shakti. We are all evolving to become world-creating beings, our own Sun with its own planets and life-forms. This is part of our eonic soul journey, of which our current life is but a brief episode—a few mere steps along the way.

This Rishi path is slowly returning, as the light of the ancients gains more respect in the modern world. As our culture slowly integrates the various paths of Yoga and spiritual traditions of humanity, out of that synthesis a new Rishi order will likely arise. We need to once more promote the Rishi ideal and should not be content with outer scientific and technological gains.

We can enter into the Rishi Yoga at any point that we have the aspiration. It is now a realistic path available in several forms, and a point of integration for many other teachings. If a Vedic aspiration arises within us, it must eventually lead us to our highest goal.

How to Practice the Vedic Yoga

There are several ways to approach the Vedic Yoga. First, we should study the Vedic teachings, starting with the *Bhagavad Gita* and classical *Upanishads*. Second, we should learn enough Sanskrit to be able to understand the Vedic deity names and qualities. Third, we should connect ourselves with one of the modern Vedic teachers and traditions, and move into its practices. In addition there are a few helpful approaches we can take:

Begin With Ayurveda

We can perhaps easiest begin to practice the Vedic Yoga and understand the Vedic deities through working with the three doshas or biological humors of Vata, Pitta, and Kapha, the biological counterparts of the Indra, Agni, and Soma energies of the *Vedas*. This will provide a practical means of encountering and learning to work with the energies of the Vedic deities.

We should then move to the subtle level of Ayurvedic practice by working to develop the higher energies of Prana, Tejas, and Ojas, the master forms of Vata, Pitta, and Kapha, which reflect the energies of Indra, Agni, and Soma as forces of healing and transformation.[403]

Energetic Yoga Practices Both Vedic and Tantric

The next step after Ayurveda is to learn to work with the corresponding Agni, Vayu, and Soma forces of Yoga through the seven chakras as taught in Hatha, Kundalini, Siddha, and Tantric Yogas. This involves learning how to raise the Agni-Kundalini fire from the root chakra for purification purposes and allowing the Soma-nectar from the crown chakra to descend for revitalization purposes. The heart as the region of the Sun or Prana is their place of unification where we can hold both forces together. Learn to work with the Vedic deities as the powers of the chakras, nadis, and subtle body.

Mantra Yoga along with Pranayama and Meditation

Once we have learned to work with the Vedic energies inside ourselves, then their specific yogas can gradually unfold for us. This can take us in the direction of any of the Vedic Yoga approaches taught in this book, either singularly or in combination. It involves specifically awakening the Vedic deities within ourselves.

An important way to approach the Vedic deities is to regularly chant a few special Vedic verses by way of Mantra Yoga and with the power of devotion. One can recite them mentally along with the breath as a kind of Vedic pranayama, and also meditate upon their meaning. Best is to start with Agni as the prime motivating power of the Vedic Yoga, then to move on to Indra as the deeper insight and Self-awakening, which develops the Sun or solar Vedic enlightenment, and the Moon or Soma as Vedic Samadhi Yoga.

A simpler way is to choose a few names of Vedic deities for chanting and meditation, either with or without additional seed mantras as *Oṁ Agnaye namaḥ*! *Or Oṁ Hūm Agnaye namaḥ*!

Regular Vedic Rituals

It can be helpful to add daily Vedic rituals like fire offerings, particularly Agni Hotra, such as is commonly performed with the Gayatri Mantra. Mantric offering of reverence (namas) to the great forces of the Sun, Moon, wind, fire, or water can be transformative. Practicing the Five Great Yajnas mentioned earlier – teaching the higher knowledge, worshipping the Divine powers, and making offerings for your ancestors, fellow human beings, and animals – is a good foundation on which to build.

****

These are but a few suggestions. Any recitation, study, teaching, or translation of Vedic mantras can energize the Vedic Yoga within us. Alternatively, we can follow our own Vedic inspiration, as the *Vedas* have many aspects and can motivate each soul in a unique manner – but we should search deeply within ourselves and not make the Vedic Yoga a mere temporary concern.

Ancient Vedic Rishis and Yogis

While the spiritual keys to the *Vedas* passed into obscurity over time, the aura of the Vedic Rishis has remained vibrant. The Rishis appear prominently in later teachings as great sages, seers, yogis, healers, and cultural guides. We find the Rishis mentioned in all aspects of Hindu literature, the *Vedas*, *Puranas*, Epics, Yoga Shastras, Dharma Sutras, *Tantras*, and Vedantic texts, where they occur as teachers, and their dialogues with each other are recorded. Many Rigvedic hymns occur in the other *Vedas*, and many verses from Rigvedic hymns occur in the *Brahmanas*. The *Upanishads* contain a number of quotes from verses of the *Vedas*, as well as paraphrases or reformulations of Vedic teachings. They prominently mention the Vedic Rishis.

The Vedic Rishis are a group of sages belonging to such an ancient era that little is known of them individually. In addition, the Rishis are not merely human figures but part of a vast cosmic and psychological symbolism, extending to the pranas, senses, lokas and chakras. The *Vedas*, particularly the *Rigveda*, have preserved the names and families of many of the great Rishis. In the *Rigveda*, the name of the Rishi of each hymn is given, and the various Vedic Rishis mention other Rishis and Rishi families (Gotras) in their hymns. This is different from the *Atharvaveda* in which the Rishis of the hymns are only mentioned generically.

In examining the content and styles of their particular Rigvedic hymns, we can learn something about the Rishis, their characters and temperaments, so that we can get a glimpse of them as individuals. In Puranic stories, the lives and characters of a number of the Rishis are discussed in detail, particularly Vasishtha, Vishvamitra, and Agastya. Agastya is prominent in South Indian and Tamil traditions. In addition, we can learn something about the Rishis from the other Vedic and yogic lines in which they were prominent. For example, Bharadvaja is prominent in early Ayurvedic teachings. Kavyakantha Ganapati Muni has done an extensive study of the Vedic Rishi lines or Gotras and classified them based upon traditional sources.[404]

Primary Rishi Lines, Families or Gotras

There are two primary lines of Vedic Rishi lines in the *Rigveda*, the *Angirasas* and the *Bhrigus*. The Angirasas are said to be born of the embers or coals of Agni or the sacred fire (as the related term *Aṅgara* means coal), while the Bhrigus reflect its flame (with *Bharga* meaning flame).[405] Of the two families, the Angirasas are most prominent and numerous in the *Rigveda*. They are legendary figures involved in the exploits of Indra, particularly in his conquest of the light and resurrection of the Sun out of darkness, which constitutes perhaps the main Vedic legend. The

Angirasas are related to Agni, who is commonly called Angiras, and constitute the original fire priests. Some equate the term Angiras of the *Vedas* with Angelos or Angel of the Greeks. Their roles as invisible guides and protectors are similar.

The Bhrigus are mentioned less often in the *Rigveda*, but in a similar way to the Angirasas. They are more prominent in the *Mahabharata, Upanishads* and in Vedic astrology, other esoteric arts and Tantra.[406] Sometimes these two Rishis families are one as Bhrigu/Angirasas, and most likely they are one in origin, as they share many common names and stories. Both Bhrigus and Angirasas are credited with bringing Agni, the Divine Fire, down to mortals and to the earth plane, and also awakening Agni in human beings to carry on the unfoldment of the Vedic work.

We can generally equate the Angirasas with the fire or "Agni line," and the Bhrigus with the water or "Soma line" because the Bhrigus are more prominent in the Soma hymns of the *Rigveda*. The Angirasas are associated with Agni while the Bhrigus are born of Varuna, the God of the sea, reflecting a watery symbolism. The Bhrigus are connected more to the south of India, like the region of Bhrigu Kachchh or Broach in the Gulf of Cambay in Gujarat. The Angirasas appear more connected to north of the country, though both lines can be found in all regions of India.

The foremost of the Angirasa Rishis is Brihaspati, the most famous and honored of the original Rishis, also identified with the planet Jupiter. Unlike the other Rishis, Brihaspati is a deity in his own right honored in many Vedic hymns. As the Lord of the Word and mantra, he is looked upon as the father of all the Vedic hymns. There are two important hymns in the tenth book of the *Rigveda* attributed to him. He is sometimes lauded as the father of all the Gods, as Divine progeneration occurs through the power of the Divine Word that he manifests. He is associated with the deity Ganesha in later times,[407] who is the primal guru and master of the Divine Word. Brihaspati is called Brahmanaspati. He represents the original Brahmin priest or the priestly order. He is sometimes equated with the deity Brahma in the later Hindu trinity.

The planet Venus, meanwhile, is connected to the Bhrigus and has Bhargava, or "of the Bhrigus," among its names. Bhrigu is called "Shukra," which is the main Sanskrit name for the planet Venus, as well as the name of a Bhrigu Rishi, also called Kavi. Ushanas of the Bhrigus, who has several hymns in the *Rigveda*, is lauded by Krishna as the greatest of the Vedic seers, as we have noted earlier. Ushanas is sometimes equated with Kavi and Shukra.

Brihaspati, or Jupiter, is the guru among the planets and represents the power of Dharma that the Angirasas represent. In Vedic thought Jupiter is the guru of the Gods or Devas. Venus is the planet of vision and inspiration, the beloved morning and evening star. Venus, or Shukra, is the guru of the Asuras or anti-gods, but sometimes a guru of the Gods as well. This makes sense astrologically as Venus relates more to the worldly force of sexuality and creativity, and Jupiter to the spiritual force of knowledge.

Yet there are Bhrigu lines associated with the Angirasas, notably the Gritsamada line of the second book of the *Rigveda*. The teaching of the *Taittiriya Upanishad* is given by Varuna to his son Bhrigu. The Bhrigus and their Venus energy are prominent in certain teachings like Ayurveda, Vedic astrology, and Tantra, where the transformative role of energy is important. The Angirasas relate to sixty-year Jupiter calendars that have dominated the calendar of India and China. The Bhrigus to forty-year Venus calendars, and to the emphasis on Venus for marking time that was common in the ancient Middle East, Egypt, and the Americas.

Hindu texts like the *Puranas* speak of a war or struggle between the Bhrigus under Shukra (Venus) and the Angirasas under Brihaspati (Jupiter), occurring at the beginning of the Treta Yuga or third world age, which was during the earlier Vedic age.[408] This involves a split in humanity between the Devic forces represented mainly by the Purus among the Vedic people, and certain fallen Vedic groups mainly the Yadus,[409] though there were later reconciliations of the Vedic people.

In addition to these two Rishi lines is the *Atharva* line that lends its name to the *Atharvaveda*. Atharva as a Rishi is mentioned in the *Rigveda* several times as a great Rishi, along with his son Dadhyak, who is very important relative to Indra and the Ashvins, and almost a deity in his own right. Generally, the Atharvans are more connected to the Angirasas as fire priests, but sometimes to the Bhrigus as well. The *Atharvaveda* is sometimes called *Bhrigvangirasa* after the two Vedic families, and can appear as a synthesis of both. The Atharva family is prominent in ancient Persian Zoroastrian lore, reflecting the term "athar" for fire. Athar occurs in the name of the country Azerbaijan, the seed (bija) of fire (athar) from the ancient fire sites in that region of greater Iran.

There are additional Rishi lines that appear to combine Angiras and Bhrigu energy, like Vasistha and Agastya, who are descendants of Mitra and Varuna, with Mitra connected to Agni and the Angirasas, and Varuna to water, Soma, and the Bhrigus. This Mitra-Varuna line is sometimes made independent of the Angirasas and Bhrigus. Sometimes it appears more related to the Bhrigus.

There is another major line of Vedic Rishis as the Kashyapas, who are related to the Sun and to Mount Kailas or Meru in Tibet, the great mountain of the Sun. Kashyapa Rishis are most prominent in the Soma book of the *Rigveda* and have connections with the Atris, the Angirasas, and the Bhrigus. In addition, Kashyapa was the name of the Buddha who is said to have lived five thousand years before Shakyamuni Buddhi. Kashyapa is associated with the land of Kashmir, that was also a famous Soma region.

The Atris appear as an ancient line connected to the Angirasas but sometimes seem to be an independent line of their own, quite ancient and also going back to Manu, with additional connections to the Kanvas, Bhrigus, and Kashyapas. The Vedic Rishi families are the basis of the Brahmin "gotras," or family lines, in India, to which many people still trace their backgrounds. New converts to Hinduism are usually placed in the Kashyapa line.

The Seven Rishis or Seven Seers

The Rishis are counted as seven, and constitute seven family lines. Usually the Bhrigus and Angirasas are not part of these seven but their descendants are. The names of these seven Rishis vary in different texts. The *Rigveda* contains seven family books (II-VIII), in which one Rishi or his family predominates.

Book II. Gritsamada (Bhrigu)

Book III. Vishvamitra

Book IV. Vamadeva (Gotama)

Book V. Atri

Book VI. Bharadvaja

Book VII. Vasishtha

Book VIII. Kanva

Gotamas, Bharadvajas, and Kanvas are usually described as diversifications of the Angirasas. Vishvamitra has connections with Bharadvajas and Kanvas, as do the Atris, which places them generally among the Angirasas. Gritsamada, though a Bhrigu, is famous for his hymns to Brihaspati, the head of the Angirasas. These seven Rigvedic families are primarily as Angirasas. The eighth, or Kanva book, contains a number of hymns of other families including Atris, Angirasas, and Bhrigus.

The first book of the *Rigveda* contains hymns of the Angirasa Rishis as the largest group (Hiranyastupa, Savya, Kutsa, Kakshivan, and Dirghatamas, which are of this line). It also has many hymns of Rishis from other diversified Angirasas including Gotamas, (Nodhas, Gotama), Kanvas (Kanva Ghora, Praskanva Kanva), Vishvamitras (Madhuchchhandas), and Bharadvajas (Paruchchhepa). Some other families appear as Vasishthas (Parashara), Kashyapa, and Agastya. The first book has hymns of some of the oldest Vedic Rishis like Dirghatamas, Kakshivan, Gotama, and Agastya, which are mentioned prominently in the other books of the *Rigveda* extending to the *Upanishads*.

The ninth, or Soma book, of the *Rigveda* contains many hymns of the Bhrigu family (Kavi) and Kashyapas (Asita and Devala), as well as Rishis from the family books, and a few hymns by groups of Rishis like the seven Rishis or the Vaikhanasas. The tenth book is more variable and contains a number of special hymns outside the usual Rishi families. Yet a number of significant hymns to the primary Vedic deities are also there from the main Vedic families.

Sometimes other Rishis are mentioned in the delineation of the seven Rishis in Vedic and Puranic texts. These include Pulastya, Pulaha, Kratu, and Agastya. The different Yugas have different lists of their seven Rishis, which are described in the *Puranas*.

Rishi-Yogis, the Rishis as Founders of the different paths of Yoga

The different branches of the Vedic teachings as Yoga, Vedanta, Ayurveda, and Vedic astrology are attributed to various Rishi lines as their founders, with the deities passing on their teachings to certain Rishis.

The usual line of the Yoga Darshana which the *Yoga Sutras* follows is from Hiranyagarbha, who relates to the solar deity, to Vasishtha, and then to his grandson Parashara. The *Yoga Vasishtha* and *Vasishtha Samhita*, though of later dates, are famous Yoga texts, indicating this Vasishtha family association to Yoga and its persistence over the centuries.

A similar line from Vasishtha to Parashara and then to Veda Vyasa relates to Vedanta, including the Advaitic form, implying an ancient connection between the Yoga Darshana and Vedanta Darshana. The Vasishtha-Parashara line is also one of the important lines of Vedic astrology or Jyotish. Parashara is perhaps the most famous teacher of Vedic astrology, as in the great compilation the *Brihat Parashara Hora Shastra*. Vasishthas were later the purohits or chief priests of the kingdom of Kosala, in which Rama was born.

Agastya, who is portrayed in the *Rigveda* as the elder brother, if not guru of Vasishtha, is famous for his founding of the Tamil language and leading Tamil group of siddhas and Yogis, much like the importance of the Vasishthas in the north of India. He is the main Vedic Rishi for South India and Southeast Asia.

Vamadeva is famous for gaining Self-realization while still in his mother's womb, and is a great figure in the Yoga of Knowledge or Jnana Yoga. His family, the Gotamas, were the Purohits of the region of Videha, from which Sita came. Their kings called "Janaka" are frequently regarded as great Self-realized sages, including the famous Janaka of the *Brihadaranayaka Upanishad* who dialogued with the sage Yajnavalkya.

There are many stories of the Vedic Rishis in the *Puranas* along with their associations with different parts of India. The main Vedic people were the Puru-Bharatas of the Sarasvati region now mainly in the Indian state of Harayana, who later shifted east to the Ganga-Yamuna area, in western Uttar Pradesh. The Rishis had associations with other Vedic peoples and their different regions of India. The Anus, associated with the Bhrigus and the Rishi Dirghatamas, were located to the northwest in the Punjab, with another group of Anus shifting to the east in Bengal. The Yadus, connected to the Bhrigus and Kanvas, were located to the south and west extending to Gujarat and Madhya Pradesh. The Ikshvakus, connected to Vasishtha, Gotama, and Vamadeva, dominated central and east India to Bihar. Vedic hymns mention the five main Vedic peoples and address all of humanity.

Kshatriya Lines/Rajarshis or Royal Seers

The two higher Vedic classes of the Brahmins and Kshatriyas, the priestly and warrior lines, are closely associated in all Vedic teachings. They intermarried and crossed over in various ways. Vedic kings like Dushyanta married daughters of great Brahmins like Shakuntala, from whom Bharata, the Vedic king from which India (Bharat) owes its name, was born. This is the subject of an important drama of the great poet Kalidas. Generally, Vedic kings had a great Brahmin as their purohit, chief priest, or chief advisor, like King Janamejaya of the *Aitareya Brahmana* and his purohit Tura Kavasheya.[410]

Krishna, himself a King or Kshatriya, in the *Bhagavad Gita* speaks of a transmission of Yoga from himself to Vivasvan, Manu, and King Ikshvaku. This is a Kshatriya Yoga line, or line of kings, who had their own special vidyas or ways of knowledge as did the Brahmins. Krishna refers to the Yoga that he teaches as a Kshatriya tradition handed down to different kings.

Yet while Ikshvaku was a king of the solar dynasty (Surya Vamsha), Krishna was a king of the lunar dynasty (Chandra Vamsha). Both solar and lunar dynasties are interrelated going back to Manu and his descendants, with many Rishis and Yogis occurring among them. Rama was of the solar line, as was Buddha, which was smaller in numbers of kings than the lunar line but stricter in its adherence to Dharma. Krishna was of the lunar line, which was larger in numbers and ruled a more extensive region.

Manu Vivasvan, the legendary first king and first Rishi, is said in the *Matsya Purana* to have been a great Yogi from Kerala.[411] When the Ice Age ended and the coastlines were flooded, the great kings and Rishis of the south moved to safer mountain regions, up to the great Himalayas in the north.

The Rishi Vishvamitra is a great teacher of Yoga and the martial arts, and of the Gayatri Mantra, that figures prominently in many Yoga and Vedantic texts. Vishvamitra is the most important of the royal seers or Rajarshis, though he also gained the status of a Brahmin, and his family now constitutes the largest Brahmin line in India. This means that the Gayatri Mantra has a Kshatriya connection. The

Kanvas and Bharadvajas were ancient Brahmins who were also Kshatriyas. If the king failed in his duty or died prematurely, sometimes his Brahmin chief priest or purohit took over the country.

The *Rigveda* mentions many great kings among its Rishis, either as patrons, Rishis, or demigods. These include Trasadasyu, Purukutsa, Mandhata, Sudas, Divodasa, Riksha, and Kuru, important figures from both the solar and lunar lines of Vedic kings. Some later kings like Suhotra appear in the *Rigveda* as Rishis of specific hymns. The *Veda* always had a Kshatriya side, which we find throughout the Hindu tradition. The *Brahmanas* and *Upanishads* contain important dialogues with King Janaka seeking instruction from the Brahmin Yajnavalkya, but also have teachings in which kings like Ashvapati appear as the teachers to Brahmins.

Traditional Yoga has Kshatriya connections, particularly those Yogas resting upon discipline, effort, techniques, and independent striving like Hatha Yoga. Yogas emphasizing knowledge, devotion, ritual, and tradition are more Brahmanical in nature. Many monastic traditions in India have Kshatriya origins as they developed as an extension of military disciplines. The two lines of Kshatriya and Brahmanical Yogas always crossed over in many ways.

Other Ancient pre-Patanjali Yogis

There are many ancient pre-Patanjali Yogis mentioned in the *Mahabharata, Puranas, Upanishads*, and Yoga Shastras, besides the many Vedic Rishis who are portrayed as great Yogis. The Yoga Sutra commentary of Vyasa mentions ancient Yogis like Jaigishavya, Asita and Devala Kashyapa (which two have hymns in the ninth or Soma mandala of the *Rigveda*). Narada is famous as the Rishi minstrel and musician. The *Bhakti Yoga Sutras* are attributed to his line. Along with his brother Parvata, both have hymns in the *Rigveda*, but Narada becomes more prominent in the *Mahabharata*. Jaimini, the founder of the ritualistic school of Vedic philosophy (Purva Mimamsa) is said in the *Puranas* to have been a great Yogi.

Most famous of the ancient Yogis is Lord Krishna. Yoga was a very common practice in Sri Krishna's time, including Bhakti Yoga, Jnana Yoga, and Karma Yoga, with the Upanishads widely studied. Prana Yoga and pranayama are mentioned in the *Bhagavad Gita* and earlier Vedic texts.

Rama is famous as an ancient Yogi as is his companion Hanuman. We do not have any specific ancient yogic teachings attributed to them but do have the *Yoga Vasishtha*, which is taught to Rama by Vasishtha. Rama is more lauded as a "Jnani" or sage in the Yoga of knowledge. Hanuman is said to have possessed all the secrets of Raja Yoga. We have already mentioned Vasishtha as a founder of lines of Yoga and other Vedic teachings.

There is a special Yajnavalkya line of Vedic and Yogic teachings that relates to the *Shukla Yajurveda, Shatapatha Brahmana, Brihadaranyaka Upanishad*, a few sections of the *Mahabharata*, and the *Yogi Yajnavalkya*, that are described as teachings that he received directly from the Sun God. Yajnavalkya is probably the most important sage in the *Upanishads* and the *Brahmanas*.

Women Rishis

In some of the lists of Rishis, like those in the *Brihadaranyaka Upanishad*, the descent is through the mother, and only the mothers' names are mentioned. While the Vedic Rishis are largely men, there are references to women Rishis, priestesses, and sages from the *Rigveda* to the *Upanishads*. These include Ghosha, Vak Ambhrini, Maitreyi, and Gargi. Wives of the Vedic Rishis are well known, particularly Maitreyi, Arundhati, Lopamudra, and Ahalya. Vedic kings often took the daughters of Rishis as their wives, as already noted.

Most notable relative to the *Vedas* in this regard is a passage from the *Jaiminiya Brahmana*, an old Vedic text of the pre-Upanishadic era. I have only the Sanskrit and don't know if there is an English translation of the text available. It contains an interesting passage on women seers. It speaks of the Atri family, one of the seven main Vedic Rishi families, as having many women seers and "mantrakrits" (makers of the mantra) among them.

> *Thus the Rishi Atri desired, "May the greatest number of Rishis be born among my progeny." He saw this trinava (twenty-sevenfold) stoma (chant). He performed that. By that he worshipped. Tejas (radiance or vigor) is the twenty-sevenfold of the chants.*
>
> *Hence among his progeny the largest number of Rishis were born. Numerous thousands of his progeny were creators of the mantras (mantra-krit). The women (or wives) of his progeny were also creators of the mantra. Therefore, whoever harms a woman in the Atri clain is despised. One is full of vigor who knows this."*

The range of feminine symbolism in the *Vedas* is vast and as extensive as the masculine. Vedic deities have consorts or feminine counterparts like Indra and Shachi. Most Vedic terms for mantra, word, and hymn are feminine in declension as Vak, Vani, and Sarasvati. The Vedic meters are feminine in nature, as are the Vedic rivers. Many Vedic Goddesses exist, though only a few have hymns directed entirely to them, notably Sarasvati and Ushas.[412] Aditi, the great mother Goddess, is the Mother of all the Adityas or Sun Gods.

The Esoteric Teachings of The Rishis

By Swami Veda Bharati

There are four *Vedas – Rigveda, Yajurveda, Samaveda and Atharvaveda* – comprising twenty thousand verses in total. But in fact, there is only one *Veda*, which means "knowledge" from the root *vid*, meaning "to know." The *Veda* is divided up into four branches or *Kāṇḍas: Jnāna*, pure or 'a priori' knowledge; *Karma*, action and ritual; *Upāsanā*, worship and direct experience; and *Vijnāna*, material science as well as direct experience of spiritual truths. These four branches are generally connected with the four Vedas (*Rigveda* with knowledge, *Yajurveda* with ritual, *Samaveda* with worship, and *Atharvaveda* with science), with the result being a differing style of language, poetry, and meter, not only between the four *Vedas*, but even within each *Veda*.

Throughout the ages, the followers of the Sanatana Dharma, the eternal path, have revered the *Vedas* as the Divine foundation of their philosophy, culture, and material sciences. They regard the *Vedas* as the first and most perfect revelation to be given to humanity at the time of the creation of the human race, and which includes all the later revelations that are fragments of the one whole. As the *Rigveda* notes:

> *This is the foremost of all speech, in which all the names and words are given through intuitive inspiration. This highest state of the Divine Word was found in the cave of the hearts of Rishis.*
>
> *Some seeing it, do not see; some, hearing it, do not hear; but to some, this speech opens up and expands itself like a well-decked, loving wife offering herself to her husband.*
>
> *Brihaspati Angirasa, Rigveda X.71.1, 4*

Manu, the first Vedic Lawgiver, echoes the same understanding:

> *In the beginning of creation, the Self-Existent Lord brought out the beginningless eternal Divine Word of the Veda, from which all actions originate.*
>
> *The Lord of all brought into manifestation the names and forms of beings and their qualities or actions from the words of the Vedas.*
>
> *All the different names and attributes of all, and the institutions also, he made from the words of the Vedas.*[413]

According to the *Upanishads*: "It is the exhaled breath of the great Being that is the *Rig, Yajur, Sama* and *Atharva Vedas*."[414] The *Vedas* are not simply a human revelation but reflect the very nature and action of the Cosmic Being.

To explain such teachings in western terms, we might say that the Logos has within its consciousness the names of all archetypes, and through that consciousness the different ideas and forms are created in all their diversity. We can see this in the statement of the *Taittiriya Brahmana*: "He saw the word *Bhūḥ* and created the earth." The *Brihadaranyaka Upanishad* says: "He diversified the speech with his mind and by so doing, created the world."

This Vedic theory of the Divine Word is called the Doctrine of *Sphota*, which has attracted the attention of modern linguists. It has been the basis of such great Indian works on philology, lost and extant, as Panini's Sutras, Patanjali's *Mahabhashya*, Yaska's *Nirukta*, and Vyadi's *Samgraha*, though this last was extinct even by Patanjali's time.

Yet let us not fall into the error of assuming that all the words used in the present day Sanskrit language indicate such Vedic revelations, with the same meanings currently as in Vedic times. Most of the words used in the *Vedas* express symbolic meanings broader than their indications in later Sanskrit. We shall explain this in detail.

Among the six traditional schools of Vedic philosophy, Vyasa's *Brahma Sutras* and Jaimini's *Mimamsa Sutras* discuss the nature of the divine revelation of the *Vedas*. A large part of Mimamsa is devoted to this subject. The approach of Vedanta is more of pure spirituality, whereas Mimamsa explains the importance of ritual, but it is also in Mimamsa that the Vedantic doctrine of the divinity of the *Vedas* is maintained logically. Shankara's commentary on the *Brahma Sutras* is worth reading regarding this connection.

According to the ancient tradition, the four Vedas were revealed to four great Rishis, who were the first humans on earth: namely *Agni* (Fire), *Vāyu* (Wind), *Āditya* (Sun), and *Angiras*. According to some explanations, these are not the proper names, but the titles of the four sages to whom this higher knowledge is revealed at the beginning of every cycle of creation. Tradition ascribes Vedic hymns to the Rishis whose names appear with each hymn in the books of the *Vedas*, reflecting various families or *gotras*.

The *Upanishads* state: "The *Vedas* are innumerable,"[415] which means that the meaning hidden behind each hymn and mantra is unfathomable and immeasurable. Different Rishis chose different hymns to express the meanings they were able to perceive in a state of samadhi or yogic realization. For instance, the *Rigveda* is said in general to be revealed to Agni, but to the Rishi Madhuchchhandas is ascribed the first eleven hymns of the *Rigveda*, with other Rishis given the remaining hymns. These Rishis also commented on the Vedic hymns, though most of their commentaries have been lost in the long course of time. Out of 1,127 explanatory versions of the four *Vedas*, only a few remain available in printed form.

"The *Vedas* are innumerable." The reason given for this statement is that the *Vedas* comprise the entire knowledge of the Universal Mind (Brahman), and incorporate all branches and aspects of that knowledge on which the entire universe is based. Shankara, commenting on the third aphorism of Vyasa's *Brahma Sutras*, says: "Brahman is the origin and cause of the great *Vedas*, beginning with the *Rigveda*. These texts incorporate all sciences, illuminate all meanings like a candle, and reflect the omniscient Being."

The importance of the *Vedas* is recognized, not only by the eastern tradition, but also by those western people who have insight into the matters of the spirit. The following words are from Rudolph Steiner in *Anthroposophy – An Introduction.*[416]

> If anyone in full earnestness extends his studies of human civilization and culture back into remote time, he finds a widespread primeval wisdom. From this is derived much that endures today and is really much "cleverer" than what our science can explore. And whoever studies, for example, the *Vedas* of India or the Yoga philosophy from this point of view will feel deep reverence for what he finds. It is presented in a more poetic form to which he is not accustomed today, but it fills him with deeper reverence the more deeply he studies it. If one does not approach those things in the dry, prosaic manner of today, but lets them work upon him in their stirring, yet profound way, one comes to understand, even from a study of the documents, what that spiritual science, Anthroposophy, must say from its own cognition: There was once a widespread primeval wisdom though it did not appear in an intellectual, but rather in a poetic form.

Another name for the *Vedas* is Brahman, the "Supreme Being." The *Veda* is *Shabda Brahman*, the Word that is God itself. The result is that anyone trying to explain the *Vedas* on only intellectual, philological, or historical grounds must fail to understand the real meaning of these profound works.

Throughout the history of *Vedic* learning, there have been three methods of translating these oldest scriptures of the world:

1. That of the Esoteric Seers, the great Rishi-yogis, from Madhuchchhandas to Sri Aurobindo. This method is followed by the translations that occur in this chapter and in this book as a whole.

2. That of the exoteric or ritualistic Indian commentators, like the celebrated teacher Sayana, who emphasized a polytheistic and sacrificial interpretation. These translators, at certain points, however, could not help seeing a deeper esoteric meaning as well.

3. That of modern western academic schools. During the past two centuries, in the words of Sri Aurobindo, "The ancient book of the *Veda* fell into the hands of that European scholarship which was hardworking, courageous in thinking…but still unable to understand the methods of the ancient mystical poets."[417] This scholarship twists and stretches the ancient poetry to prove certain modern philosophical and historical assumptions, missing its spiritual essence and yogic implications.

Decline of the Esoteric Tradition

The esoteric or yogic system of Vedic interpretation prevailed throughout the ancient or legendary period of the Vedic Rishis. Even apparently mere ritualistic Vedic hymns are sometimes explained at a spiritual level in the *Brahmanas*, texts that usually emphasize a ritualistic interpretation. By the time of Lord Buddha, some twenty five hundred years ago, it seems that the deeper Vedic tradition had already been lost. Yet even then, many Vedic terms were not given the limited outer meanings ascribed to them by later interpreters of mythology and by modern scholars.

Let us take an example. There is a well-known legend in Indian mythology that Indra, the Lord of the heavenly gods, had a thousand eyes. But Chanakya, in his well-known work on the science of politics, about two centuries after the birth of Buddha, in discussing the number of ministers of a king, says that the council of ministers in the court of Indra numbers one thousand; therefore Indra, though having only two eyes is called *Sahasraksha* or "one-thousand-eyed." Strangely enough, other deities of the Vedas are also called Sahasraksha and this cannot be properly explained at a literal level.

By studying the *Mahabharata*, we learn that certain great kings or Rishis ascended to and fell from the post of Indra from time to time, which indicates that "Indra" is more a degree or rank than a term for one deity only. Ultimately Indra stands for the supreme principle of truth.

Although the mythology of the *Puranas*, emphasizing deities like Vishnu and Shiva, prevailed from the period of the *Mahabharata*, the esoteric Vedic tradition was never completely lost. Great scholar saints like Shankara, a devotee of Shiva, in spite of adhering to one primary deity form, understood the ultimate reality engulfing all differences. Such spiritual scholars quoted the *Vedas* not to prove the supremacy of the God-manifestation of their particular choice, but rather to show the supremacy of the supreme Deity or Brahman as the Self of all. Shankara commented on the *Upanishads* but not specifically on the *Vedas*; yet he did quote older Vedic mantras to prove the unity of Brahman, such as we find commonly in the *Upanishads*. The scholar-mystics never forgot the following verse of the *Rigveda*:

> *He is called Indra, Mitra, Varuna...the seers call that One Reality by different names like Agni, Yama and Matarishvan.*
> *Dirghatamas Auchatya, Rigveda I.164.46*

The only esoteric commentary on the *Rigveda* that remains from the medieval period that is available for us is that of *Ananda Tirtha* or *Madhvacharya* who lived from 1119-1197 A.D. His commentaries on the *Upanishads* and related works are widely studied, not only by the followers of dualist Vedanta school that he founded, but also by all those who are interested in comparative Indian philosophy. Traditionally, according to the followers of Madhva's (Ananda Tirtha's) school, he commented on the entire *Rigveda*, but only the first three chapters (forty of the thousand hymns) are available today.

The main commentary on the *Vedas* that we have from this period was of an exoteric nature by *Sayana*, who was the Prime Minister of the great Vijayanagar Empire of the fourteenth century. In Sayana's work, there is some inconsistency, and many scholars have concluded that his voluminous commentary extending to many thousands of pages could not be entirely his own, but were written for him by different pandits employed specifically for that purpose, reflecting their different views. Curiously, Sayana's introduction to the *Vedas* seems to advocate the esoteric system of interpretation and expands the doctrine that the different deities belong to the One Essence or Brahman. Unfortunately, most of Sayana's commentaries take the outer meanings only of the Vedic mantras. Modern western scholars have also emphasized the ritualistic views of Sayana over the esoteric views of other older Vedic scholars and teachers.

Revival of the Esoteric Tradition

The esoteric tradition of Vedic interpretation, though not completely lost, was marginalized and known only to very few. In recent centuries, however, it has also undergone a great revival, paralleling but different from the contemporaneous Vedic studies of western scholars.

Swami Virajananda, a blind hermit in *Mathura* in the nineteenth century, challenged scholars to accept the deeper yogic meanings of the *Vedas* and to reject the ritualistic interpretation of Sayana. Swami Virajananda had a famous disciple called Swami Dayananda Saraswati, one of the most important spiritual teachers to come out of modern India, about whom Madame Blavatsky, the founder of the Theosophical Society, wrote:

> It is perfectly certain that India never saw a more learned Sanskrit scholar, a deeper metaphysician, a more wonderful orator and a fearless denunciator of an evil than Dayananda, since the time of Shankara.

Swami Dayananda's contribution to understanding the *Vedas* is well expressed in the words of the world-famous mystic and Mahayogi of the twentieth century, Sri Aurobindo:

> The ancient civilizations did possess secrets of science some of which modern knowledge has recovered, understood and made more rich and precise, but others now not recovered. There is then nothing fantastic in Dayananda's idea that the *Veda* contains truth of science as well as religion. I will even add my own conviction that *Veda* contained the other truths of a science the modern world does not at all possess, and in that case, Dayananda has rather understated than overstated the depth and range of the Vedic wisdom.[418]
>
> In the matter of Vedic interpretation, I am convinced that whatever may be the final, complete interpretation, Dayananda will be honored as the first discoverer of the right clues, amidst the chaos and obscurity of old ignorance and age-long misunderstanding, his was the eye of direct vision that pierced to the truth – fastened to what was essential. He found the keys of the doors that time had closed and rent asunder the seals of the imprisoned fountains.[419]

Swami Dayananda lived from 1824-1883 and spread his teachings throughout India, gaining a great following for his movement of returning to the *Vedas* called the *Arya Samaj*. Apart from the many major social and religious reforms that he and his organization promoted, he left for India and for the world a great heritage in the form of his commentary on the *Yajurveda* and on certain books of the *Rigveda*. Not unexpectedly, Dayananda's translations and interpretations were rejected by contemporary western scholars. They are still ignored by many westernized academic institutions in India. Yet since India's independence, Dayananda's views have been given recognition by many Indian universities, where the student is often free to choose either a study of the esoteric translation of Dayananda or exoteric translations of Sayana and western scholars.

In the West, it was the Theosophists who, in spite of the absence of a correct esoteric Vedic translation in English, broke the ice and prepared a field in which the seed of the right understanding of the *Vedas* could be sown. It was in the nineteenth century that Madame Blavatsky wrote in the *Secret Doctrine*:

> For have not even the *Vedas* been derided, rejected and called a 'modern forgery' even so recently as fifty years ago? ......About 1820, as Prof. Max Muller tells us, the sacred books of the *Brahmans*, of the *Magians*, and of the *Buddhists*, were all but unknown, their very existence was doubted, and there was not a single scholar who could have translated a line of the *Vedas*...... and now the *Vedas* are proved to be a work of the highest antiquity, whose preservation amounts almost to a marvel.[420]

> The *Veda* of the earliest Aryans, before it was written, went forth into every nation......and sowed the first seeds of all the now existing religions. The offshoots of the never dying Tree of Wisdom have scattered their dead leaves even on Judeo-Christianity.[421]

The early twentieth century witnessed another great mystic scholar, Sri Aurobindo, who developed the same esoteric lines of Vedic interpretation as Swami Dayananda. At his disposal, he had not only the insight of his practice of Raja Yoga and a deep scholarship in the Sanskrit language, but also the comparative study of Greek and Latin gained during his younger student years at Cambridge. Aurobindo came to recognize an affinity between the Orphic and Eleusinian mysteries on one side, and Vedic realization of Brahman on the other. In his words:

> The *Rigveda* itself is a great book. Various sermons have descended from the beginning of human thought of which the historical Eleusinian and Orphic mystery sayings were mere broken fragments.[422]

Like Dayananda, Aurobindo based his understanding of the *Vedas* on his yogic experiences, with the result that he too rejected the views of Sayana. On this point he says: Sayana's commentary "is a key that has double locked the inner meaning of the *Veda*." To understand Sri Aurobindo's views on the *Veda*, his work *The Secret of the Vedas* is well worth reading. It not only explains the esoteric and yogic meaning in the traditional sense, but also refutes the philological theories of Western scholars on the basis of their own logic and their own research.

Nature of Vedic Sanskrit

Here we must enter into a more technical discussion. The Sanskrit language is different from other languages in its quality of having all words based upon inherent root meanings. All nouns derive from a root verb that describes the functions and actions of the object designated by the noun. For instance, the word *manushya*, "man", reflects its verb root man that expresses the function of intelligent thought, meaning "the thinker." There are relates terms like *manas* for mind that reflect the same root sound and its meaning.

In the ancient development of the Sanskrit language, all words were divided into two primary categories: (1) *Yaugika*, which indicates quality, function or action, rather than a specific object. (2) *Rudhi*, which indicate a specific object. Yaugika affords words a greater symbolic, analogical, or descriptive value beyond any fixed outer meanings. Most Sanskrit words are not purely Yaugika, otherwise Sanskrit could never have been a spoken language for ordinary activities. But the Vedic language is predominately Yaugika, meaning that Vedic terms cannot be simply regarded as indicating particular objects. All apparent substantive nouns in Sanskrit have a broader descriptive or adjectival value.

Even though a Vedic word can indicate a specific object, it can also indicate any number of other objects having similar actions as described by the root verb. A generic and symbolic meaning prevails over a specific indication for the words of the *Vedas*. Even in later Sanskrit a term like Manu, meaning the first man or law-giver also means a "mantra," reflecting such inner meanings in the language.

Let us take the first word of the *Vedas* as an example. Agni in later classical Sanskrit usually designates "fire" as an object, such as the word means to us today. The term has not lost contact with its root meaning, but has been fixed to mean primarily an object in nature. The word Agni derives from the root *anch*, with the result that in the older more symbolic Vedic language, it may mean "fire", but its broader indication is relative to the quality of leading, of motion, action, enlightenment, and illumination that can apply to many other things as well both concrete and abstract. This makes it very difficult to translate the *Vedas* in any single manner only. It is particularly challenging for our modern English language in which precise outer meanings of words prevail. For us fire is primarily the material fire, not a metaphor for universal energy and consciousness. Swami Dayananda Saraswati provided four hundred different renderings of the word Agni in his partial commentary on the *Vedas*. Even exoteric translators of the *Vedas* are compelled to translate certain Vedic terms in several different ways in order to have them make sense in the context of different Vedic hymns, although these scholars may not accept the deeper yogic implications of Vedic terminology.

There have also always existed differences of opinion among the ancient Indian grammarians and philologists on interpreting the *Vedas*. In the view the Vedic Rishis, Vedic mantras were cognized in the state of samadhi, from which the relationship of a root verb with its derivative terms was established according to the spiritual principles of cosmic sound vibration. But this relationship was never taken to be final, for it was quite possible, in harmony with the principles of the Vedic language, that another Rishi would understand the same word with a different meaning according to a different context. Eventually schools of grammar arose in

India that standardized the Sanskrit language in order to make the relationship of words and meanings fixed and stereotyped. This caused students of later Sanskrit to have difficulty understanding the fluidity of the Vedic language and its many levels of meaning. There is an interesting passage on this subject in the first book of the *Gopatha Brahmana*:

> The ancient Acharyas understood the language through the oral tradition and did not reason about it. But those who originated the six *Vedangas* or limbs of the *Vedas*, such as grammar, said "We shall reason; this should happen thus to these letters."

In this rational intellectual tradition were born the later Sanskrit grammarians like *Shakatayana, Yaska, Apishali, Vyadi, Panini, Vararuchi* and *Patanjali*. But they clearly recognized that the language of the *Vedas* was an exception to the rules set down by them and transcended these. *Panini* has repeated one of his aphorisms five times in his work "Bahulam Chandasi," and total of eleven times in other phraseology: "In the *Vedas*, it happens in a variety of ways".

The *Nirukta* of Yaska, the greatest Vedic work on etymology, is regarded as the key to the *Vedas*. Unfortunately, it is seldom consulted by modern scholarship. This work, on which have been written such great commentaries as that of Skanda Swami, states: "In the study of the *Vedas*, one should not respect the interference from the set rules of grammar." In other words, the *Vedas* do not conform to later Sanskrit grammatical rules and cannot be understood according to them.

It is the symbolic quality of the Vedic language that supports the traditional view as mentioned in the *Brihad Devata* of the Rishi Shaunaka. This is the most authentic work on the subject of Rishis and Vedic deities (Devatas) to whom different mantras are attributed. Here the word "Devata" is translated as "god", but in fact, it only means a subject of a mantra. I feel it is not out of place to quote some verses from the first chapter of this book as translated by A.A. Macdonnell.[423]

1. In every formula (Vedic hymn) one should know the divinity (Devata) with exactness; for he who knows the divinities of the formulas, understands their objects.

3. He is capable of giving an (authoritative) opinion as to their intentions which were contained in them at the time formulas were revealed to the seers, (and) as to the correct understanding (of them) and the various sacraments (connected with them).

10 But whether the seers who discern the truth either praise or state (an object), they express both, for both are in reality the same.

Verse 10 reflects another key difference between Vedic levels of statements. In offering praise or worship to a certain god that god is eulogized in the second person (as "thou"). As a statement in terms of fact or science, merely the attributes of the deity or object are stated, which occurs in the third person (as "that"). For instance, in the second person, "O Agni, Thou art a leading force:" is a eulogy. Taken in the third person, "Agni is a leading force" is a scientific or objective statement.

Yet Verse 10 goes further and connects the two and indicates that in the case of objects of the hymns (Devatas), even a eulogy can be considered as a statement. The praise is describing the nature of the deity involved, and this deity is ultimately within ourselves!

Here we must remember another rule of esoteric Vedic translation, that all names are ultimately names of Brahman (names of God). Therefore, when an inanimate object is apparently eulogized, it is Brahman that is indicated according to the symbolism involved. Let us take again as an example the above sentence, "O Agni, Thou art a leading force." As we have explained Agni means "fire", but also because of the implied root meanings it can be one of the names of Brahman, particularly as the original power of light and transformation, the flame of God.

If a translator intends to attribute this mantra to the inanimate fire only, he should take the sentence not as a eulogy to an imaginary god of fire, but as a statement. Another translator, intending to attribute the hymn to the Ultimate Brahman, may take it as a eulogy or as a statement about the nature or qualities of Brahman. Referring to these facts, the sixth verse says:

6. Whatever god a seer desiring an object mentions, let that one, it is said, be (the god of the formula). A formula predominantly praising (a god) with devotion, is addressed to that same god.

Verse 12 indicates that not only are Vedic deities different names of the One Deity, each Vedic deity itself can have a number of names. Sometimes when a different aspect of the same deity is explained, there are other hymns written on it, having different Devatas as their object.

12. Therefore one familiar with the application (of formulas) should in every formula carefully observe the deity, with regard to name, and the multiplicity of the designations (of deities).

For instance, hymns to Agni are divided into three: some are devoted to pure Agni, some to Vaishvanara (the fire that dwells within all beings, often identified with the sun) and some to Jatavedas (the life-fire that knows all beings, which is usually placed in the atmosphere). These three divisions refer to the different aspects of Agni and are not separate god or deities. That is what is explained in the below reference from the *Brihad Devata*.

91. Because this (terrestrial Agni) is led by man, and that (celestial Agni) leads him from this (world), therefore these two (Agnis) while having the same name, have performed their work separately.

91. Because he is known when born, or because he is known here by creatures, therefore these two, while having an identical name pervade both worlds (separately).

96. It is impossible to explain their production or their power, sphere, and birth; for the whole of this world is pervaded by them.

97. Agni is contained in Vaishvanara, Vaishvanara is contained in Agni; Jatavedas is in these two; thus these two (lights) are two (forms of) Jatavedas.

98. The divine nature of each god here (is derived) from their belonging to the same world, from their having one and the same birth, and from brilliance being inherent in them; at the same time they appear praised separately.

104. Just as this has been said of these (three) as arising from (their different) powers or spheres, so it also appears here in its respective place (as applicable) to the god of gods (Prajapati).

Regarding the last three verses, although literal translators take Vaishvanara in the sense of a material fire, in the *Upanishads, Brahmanas, Bhagavad Gita*, and Shankara's commentaries, it is clearly interpreted to mean the mystic fire of the universe. In the *Bhagavad Gita*, Lord Krishna says: "I enter into and stay in the bodies of creatures as Vaishvanara fire, and with prana and apana, operate the digestive system."[424] In the *Chandogya Upanishad* a disciple asks his guru to explain to him the Vaishvanara, the Self or Atman.[425] In the *Shatapatha Brahmana* it is said: "The Eternal Purusha as individual soul is the Vaishvanara fire; one who knows this Vaishvanara fire knows the Eternal Purusha."[426] In the *Brahma Sutras*, Vaishvanara is said to be one of the names of Brahman.[427] Shankara's commentary on this aphorism explains it in detail.

For a further illustration of this point, I would like to quote a western translation of one of the *Vaishvanara* hymns by Hermann Oldenberg.[428] The translator has obviously failed to reconcile his words with the real spirit of the hymn; still that meaning shines through.

> *By his birth he has given splendor to both worlds (heaven and earth). He became the praiseworthy son of this parent, Agni, the carrier of oblations, never aging, with satisfied mind, undeceivable, the guest of men, rich in light.*
>
> *Through the power of their mind, with the sphere of their superior strength, the gods have procreated Agni by their thoughts. Desirous of winning, I address him who shines with his splendor, who is great in his light as*

(one who desires to win the prize addresses his racehorse.
Maitravaruni Vasishtha, Rigveda III.2.2-3. Oldenburg Translation

The esoteric understanding applies not only in the case of Agni, Vaishvanara, and other mystical fire deities, but is true of all deities in the *Vedas*. Let us illustrate the meaning of the word *Aditi*. In academic mythological translations, Aditi is sometimes taken as the earth, sometimes as the mother of the Adityas or Sun Gods. Esoterically, the term is *a-diti* or "non-diversity," which is the force of unity. In Vedic terminology *diti* and *aditi* are terms for the forces of diversity and unity. It is Aditi that is the earth, the widespread ground of being, the mother of all gods, and the nourisher of all the forces of light. There are twelve Adityas, corresponding to the twelve months of the year, and this Aditi is not only the mother of substance in space, but also of all the divisions in time.

Here we touch the word *Varuna* also, a name of one of the Sun Gods. The 24th hymn of the first book of the *Rigveda* is most poetic and beautiful in its devotion, wonder, and awe. It is addressed to the forces of nature and their creator. Shunashepa, a soul in bondage, taken in literal translations as a person bound for human sacrifice, prays to the Lord Prajapati, the God of gods, to enlighten him as to which form of worship to take in order to be returned to Aditi, the state of unity beyond all bondage.

It is a great temptation to quote here the translation of the Shunashepa hymn by Ananda Tirtha and the commentaries on it by Jayatirtha and Roṭi-Venkatadri, but limitations of space prevent this. We paraphrase Ananda Tirtha: "Being greater than all the immortal liberated souls, being eternal in space and indivisible in time, it is the Supreme God who is called Aditi, Mother and Father, in this hymn." Among the available translations of the *Vedas*, only Ananda Tirtha in the eleventh century and Swami Dayananda in the nineteenth century have translated all deity names as the names of Supreme God, although Ananda Tirtha's term is Vishnu.

Paul Deussen, a western Vedic translator, explained Varuna as the supreme godhead of the *Vedas*, who is referred to as the controller of *Rita* (truth or dharma) in the hymns like that of Shunashepa. We can easily join the ancient poet in singing the praise of this Varuna when he says:

These birds flying in the sky cannot touch thy splendor, power, and glory, nor can these waters, flowing perpetually, nor these wafting breezes.

These stars shining high in the sky are seen during the nights. Where do they disappear during the day? Unsurmountable, verily, are the laws of Varuna. Lo! the moon comes glittering through the night.

Ajigarta Shunasepa, Rigveda I.24.6, 10

Let us now see the splendor of this *Varuna* in this hymn of the seventh book of the *Rigveda*, translated by H.D. Griswold.

1. I do not wish, King Varuna to go down to the house of clay[429]

O, Lord, have mercy and forgive.

2. When tottering I move about, O, like a bellow puffed up,

O Lord, have mercy and forgive.

3. Somehow through lack of insight I have gone astray, O shining one,

O Lord, have mercy and forgive.

4. Thirst finds thy worshipper even when he in the midst of water stands,

O Lord have mercy and forgive.

5. Whatever wrong against the race of gods we do, Being but men, O Varuna, whatever law of thine we may have broken in thoughtlessness,

For that transgression do not punish us, O God.
Maitravaruni Vasishtha, Rigveda VII.89

Rishis and Devatas

Each Vedic hymn refers to the Rishi and Devata, its seer and intended deity. In the *Gopatha Brahmana* and Katyayana's *Sarvanukramani*, there are almost identical passages saying: "One who studies or teaches the *Vedas* without knowing the Rishis and Devatas falls, destroys himself and becomes impure."

As for the Rishis, we have pointed out that they were the vehicles, the seers of the hidden meaning behind the hymns. In the ancient commentaries and indices of the Vedic Rishis and Devatas, it is repeated again and again: "The Rishi saw this hymn." Saw or perceived is primarily indicated, a state of perception or cognition, not "composed" or "created" in a personal or intellectual sense. To know the Rishi implies not just knowing the name of the particular Rishi of a hymn but to have the same level of Rishi consciousness to which the hymn was revealed.

It is not possible to ascertain the historical existence of all the Rishis mentioned in the *Vedas*, but there is no doubt that their names are a great help in understanding the meaning of the hymns. Some of these Rishis took their names in accordance with the hymns of their choice. For instance, the Rishi of the *Shraddha* hymn (on Right Faith) is called *Shraddha*.[430] Many such names occur in the *Vedas*. We may never know the real names of the Rishis of all the hymns.

Two additional points should be brought out in regard to the above: (1) If the school of a certain Rishi is not known, he is taken as belonging to the Angiras school. Let us not forget that the whole of the *Atharvaveda* has its origin in the school of Angiras and is also called *Angirasa-veda*. (2) This suggests that the Rishis mentioned in *Anukramanis* or Vedic indexes are not always the original authors of the hymns. There are some instances in *Anukramanis* where the change of name of a Rishi is clearly mentioned. For instance, "Gritsamada, who was Shaunahotra of Angiras school and later became Shaunaka of Bhrigu school saw the second book (of the *Rigveda*)". The Rishis often appear part of a cosmic and psychological symbolism rather than as only individual human beings.

Hindu mythology as occurring in the *Puranas* is of a date much later than the *Vedas*, and it can be a great injustice done to the *Vedas* by many translators to interpret the Vedic deities according to Puranic mythology. Even Western scholars could not help noticing such errors. As Griffith says in his preface to the translation of the *Rigveda*:

> The very qualities which have made those commentators excellent guides to be unsuitable conductors on the far older and quite differently circumstanced domain. As the so-called classical Sanskrit was perfectly familiar to them, they sought its ordinary idiom in the Vedic hymns also. Since any difference in the ritual appeared to them inconceivable and the present forms were believed to have existed from the beginning of the world, they fancied that the patriarchs of the Indian religion must have sacrificed in the very same manner. As the recognized mythological and classical systems of their own age appeared to them unassailable and revealed verities, they must necessarily (so the commentators thought) be discoverable in that centre point of revelation, the hymns of the ancient Rishis, who had, indeed, lived in familiar intercourse with the Gods, and possessed far higher wisdom than the succeeding generation ....It has never occurred to anyone to make our understanding of the Hebrew books of the Old Testament depend on the Talmud and the Rabbis, while there are not wanting scholars who hold it as the duty of a conscientious interpreter of the *Veda* to translate in conformity with Sayana, Mahidhara, etc.

Puranic scholars have tried to support their mythological beliefs on the grounds of their origin in the *Vedas*, but not always wisely so. For instance, let us take the story of the Vamana avatara, in which Lord Vishnu incarnated as a dwarf at the request of the gods, and begged Bali the Demon-King who ruled all regions, for as much land as could be covered by three steps. Bali, thinking that the dwarf's three steps could not cover much land, granted the request. The dwarf expanded and covered the whole sky with his first step, the earth with his second, and his third step he placed on the head of Bali and sent him to Patala or the antipodean world.

Allegorically, the story expresses the phenomenon of the dwarf sun rising every day while Bali, or darkness has been ruling the regions of sky and earth. The sun extends his rays and covers the sky with his first step, earth with his second, and sends darkness to the other side of the world with his third. Esoterically, this story explains the elimination of inner darkness as well and stages in chakra awakening. But Puranic scholars sometimes take it literally and try to prove it by quoting verses of the *Rigveda*. In this hymn there is no mention of the Bali story, but only the verses:

> *Vishnu moved, placed, and established his step in three ways.*
>
> *The insurmountable protector of movement, Vishnu moved three steps, sustaining the laws in this way.*
>
> *See the doings of Vishnu with which he spread his laws, the friend of the soul in union.*
>
> *Learned people always see the extended step of Vishnu as the vision of the eye depends on the sun.*
>
> *The alert, wise men kindle that which is Vishnu's ultimate step.*[431]
> *Medhatithi Kanva, Rigveda I.22.16-21*

According to Ananda Tirtha, these three steps are the three aspects of the Veda, the three divisions of time, and the three gunas or aspect of Nature (Prakriti). They are the three realms: of humans, devas, and lower beings; animate, inanimate, or mixed forms of creation. These are the three steps taken by the Supreme Lord in the process of creating this universe. In the phrase, "the friend of the soul in union," I have translated the word Indra as "soul" following Swami Dayananda, but Ananda Tirtha translates it as Prana or Life Breath. The two are not fundamentally different as the soul is the supreme Prana. This is another indication of the way the deity names like Indra are to be understood wherever they occur. Even Sayana translates one of the verses of this hymn as follows: "Learned men are, from the view of the scriptures, that ultimate point of God."

In the *Katha Upanishad* the same meaning is given to the word Vishnu, and the first line of the twentieth verse, *Tad Viṣṇoḥ paramam padam* shows exactly the same form without reference to the *Veda*. The entire stanza is as follows:

> *One whose charioteer is knowledge and who holds fast the reins of his mind attains the end of the path, which is Vishnu's ultimate step.*
> *Katha Upanishad 1.3.9*

It would require voluminous writing and research in order to explain the deeper meanings of all the Vedic deities. There are very few abstract deities in the *Vedas* named without any symbolic covering.[432] We have illustrated the fact that Devatas in the *Vedas* are not necessarily otherworldly beings, but simply the subject titles of the mantras. It is even a mistake even to translate the word mantra as "hymn." It comes from the root man (process of deep silent thought and meditation) and suggests an esoteric secret, not just an ordinary hymn of praise. In summing up this topic of Rishis and Devatas, let us quote from Rishi Katyayana in the *Sarvanukramani*, the most authentic index of Rishis and Devatas:

> *The Creator is the Devata of all Vedic mantras, i.e. One, that engulfs all Devatas, the ultimate Brahman, is the one Spiritual God. Other Devatas are only his powers and they are praised separately because of the different actions of the One. Only the one Great Atman is the real Devata.*

Historical Interpretations – Seven Rivers and Seven Chakras

It might be well here to say a few words about the historical interpretation of the *Vedas*. There is no doubt that some of the words occurring in the Vedas correspond to names of rivers or other outer aspects of life and can help us reconstruct the location and time of the Vedic era. But these terms are also to be understood as symbolic and cannot be regarded as just referring to outer objects. For instance, let us take the word Ganga. According to the Yaska's *Nirukta*, the root meaning of this word is "something that goes on incessantly".

The word Sarasvati later refers to the Goddess of Wisdom. There are several hymns eulogizing Sarasvati as a river in the *Rigveda*, but is the Sarasvati River only an outer stream? Is it only a river that is mentioned the "inspirer of true speech and kindler of good, deep thoughts"?[433] Sri Aurobindo tells us that, "the ocean is a symbol of immeasurable and eternal existence. The allegory of a river or a flowing stream is used as a symbol for the flow of conscious existence." Sarasvati is one of the seven rivers, the river of inner inspiration that emanates from the consciousness of truth. So we have every right to assume that the other six rivers should be translated symbolically. The *Hatha-Yoga-Pradipika* states: "Those who take a dip at the point where the rivers *Sita* and *Asita* converge, they attain liberation."

Perhaps it is not known to academic scholars that in the tradition of the Himalayan Yogis of India, Ganga, and Yamuna (names also of two geographical rivers) are synonyms of *Sita* and *Asita*, which are the two streams of consciousness. They are called also *Pingala* and *Ida Nadis*, flowing on the right and left sides of the *Sushumna*, the stream of consciousness in the spinal chord. In the *Rigveda* these three streams are called *Ida, Sarasvati,* and *Mahi* (or *Bharati*) the later two being the names of Sushumna and Pingala respectively.[434]

The converging point of these rivers is the *Ajna chakra* or Third Eye, the sixth of the seventh chakras. The *Jabala Upanishad*[435] says that the meeting place of Prana between the eyebrows is the converging point of heaven and earth. That is why, even in mythology, the river *Ganga* has come from the feet of *Vishnu* in the sky.

Other names of geographical rivers in the *Vedas* have similar deeper meanings. For example, *Vipasha*, literally means "free of ties and bonds." Vipasha helps a Rishi to cross over it, but it also helps to untie another's ties.[436] There is another word, *Shutudri*, that occurs with Vipasha in the above hymn, and also with Ganga, Yamuna, and Sarasvati in the tenth book.[437] The foregoing explanations suggest that the word Shutudri should also be understood in its root meaning. Vipasha and Shutudri are two aspects of the three-fold stream of consciousness of the spinal cord. Shutudri means "that runs in a hundred ways". So Shutudri is the consciousness divided into the hundred of streams in the nervous system, like the vagus nerve that is called the wandering nerve, whereas Vipasha, as already mentioned, is the quality of consciousness that unties the ties of bondage.

It was natural for such a spiritual people as the Vedic Indians to see the macrocosm in the microcosm, and so give names of the rivers of spiritual consciousness to the geographical rivers of their country. There are many examples of this fact. In the *Atharvaveda*, there is the verse:

> *"There is the city of Devas called Ayodhya*[438] *with eight chakras and nine doors and in which there is a golden treasure surrounded by brilliant light."*

The *Upanishads*, explaining this idea say, "In the ultimate golden treasure, there is the undivided pure *Brahman* which is the brilliant light of all lights known by those who know the Atman."[439] This verse from the *Upanishads* has been quoted to show that the terminology of the above mantra of *Atharvaveda* is also yogic. We know that there was a city called Ayodhya over which the whole dynasty of Ikshvakus ruled. The epic *Ramayana* is woven around this city. Does that mean that the above verse of the *Atharvaveda* was written after the city had been built? Or was the name of the city taken from the *Vedas*? Let us not forget, in making our judgment, that according to the *Ramayana*, the Ikshvakus were well versed in the *Vedas*.

There is another important point that has been ignored by most translators. Every hymn of the *Vedas* according to the *Nirukta* tradition should be explained in three aspects: (1) *Adhyatmika*, spiritual or psychological, (2) *Adhidaivika*, pertaining to devas or conscious and live forces of nature, (3) *Adhibhautika*, pertaining to Bhutas, the elements and the external world. Exoteric Indian scholarship and western academics focus on the third level and do not afford adequate emphasis to the other two. In addition, there are some hymns that scholars find difficult to translate in all three aspects. For example, the 24th hymn of the tenth book of the *Rigveda* is called *Dyuta-Sukta* or the "Hymn Against Gambling." The spiritual translation of this hymn is available with this writer.

Western Academic Views of the *Vedas*

This discussion would be incomplete without taking into consideration Western academic researches on the period of the *Vedas*. An interesting passage from one of Sri Aurobindo's earlier works brings into focus some important questions of this topic.

> This everlasting rock of the *Veda*, many assert, has no existence, there is nothing there but the commonest mud and sand, it is only a hymnal of primitive barbarians, only the rude worship of personified natural phenomena, or even less than that, a liturgy of ceremonial sacrifice, half religion, half magic, by which superstitious animal men of yore hoped to get themselves gold and goods and cattle, slaughter pitilessly their enemies, protect themselves from disease, calamity and demoniac influences and enjoy the coarse pleasure of a material Paradise. To that we must add a third view, the orthodox, or at least that which arises from Sayana's commentary. His view admitted, practically, the ignoble interpretation of the substance of the *Veda* and yet exalts the primitive farrago as holy scripture and a Book of Sacred Works……
>
> But there has always been this double and incompatible tradition about the *Veda* that is a book for ritual and mythology and it is a book of divine knowledge. The *Brahmanas* seized on the one tradition, the *Upanishads* on the other. Later, the learned took the hymns for a book essentially of ritual and works, they went elsewhere for pure knowledge but the instinct of the race bowed down before it with an obstinate, inarticulate memory of a loftier tradition……
>
> In any case, we have to make one choice or another. We can no longer securely enshrine the *Veda* wrapped up in the folds of an ignoble reverence or guarded by a pious self-deceit. Either the *Veda* is what Sayana says it is and then we have to leave it behind for ever as the document of mythology and ritual which has no longer any living truth or force for thinking minds, or it is what the European scholars say it is and then we have to put it away among the relics of the past as an antique record of semi-barbarous worship; or else it is indeed *Veda*, a book of divine Knowledge, and then it becomes of supreme importance to us to

know and hear its message…

> …if ever there was a tool of interpretation in which the loosest vein has been given to an ingenious speculation, in which doubtful indications have been snatched at as certain proofs, in which the boldest conclusions have been insisted upon with the scantiest justification, the most enormous difficulties ignored and preconceived prejudice maintained in the face of the clear and often admitted suggestions of the text, it is surely this labour, so eminently respectable otherwise for its industry, good will and power of research, performed through several centuries by European Vedic scholarship.

On this last question hinges the whole Hindu cosmology, the creation of man and the time of the revelation of the *Vedas*. The discussion must be limited to a short criticism of western academic theories related to this. There has been a very widespread tendency among western scholars to prove that hymns involving deep philosophical truths were of a more recent period than other hymns. This stand is taken because they cannot help seeing these profound truths in some of the hymns. The whole conception, in the West, of the historical intellectual evolution of man and the western concept of progress, blinds these scholars to the fact that human beings were capable of understanding deep spiritual truths at an early date, as these relate more to intuition than to intellect. Many of the Vedic hymns are couched in a deep symbolic terminology through which the inner meaning does not readily appear, and these scholars, honest and courageous as they are, cannot be blamed for lack of insight into the matters of divine experience. However, if research is done following such outer methods only, the inner truth of the *Vedas* will not be revealed.

The following is an example of the type of reasoning followed in these studies. The *Rigveda* is divided into ten books. Some of the hymns in the first and the tenth book are, even to the eye of a materialist, clearly spiritual and deeply philosophical. But many western academic scholars have worn themselves out trying to prove that the first and tenth books are of a later date for this reason. Understanding Vedic symbolism we can find such deep meanings even in the symbolic hymns of all the other books of the *Rigveda*.

Some of the hymns of the other books of the *Rigveda* have also been considered as the basis of Vedantic thought. For instance, the hymn of the Rishi Vamadeva from the fourth book of the *Rigveda* states:

> *I have been Manu and the Sun, I am the learned Rishi Kakshivan;*
> *I have given the earth to the noble, I have given rain to the charitable man;*
> *I have led gleaming waters and all the Gods have come to take*

refuge in my knowledge...
Vamadeva Gautama, Rigveda IV.26.1-2

An aphorism in the *Brahma Sutras* of Vyasa says that enlightenment comes to people as it came to the Vedic Rishi Vamadeva. Shankara, commenting on this aphorism, says:

The Self of the Deva Indra realized and saw the vision of the Ultimate as a Rishi, and preached, "Know Me." In the same way, the Rishi Vamadeva had the realization of the Universal One and felt himself being expanded into all.[440]

This is the real meaning of Vamadeva's hymn. Its Devata is Indra as Atman, the Supreme Self, not Indra as a mere king of the Gods. An esoteric scholar has no hesitation in saying that exoteric scholarship dare not reject all these hymns as later interpolations, or they will end up rejecting most of the *Rigveda*, which has many such symbolic utterances in all of its books, as an interpolation.

When the authorship of the Rishis mentioned with each hymn is taken literally, exoteric scholarship finds itself confronted by strange phenomena, and postulates many different possible meanings, each as difficult to understand as the next. For instance, in *Rigveda VIII.67.8*, the Rishis of this hymn are described as "many fish caught in a net." A person of spiritual insight does not have to speculate as to the possibility of fish in a net singing out a hymn of the *Rigveda*. Its spiritual significance is clear. The Devatas of the hymn are unity and the forces of unity, Adityas and Aditi. It is obvious that the souls caught in the net of karmic reactions have cried out in this hymn. These are the fish referred to. One might ask why the allegory of fish was chosen. The answer is that the image of being in the midst of waters is a favorite one for expressing spiritual unrest. A Vedic hymn to Varuna says:

The devotee is standing in the midst of water, dying of thirst.

Have mercy, O Healer of Wounds!
Maitravaruni Vasishtha, Rigveda VII.89.4

It is not possible to compare all the exoteric translations with the esoteric ones as we envision them. It will suffice to give one example. The esoteric translation refers to the Life Breath or Prana inherent in the whole Universe; but modern translators see Vata, the Devata of the hymn, as the deity of Wind, a eulogy of the Wind God. This is a representative specimen of other outer interpretations as well. Here is the translation of Hermann Oldenberg.

1. Now for the greatness of the chariot of Vata! Its roar goes crashing and thundering. It moves touching the sky creating red streams, or it goes scattering the dust of the earth.

2. Afterwards there rise the gusts of Vata, they go towards him like women to a feast. The god goes with them on the same chariot, he, the king of the whole of this world.

3. When he moves on his paths along the sky, he rests not even a single day; the friend of the waters, the first born, the holy, where was he born, whence did he spring?

4. The breath of the gods, the germ of the world, that god moves wherever he listeth; his roars indeed are heard, not his form – let us offer sacrifice to Vata.

Anila Vatayana, Rigveda X.168.10

The reader is invited to compare the above with our translation below:

1. We think of the greatness of the chariot of the Life Breath. Its roar comes breaking through. Touching the insides of the heavenly region, it moves, creating the colors of the dawn and throwing the dust off the earth.

2. The states of the Life Breath harmoniously inspire, and the feminine aspects follow it as if in a battle. United with the states of the Life Breath on the chariot (the body) the Divine is attained, the ruler of this whole universe.

3. Passing the paths of inner sight, it does not enter the outer light. This friend of the waters of peace, the first-born, the conveyor of the Absolute Truth, where was it born and whence?

4. This Atman or spirit of the Devas, this womb of the universe moves freely. Its roarings are heard but its form is unseen. For such is Life Breath we sacrifice to with the oblations of action.

Anila Vatayana, Rigveda X.168.10

Let us take the second half of the second verse. Esoterically it states, "united with the state of Life Breath on the chariot, (the body) the Divine is attained." But to Oldenburg, it is only the God of Wind that goes with gusts in his chariot, like women to a feast. Although Oldenberg clearly sees the word *sayuj* (which refers to one of four categories of *Mukti*, liberation) and the words "the ruler of this whole universe" does not seem to understand their real significance. The Atman or Self is the universal breath.

There is an interesting series of paradoxical questions and answers in the *Rigveda* and also the *Yajurveda* as follows:

> *I ask you, "What is the ultimate end of the earth?" I ask you, "What is the centre of the universe?"*
>
> *I ask you, "What is the semen of the powerful Ashva"? I ask you, "What is the ultimate abode of Speech"?*
>
> *"This center (fire altar of sacrifice) is the ultimate end of the earth. The sacrificial act is the center of the universe."*
>
> *"Soma is the semen of the powerful Ashva. Brahman (or the Veda) is the ultimate abode of Speech."*
>
> *Dirghatamas Auchatya, Rigveda I. 164.34-35, Shukla Yajurveda 23.61, 62*

The word *ashva* is exoterically translated as "horse", but if the grand symbol of Soma as described in the many hymns of the ninth book of the *Rigveda* is the semen of an ordinary animal, the whole thing makes no sense.[441] In the above sentence, a clue has been given as to the meaning of ashva. The scholars should note that one of the names of *Soma* that occurs in the *Veda* is *vājin*, which is also a synonym of ashva. This ashva is the symbol of animality and of Prana, and represents the beast-man that is, the man before his full spiritual development. We find both in the *Bhagavad Gita* and in the *Upanishads* that the senses are called "horses" and the mind, the "reins."

Esoteric Translations of the Vedic Hymns

I have only the photocopy of a translation of fifty-nine hymns of the ninth book of the *Rigveda* by one MSI who went by the name of *Ishaya* (literally "for God") and all his followers carry the surname Ishaya. An American, he found some unknown master who showed him the path and gave him insight into the *Veda*. I do not know if he translated any other hymns of the *Veda*.

The ninth book of *Rigveda* is dedicated to Soma, the Vedic symbol of Ananda or bliss on all levels of existence. Ishaya's translation of the very first Soma mantra takes into account the ideas of Soma and Indra that are parallel to what Vamadeva presents in this book. Here is Ishaya's translation and comments on the first hymn of the soma book of the *Rigveda*:

> *Oh Soma, purify with sweetest and most exhilarating shower. Effused for Evolving Consciousness, for the Guardian.*
>
> *Madhuchchhandas Vaishvamitra, Rigveda IX.1.1*
>
> The first syllable of the first word of the first verse begins with Sva, which also means the soul or the Self. All the movements of growth of consciousness come out of the Self. The entire *Veda* describes the movements of consciousness within the Self. The ninth mandala describes the transformations of Soma that generate Exalted Consciousness. This is the Holy Spirit moving in creation.
>
> "Evolving Consciousness" translates as *Indra*, called the "King of the Gods." Consciousness evolving is the root or basis of all higher transformations of sensual perception and mental experience that are symbolized by the gods. "The Guardian" or Evolving Consciousness supports, nourishes and protects everything in Creation.

This is just a taste of what Ishaya saw of the *Vedas*. I have not come across many who have this spiritual vision of the Vedic meaning arising out of meditative consciousness.

Below is a translation of one of the Vedic hymns as an example of the wisdom of the Vedas. Some day it is our hope to publish many more hymns and their translations. Some of these translations have been lying with us since 1946, first in Hindi and then in English from 1956 onwards.

1. *For protection and inspiration, each day we call upon the creator of good and beautiful forms, as a good milking cow calls the milkman at the time of milking; as that speech, capable of giving out great value, calls to itself one able to draw it forth.*
2. *Protector and drinker of Soma, come to our sacrifices of extracting soma juice and drink of it. The joy of one with wealth is the gift of the Word.*
3. *And may we know of thy intimate ideations. Mayst Thou come, but never to condemn us.*
4. *Go and ask Indra who speaks with discrimination, who has no thought-coverings, who awakens speech with his discriminating vision; who brings all that is desirable for your friends, for those who share your space in equality.*
5. *And let them speak who despise or censure us and who have the source of their movements elsewhere, but, O Indra, who have Thee at worship.*
6. *May all people, the cultivators of good, speak beautifully for that which is desirable. May we all take refuge in Indra.*

7. *Bring quickly this Soma for the initiate whose speed of progress is rapid; this Soma which is the glory of sacrificial acts, which gives joy to all humans, which is the friend of all joyful ones.*
8. *One with a hundred sacramental acts, by drinking it thou hast become the destroyer of evils and hast protected in struggles the swift and strong one.*
9. *Indra, O One with a hundred sacramental acts, O strong and swift one, possessor of great prowess, in struggles we follow Thee in order to attain a share of wealth.*
10. *People, sing for that Indra who is the sharer of wealth, who is great; who is good in taking one across (the ocean); who is a friend to those who extract Soma for sacrificial acts.*

Madhuchchhandas Vaishvamitra, Rigveda I.4.1-10.

This hymn is addressed to Indra in a Soma sacrifice. The inner meanings of both Indra and Soma have been clearly explained by Pandit Vamadeva Shastri (David Frawley) in the present book. If the meanings of these two words, Indra and Soma, are properly understood, the rest is crystal clear. This hymn sheds some light on important spiritual problems. Let us take each verse into consideration:

1. God is the creator, the creator of forms. He does not create out of non-existence but only carves out the forms. He is an architect or carpenter, following a plan. In many hymns he is called *takshan* or "one who carves out." Such hymns are the basis of Samkhya philosophy according to which the world is created out of the subtle substance of Prakriti or Nature. The point of discussion here, however, is not whether the world is actually created out of a substance called Prakriti or is just a manifestation of Brahman's abstract will. The whole point of the verse is that these manifested forms are not original but a creation. These forms are good and beautiful, but not ultimately true, because they are transitory. The suffix *su* denotes goodness and beauty, but not always truth. In order to understand these forms, we have to call upon the Creator. He only is capable of "milking" speech, the word (i.e. all things) and knowing its relation with the meaning denoted within. The meaning is hidden inside everything and inside us. If a milker does not come to milk a cow at the required time, the cow calls out for him. In the same way, all we beings on earth in different outer forms have the true meaning of God within us and are calling upon Him to reveal it. That is why in the fourth verse he is spoken of as one who is uncovered.

2. The second verse explains the meaning of the first verse more explicitly. There is no doubt that a milkman milks the cow, but there must be some milk in the udders. Similarly, to be responsible for extracting the juice of Soma, we have to see the true Reality in the state of samadhi. The value of food is extracted in a long digestive process; the joy of extracting Soma is to give the Word out. The great masters see the truth and cannot help singing out of this joy. Their word is the eternal poetry. The Vedas are called "Divine poetry that never dies and never decays."[442]

3. The word *antama* in the third verse means "intimate" or "the one that is the end or ultimate." The understanding of God's Word and the realization of the Supreme Idea (the archetype of all) is the most intimate form of all knowledge and also the ultimate end of all thoughts. That is why we are told in the *Upanishads*, "By knowing that, all becomes known."[443]

4. In the fourth verse, only one sentence requires clarification, friends, those who share your space in equality." The word *sakhi* means "friend" but the root meaning is "one with equal or common space."[444] Space here is not meant in the general sense of the word, but denotes equal and common standing. The aim of life is to attain friendship with the Ultimate Reality. In highest states of meditation the individuated consciousness experiences sharing the same space as the infinite Divine being.

5. The fifth verse teaches that other paths can also lead toward the Supreme Idea as beautifully as one's own.

6. The word *kṛṣṭi* has the inherent meaning of "cultivation." The word often means "the people" but the root *kṛṣ* means "to cultivate." The Latin cultare is its cognate, and from it our word culture is derived. This one word explains a very important factor of the anthropology and social history of humanity. The spiritual culture of humanity begins with humans settling down in sedentary groups to cultivate the land. In such a community there is more time for leisure, and a human is able to cultivate the spirit. The most suitable word to describe such a people is *kṛṣṭi* because it conveys the idea of an established society of those people who, in addition to cultivating the land, cultivate themselves spiritually as well. The direct contact of the human soul with outer nature creates the link between those artificial divisions usually called "metaphysics" and "ethics." The institution of the modern city in no way allows people to become *kṛṣṭi*. In the verse, the word *kṛṣṭi* speaks

beautifully and brings about everything that is good and desirable. This combination of truth, goodness and beauty can be manifested only in a society in which every individual has cultivated himself. Such a society takes refuge in Indra, the one who has given it all to us.

7. The seventh verse answers a question that is generally asked by the novice. "How long will it take before I reach the goal?" The answer is that it depends on how quick you are.[445] One of the names of Soma is quick one (āśu, vājī). One's speed of spiritual attainment, of course, is an outcome of the accumulations of previous memories and samskaras. The more one purifies oneself, the friendlier the attitude of Soma and the greater the bliss of samadhi becomes.

This is but a typical example of a spiritual, yogic, or esoteric interpretation of a typical Vedic hymn that could easily be extended to all the Vedic hymns.

APPENDICES

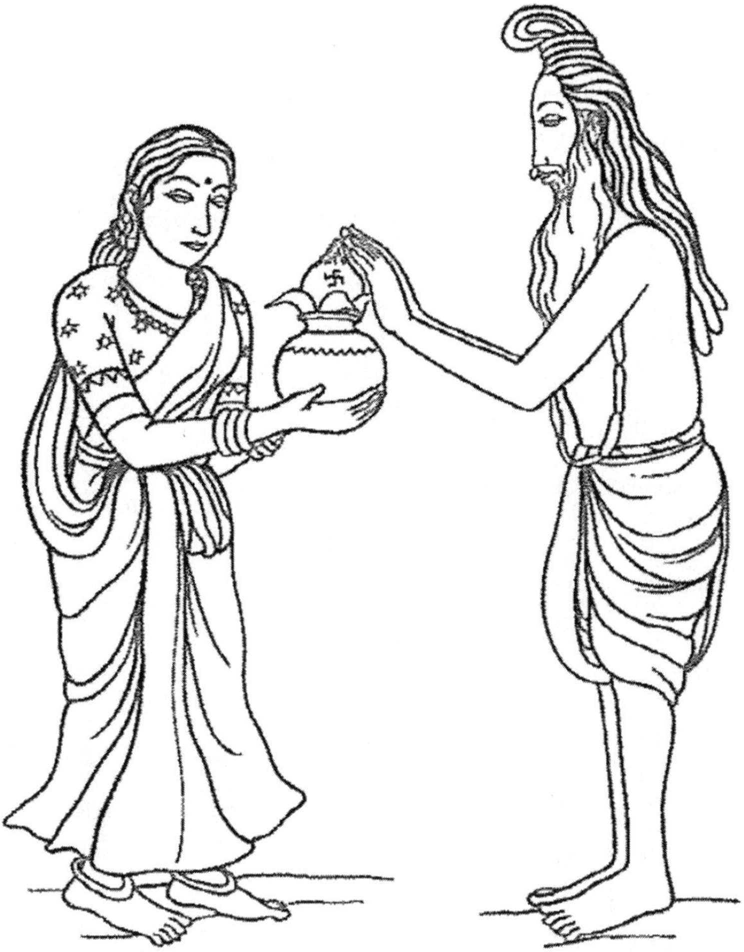

Sanskrit Terms

A

Adhibhutic – relative to the elements

Adhidaivic – relative to the Gods or cosmic powers

Adhvaryu – priest making the offerings, symbolic of mind or prana

Adhyatmic – relative to the self or psychological dimension

Adhyayana – study of the Vedas

Aditi – the Unbounded, Vedic name for the Mother Goddess

Aditya – Sun God as power of primal intelligence

Adityas – Sun Gods

Advaita – non-duality

Akshara – Divine word, Mantra Yoga

Agastya – Rigvedic seer connected to South India, older brother of Vasishtha

Agni – Vedic sacred fire, cosmic fire, light of the soul. fire of yoga, fire of prana, fire of intelligence (dhi or buddhi), fire of consciousness, fire of Brahman

Ahamkara – ego

Aja – goat or unborn as the higher Self

Ananda – bliss

Angiras – original Vedic Rishi born of the coals of the sacred Fire

Angirasa Rishis – Rishis in the line or family of Angiras

Antariksha – atmosphere

Antar yajna – inner sacrifice

Anubhuti – inner flow of Self-awareness

Anveshana – inner search

Aparoksha – direct knowledge of the Self

Apas – waters as a cosmic principle, literally the waves, often the ocean of air, ocean of space, or field of prana

Aranyaka – third division of Vedic texts as forest texts, meditational in nature

Aryaman – Vedic Sun God as the meditator

Asana – Yoga postures

Ashva – horse as power of prana

Ashvins – Twin horseman deities

Asura – anti-God

Atharva-veda – last of the four *Vedas*

Atman – higher Self

Atri – Vedic Rishi family line

Ayurveda – Vedic medicine and healing system for body and mind

B

Bahir yajna – outer sacrifice

Bhaga – blissful form of Vedic Sun God

Bhagavan – Divine Lord

Bhakti Yoga – Yoga of Devotion

Bharadvaja – Vedic Rishi family line

Bhishma – Great teacher and elder in the Mahabharata

Bhrigu – one of the two oldest families of Rishis, born of the flame of the sacred Fire

Bhrigu Rishis – Bhrigu family of seers

Bindu – central point behind all time and space

Brahma – creator among the Hindu trinity

Brahma Sutras – Sutra texts of the Uttara Mimamsa or Vedantic school among the six schools of Vedic philosophy, by Badarayana

Brahman – Godhead or Absolute

Brahmin – member of the Brahmin class

Brahmanas – Vedic ritualistic texts

Brahmanaspati – same as Brihaspati

Brihaspati – Vedic deity of speech

Buddhi – higher mind or awakened intelligence; Dhi

C

Chakra – energy centers of subtle body, wheels of the Sun or prana

Chhandas – Vedic meters

Chitta – mind in the general sense

D

Daksha – discernment, yogic viveka

Deva – deity, God

Devata – Deity, divine or cosmic principle

Dharana – concentration

Dhara – flow of Soma, as flow of bliss or samadhi

Dharma – natural law or way of truth, Yoga Dharma

Dhi – higher mind, buddhi

Dhyana – meditation

Diksha – initiation

Dvaita – duality

Dyaus – heaven

G

Ganapati, Ganesha – Elephant-headed God of wisdom

Gaveshana – search for the cows; the light or the origin of the soul

Gayatri – Vedic verse to awaken the higher light within us; Vedic meter

Gotama – Vedic Rishi and Rishi line, father of Vamadeva of the fourth book of the *Rigveda*

Go – cow, ray of light, the sense organs, the soul; what is hidden

Gotra – Vedic family line

Gritsamada – Vedic Rishi of second book of the *Rigveda*, of the Bhrigu family

Ghrita – clarified butter; clarified mind or perception

Guha – secrecy, cave of the heart, name of Agni Vaishvanara

H

Hanuman – monkey companion of Lord Rama

Havan – Vedic fire sacrifice

Hatha Yoga – Yoga of effort and pranic practices

Hiranyagarbha – Vedic solar deity/sage; founder of Yoga Darshana

Hota – priest who recites the invocation, identified with Agni or the sacred Fire

Hridaya – the spiritual heart

I

Īṁ – Vedic Pranava or Divine Word

Indu – Soma as a drop or sphere

Indra – Self as seer; higher prana

J

Jatavedas – Agni as the Knower of all births or indwelling soul and life-principle

Jatharagni – digestive fire

Jnana Yoga – Yoga of knowledge

Jiva – soul as reincarnating entity

Jivatman – individual soul

Jyotisha – Vedic astrology

K

Kaivalya – liberation

Kanvas – Vedic Rishi family line, relate to the eighth book of the Rigveda

Kapha – biological water humor

Karma – Karma Yoga or rituals; Yoga of action

Kashyapa – ancient Rishi and Rishi family; Buddha prior to Shakyamuni who taught the Vedas

Kavi – seer or seer-poet; one who has the vision of Yoga

Kratu – will power, samkalpa

Krishna – ancient avatar of Vishnu and avatar of Yoga

Kumara – Agni as the child of the inner rebirth; Lord Skanda

Kundalini – root Shakti of sound and light in the subtle body

M

Madhu – honey-wine, bliss

Mahabharata – epic of Krishna and the Pandavas

Mahayajna – great sacrifice

Manas – mind in the general sense, outer aspect of mind connected to the senses

Mandala – book of the *Rigveda*, of which there are ten

Manisha – inspired intelligence

Mantra – Mantra Yoga

Manu – first sage and king of this yuga or world-age

Maruts – Vedic storm Gods connected to Indra and Rudra

Mati – thought power

Maya – negatively the power of ignorance (Asura Maya), positively the power of knowledge (Deva Maya)

Medha – wisdom, Goddess

Mitra – Vedic solar deity of friendship and compassion

Moksha – liberation of the Spirit

N

Nada – Nada Yoga or Yoga of the sound current

Namas – Surrender or Bhakti Yoga

Nama – recitation of Divine names

O

Ojas – primary vitality

Oṁ – Divine word

P

Paramam Vyoma – the highest space of the heart

Paramatman – supreme Self

Parashara – great Vedic Rishi and astrologer

Parashurama – sixth avatar of Lord Vishnu

Parayana – recitation of the *Vedas*

Paroksha – Vedic intuitive knowledge

Patanjali – great sage and compiler of the *Yoga Sutras*

Pitta – biological fire humor

Prakriti – nature, matter, process or basis of all outer manifestation

Prana – life-force; cosmic life-force

Pranava – primal sound, Divine word, Oṁ or bija mantras

Pranayama – Yogic practice developing the higher energy of prana

Prarthana – prayer or supplication

Pratyahara – Yogic internalization of the mind, prana, and senses

Pratyaksha – knowledge born of direct perception, generally through the senses

Prithivi – earth

Puranas – Hindu sacred texts, encyclopedic in nature

Purusha – cosmic person

Pushan – perceptive and nourishing form of the Solar Deity

R

Raja Yoga – royal or integral Yoga

Rama – seventh avatar of Vishnu

Rasa – essence

Ratha – chariot, term for the Yoga of the chakras and the subtle body

Rigveda – oldest, largest and most central of the Vedas

Rishi – Vedic seer or sage

Ritam – truth and law

Rudra – fierce form of Shiva and Agni

Rudram – famous Yajurveda chant to Rudra

Rudras – sons or manifestations of Shiva, usually same as Maruts

S

Samadhi – yogic state of higher consciousness

Samhita – mantra portion of the four *Vedas*

Samkhya – Vedic philosophy of twenty-five principles, founded by Kapila; along with Yoga an important one of the six schools of Vedic philosophy

Samkhya Karika – main Sutra texts on the Samkhya school; one of the six schools of Vedic philosophy, compiled by Ishvara Krishna

Sanatana Dharma – the Eternal Dharma

Sara – essence

Sarasvati – Goddess of wisdom

Sat – Being

Satya – truth

Savita – solar enlightenment power

Shakti – energy or power; the Goddess

Shankara – name of Shiva, great teacher of Advaita Vedanta

Shanti – peace

Shantipatha – Vedic peace recitations

Shastra – definitive text of Vedic knowledge

Shiva – dissolver of the Hindu trinity

Skanda – Second son of Shiva and Parvati, connected to Agni or fire

Soma – nectar of devotion, samadhi, bliss or ananda

Stotra – hymns in classical Sanskrit

Stuti – praise as part of Bhakti Yoga

Sukta – Vedic hymn or mantric verse

Surya – Sun; principle of truth and illumination

Svadhyaya – study of the teachings relevant to oneself

Svaha – Vedic fire offering mantra; consort of Agni

Svara – mantra sound vibration or Mantra Yoga, essence of sound

T

Tantras – Medieval teachings relating to Shiva and Shakti

Tejas – fire as a vital principle of positive energy and light

Tapas – tapas or concentrated energetic practice as a yogic principle

Tat – cosmic consciousness

Tvashta – solar deity as master craftsman

U

Udgata – singer among the Vedic priests

Upanishads – Philosophical portion of the Vedas, foundation of Vedanta and Jnana Yoga

Ushanas – famous Vedic seer-poet

Ushas – Dawn Goddess, aspiration to the higher knowledge and Yoga

V

Vaishvanara – Agni as the universal soul

Vak – higher speech or Mantra Yoga

Vamadeva – Rishi of the fourth book of the *Rigveda*, of the Gautama line

Varuna – Vedic deity of the cosmic waters and the setting sun

Vasishtha – Rishi of the seventh book of the *Rigveda* and Rishi family line

Vata – cosmic life-force of Prana Yoga

Vayu – cosmic spirit of Prana Yoga

Vipra – enlightened sage; Rishi

Veda – spiritual knowledge

Veda Vyasa – compiler of the *Vedas*, also known as Krishna Dvaipayana

Vedas – Vedic texts

Vedanta – Vedic philosophy rooted in *Upanishads* and *Bhagavad Gita*

Vidya – way of knowledge

Vidyut – lightning or electrical energy

Vishnu – the preserver aspect of the Hindu Trinity

Vishvamitra – Rishi of the third book of the *Rigveda* and Rishi family line

Vishvedeva – universal deities; a class of Vedic deities

Vivasvan – solar deity who taught Manu

Vyoma – space, including the space within the heart

Y

Yajna – sacred offering, worship, or consecration; Yoga as the inner sacrifice

Yajnavalkya – great later Vedic, Upanishadic and Yogic sage

Yajurveda – *Veda* of sacrificial action or worship

Yoga – yoking or coordinating of higher powers

Yoga Darshana – Yoga as one of the six schools of Vedic philosophy, in the Smriti literature

Yoga Sutras – main Smriti and Sutra text on Yoga Darshana, compiled by Patanjali

Yogi Yajnavalkya – important ancient Yoga text

Sanskrit Diacritical Marks Pronunciation Guide

From 108 Sanskrit Flashcards w/CD,
by Nicolai Bachman/The Ayurvedic Press.

14 Vowels

a	another
ā	father (2 beats)
i	pin
ī	need (2 beats)
u	put
ū	mood (2 beats)
ṛ	macabre
ṝ	trill for 2 beats
ḷ	table
e	etude (2 beats)
ai	aisle (2 beats)
o	yoke (2 beats)
au	flautist (2 beats)

2 Special Letters

aṃ	hum (also ṃ)
aḥ	out-breath

33 Consonants

ka	paprika
kha	thick honey
ga	saga
gha	big honey
ṅa	ink
ca	chutney
cha	much honey
ja	Japan
jha	raj honey
ña	inch
ṭa	borscht again
ṭha	borscht honey
ḍa	shdum
ḍha	shd hum
ṇa	shnum
ta	pasta
tha	eat honey
da	soda
dha	good honey
na	banana
pa	paternal
pha	scoop honey
ba	scuba
bha	rub honey
ma	aroma
ya	employable
ra	abra cadabra
la	hula
va	variety
śa	shut
ṣa	shnapps
sa	Lisa
ha	honey

Bibliography

Aurobindo, Sri. HYMNS TO THE MYSTIC FIRE. Twin Lakes WI: Lotus Press 2001.

Aurobindo Sri, THE LIFE DIVINE. Twin Lakes WI: Lotus Press 2001.

Aurobindo Sri. SAVITRI. Twin Lakes WI: Lotus Press 2001.

Aurobindo, Sri. SECRET OF THE VEDAS. Twin Lakes WI: Lotus Press 2001.

Dayananda Sarasvati, Swami. SATYARTHA PRAKASH. New Delhi, India: Savradeshik Arya Pratinidhi Sabha 1994.

Daivarata, Brahmarshi, CHHANDODARSHANA (out of print).

Daivarata, Brahmarshi, INDRA YAJNA (out of print).

Daivarata, Brahmarshi, VAK SUDHA (out of print).

Kak, Subhash. THE ASTRONOMICAL CODE OF THE *VEDAS*. Delhi, India: Munshi Manorharlal, 2000.

Kavyakantha Ganapati Muni, COMPLETE SANSKRIT WORKS IN TWELVE VOLUMES. K. Natesan, editor. Dr. Sampadananda Mishra, Associate Editor. Thiruvannamalai, India: Sri Ramanasramam, 2007.

Mishra, Sampadananda. THE WONDER THAT IS SANSKRIT. Pondicherry, India: Sri Aurobindo Society, 2010.

Mishra, Sampadananda. SANSKRIT AND THE EVOLUTION OF HUMAN SPEECH. Pondicherry, India: Sri Aurobindo Society, 2010.

Pandit, M.P. ADORATION OF THE DIVINE MOTHER. Ganesh and Company: Madras, India 1973.

Pandit, M.P. VEDIC DEITIES. Twin Lakes WI: Lotus Press 1989.

Pandit, M.P. WISDOM OF THE VEDA. Twin Lakes WI: Lotus Press 1990.

Lal, B.B. THE OLDEST CIVILIZATION IN SOUTH ASIA. Delhi, India: Aryan Books International, 1997.

Lal, B.B. THE SARASVATI FLOWS ON. Delhi, India: Aryan Books International, 2002.

Rao, S.R. DAWN AND DEVOLUTION OF THE INDUS CIVILIZATION. New Delhi, India: Aditya Prakashan 1991.

Sastry, T.V. Kapali. Siddhanjali. COLLECTED WORKS OF T.V. KAPALI SHASTRY, volumes one to four. Pondicherry, India: Dipti Publications 1983.

Subramuniyaswami, Satguru Sivaya. DANCING WITH SIVA. India, USĂ Himalayan Academy, 1993.

Swarup, Ram. THE WORD AS REVELATION: NAMES OF GODS. Delhi, India: Voice of India 2001.

Tilak, B.G. ORION OR RESEARCHED INTO THE ANTIQUITY OF THE VEDA. Poona, India: Shri J.S. Tilak 1986.

Veda Bharati, Swami. DIVA DUHITA (contains Chhandasi). Delhi, India: Chaukhambha Books 2012.

Yogananda, Paramahamsa. AUTOBIOGRAPHY OF A YOGI. Los Angeles CA: Self-realization Fellowship, 1976.

Relevant Books by the Author – David Frawley (Vamadeva Shastri)

ASTROLOGY OF THE SEERS: A COMPREHENSIVE GUIDE TO VEDIC (HINDU) ASTROLOGY. Twin Lakes WI: Lotus Press 2001.

GODS, SAGES AND KINGS: VEDIC SECRETS OF ANCIENT CIVILIZATION. Twin Lakes WI: Lotus Press 2012.

HIDDEN HORIZONS: UNEARTHING 10,000 YEARS OF INDIAN CULTURE. Ahmdavad, India: Swaminarayan 2006.

IN SEARCH OF THE CRADLE OF CIVILIZATION (with Georg Feuerstein and Subhash Kak). Wheaton IL: Quest Books 1995.

MANTRA YOGA AND PRIMAL SOUND. Twin Lakes WI: Lotus Press 2010.

MYTH OF THE ARYAN INVASION OF INDIA. Delhi, India: Voice of India 1994, 2005.

RIG VEDA AND THE HISTORY OF INDIA. Delhi, India: Aditya Prakasha, 2001.

SOMA IN YOGA AND AYURVEDA: THE POWER OF REJUVENATION AND IMMORTALITY. Twin Lakes WI: Lotus Press 2001.

WISDOM OF THE ANCIENT SEERS: SELECTED MANTRAS FROM THE RIGVEDA. Twin Lakes WI: Lotus Press 2001.

YOGA AND THE SACRED FIRE. Twin Lakes WI: Lotus Press 2001.

Sanskrit Texts

Aitareya Aranyaka

Aitareya Brahmana

Atharvaveda Samhita

Bhagavad Gita

Brahma Sutras Of Badarayana

Brihadaranayaka Upanishad

Brihad Devata Of Shaunaka

Brihad Yogi Yajnavalkya Smriti

Chandogya Upanishad

Hatha Yoga Pradipika

Kaushitaki Upanishad

Mahabharata

Mahanarayana Upanishad

Rigveda Samhita

Samaveda Samhita

Samkhya Karika Of Ishvara Krishna

Shatapatha Brahmana

Shvetashvatara Upanishad

Taittiriya Aranyaka

Taittiriya Brahmana

Taittiriya Upanishad

Vasishtha Samhita

Yajurveda Samhita, Shukla

Yajurveda Samhita Krishna
Or Taittiriya Recension

Yoga Sutras Of Patanjali

Resources

Vedacharya David Frawley (Pandit Vamadeva Shastri)

David Frawley (b. 1950) is the author of more than thirty books and several distance learning courses written over the past thirty years. His books are available in twenty different languages and include important publications in the fields of Ayurvedic medicine, Vedic astrology, Raja Yoga, Veda, Vedanta, and Tantra. His works are noted for their depth and specificity and often serve as textbooks in their respective fields.

Vamadeva is one of the most respected *Vedacharyas* or teachers of the ancient Vedic wisdom in recent decades, East and West. He is honored in traditional circles in India, where his writings are well known and frequently quoted. He is also regarded as a teacher or acharya of Yoga, Ayurveda and Vedic astrology, reflecting his rare ability to link different Vedic disciplines together and teach them in an integral manner. He works with several Vedic and yogic groups worldwide.

Vamadeva's first works of translations and interpretations of the *Vedas* and *Upanishads* were written in the period of 1978-1984, and included extensive studies of the classical *Upanishads, Yajurveda*, and, most notably, the *Rigveda* in the original Sanskrit published through the Sri Aurobindo Ashram and Motilal Banarsidass (MLBD) in India. He is better known in the West through his popular books on Ayurveda, Yoga, and Vedic astrology, but all of these reflect an earlier and continuous study of the *Vedas*, such as occurs in the present book. He views the *Vedas* as the foundation of all these later teachings and as the most important texts for humanity today as well.

American Institute of Vedic Studies, *www.vedanet.com*

The American Institute of Vedic Studies is an internationally recognized center for Vedic learning, with affiliated organizations worldwide. Directed by Acharya David Frawley (Pandit Vamadeva Shastri) and Yogini Shambhavi, the Vedic institute serves as a vehicle for their work, books, CDs, programs, and activities. The institute, which is now primarily web-based, offers in depth training, including distance-learning programs in Ayurveda, Raja Yoga, and Vedic astrology. Its courses are available in a number of different languages and through several affiliated organizations worldwide.

The institute participates in regular retreats in different countries in order to bring students from all over the world for a deeper level of instruction with Vamadeva and Shambhavi. It also participates in various international programs, events and conferences. The institute website features extensive on-line articles, on-line books, and a full range of Vedic resources for the serious student, including a regular newsletter.

Yogini Shambhavi

Yogini Shambhavi Chopra is one of the foremost traditional women teachers coming out of India today. She is the author of several important books on the Goddess (*Yogini: Unfolding the Goddess Within* and *Yogic Secrets of the Dark Goddess*), noted for their experiential approach to higher consciousness. Her *Yogini Bhava* and *Jyotish Bhava* CDs provide powerful guides for traditional chanting and mantra sadhana, invoking the Divine presence and power of Shakti in our lives.

Shambhavi offers consultations in Vedic astrology and spiritual guidance, reflecting her understanding of the Divine powers of the planets and their karmic connections. She also offers special initiations into Shakti Sadhana and Shakti Dharma for select students from all over the world who seek her guidance. She has a proficiency in both Vedic and Tantric mantras that she shares with her students. She is a great inspiration for all who come into contact with her.

Sampadananda Mishra

Sampadananda Mishra is one of the leading Vedic and Sanskrit scholars and teachers in the tradition of Sri Aurobindo. He has completed several important projects on Sanskrit and Indian culture including such books as *The Wonder That is Sanskrit, Sanskrit and the Evolution of Human Speech, Sri Aurobindo and Sanskrit, and Srimad Bhagavad Gita in the Light of Sri Aurobindo*, and several multimedia CD-Roms including *Devabhasha, the Language of Gods*, and *Ashtavadhanam* or *Eightfold Concentration*.

Most notably for the present book, he taken up another project titled *Vedas in the Light of Sri Aurobindo*. The aim of this project is to explore the secret of the *Vedas* and make the study of the Vedas more relevant to the present age. His website is http://aurosociety.org/focus-area/indian-culture.aspx. He also has a special blog on Ganapati Muni at http://kavyakantha.blogspot.in.

Mahamandaleshwara Swami Veda Bharati

Swami Veda Bharati was born in a Sanskrit speaking family in 1933. He taught the *Yoga Sutras* of Patanjali to classes from 1942, at the age of nine. In 1946 a number of articles appeared in the Hindi press proclaiming this child prodigy's exceptional knowledge of the *Vedas*, with his ability to instantly provide a threefold translation of any of the four *Vedas*. He then began to be invited to address crowds of thousands as well as colleges and universities throughout North India.

Between 1965 and 1967-68 he also obtained all his degrees: B.A. (Honours) London, M.A. (London), D.Litt. (Holland), and is F.R.A.S. He has varying degrees of access to seventeen languages. He runs over sixty meditation groups and centers in twenty-five countries.

Swami Veda has written eighteen books, including a fifteen hundred page commentary (so far in two volumes) on the first two padas (quarters) of the *Yoga Sutras*, which is proclaimed by scholars as a highly scholarly and meticulous work. The work on third pada is now in progress.

He holds the prestigious title of "Mahamandaleshwara" in the community of the Swami Order of monks. He is the spiritual guide to two Ashrams in Rishikesh: Sadhana Mandir, the Ashram of Swami Rama, and now also Swami Rama Sadhaka Grama of which is the founder, where seekers from throughout the world come to learn meditation. Now at the age of eighty, from March 2013, he has entered a five year mauna vrata (vow of silence).

For further information please inquire from Association of Himalayan Yoga Meditation Societies International (www.ahymsin.org) of which he is the founder. A list of his inspirational and spiritual works may also be obtained from:

ahymsinpublishers@gmail.com

www.swamiveda.org

www.swamivedablog.org

www.swamiveda.org

www.swamivedablog.org

Quotes about the Book

Philip Goldberg, Hinduism Today, Deepak Chopra, Subhash Kak, Jnana Deva, Swami Sitaramananda

David Frawley is one of the most important voices in the ongoing transmission of Vedic knowledge that has already transformed the spiritual landscape of the West. This book is a sparkling gem in his necklace of trenchant commentaries; it will doubtless leave a profound and enduring mark on religious history. It could not come at a better time. The extraordinary popularity of Yoga has brought enormous benefits to millions of people, but it comes at a price: the growing tendency on the part of practitioners and teachers alike to equate the word 'Yoga' with the familiar postures, bends and stretches called *asanas*. This threatens to reduce a rich, complex philosophical and spiritual system to a form of physical fitness. By interpreting the most ancient of sacred texts in the light of modern knowledge and contemporary needs, *Vedic Yoga* connects today's yogis to the legendary rishis whose Himalayan insights formed the foundation of India's glorious spiritual heritage. Thought-provoking, revelatory, and pregnant with practical implications, Frawley's brave book should be cherished by spiritual aspirants of all traditions and paths.

Philip Goldberg, author of *American Veda: From Emerson and the Beatles to Yoga and Meditation, How Indian Spirituality Changed the West*

Vedic Yoga: The Path of the Rishi is a masterful book that takes the reader back to the earliest original sources of the Yoga tradition and in the process presents unexpected pathways of understanding and self-examination. David Frawley is one of the world's foremost authorities on the Veda and his search for the Vedic roots of Yoga breaks much fresh ground. This new light on Yoga comes at a very good time as practitioners of Yoga around the world are beginning to seek its deeper dimension beyond *asanas* and meditation to a direct apprehension of reality.

Vedic Yoga is not a mere academic exercise since it is informed by Frawley's own personal spiritual journey which is described charmingly in the autobiographical sections of the book. Frawley came to know some of the leading masters and scholars of Yoga and the account of these encounters is very instructive. The book will benefit both the scholar and the layperson.

Subhash Kak, Regents Professor at Oklahoma State University and author of *Mind and Self*.

Vedic Yoga is a treasure for every serious practitioner of Yoga. With profound insight, Acharya Vamadeva (Dr. Frawley) reveals the practical yogic secrets hidden within the symbolism of the *Vedas*, and brings forth the power of the Vedic mantras for developing the cosmic forces of higher awareness within each person. *Vedic Yoga* is an authoritative, eye-opening journey into the core of this time-honored science for experiencing our true, divine nature.

Gyandev McCord, author of *Spiritual Yoga: Awakening to Higher Awareness*
Co-founder of Yoga Alliance

In this new book on Vedic Yoga, Acharya Vamadeva Shastri David Frawley, a Vedic rishi in his own right, once more goes back to the depths of Vedic knowledge from the *Rigveda*. Exploring this largely uncharted territory, he brings to life and makes relevant for our modern yoga times and current environmental crisis the Sadhana of contemplation on the Vedic deities and the world of Nature they represent, and on the Rishis' path itself. Acharya Vamadeva Shastri not only enhances our understanding of the classical paths of Yoga, but also opens us to inspiring hopeful possibilities for a new human consciousness.

Swami Sitaramananda
Acharya, International Sivananda Yoga Vedanta Centers and Ashrams

This profound and intricate book from a great Vedic master can serve as a guide to total well-being and complete enlightenment.

Deepak Chopra, M.D.

David Frawley is one of the most important voices in the ongoing transmission of Vedic knowledge that has already transformed the spiritual landscape of the West. This book is a sparkling gem in his necklace of trenchant commentaries; it will doubtless leave a profound and enduring mark on religious history.

It could not come at a better time. The extraordinary popularity of Yoga has brought enormous benefits to millions of people, but it comes at a price: the growing tendency on the part of practitioners and teachers alike to equate the word 'Yoga' with the familiar postures, bends and stretches called asanas. This threatens to reduce a rich, complex philosophical and spiritual system to a form of physical fitness. By interpreting the most ancient of sacred texts in the light of modern knowledge and contemporary needs, Vedic Yoga connects today's yogis to the legendary rishis whose Himalayan insights formed the foundation of India's glorious spiritual heritage. Thought-provoking, revelatory, and pregnant with practical implications, Frawley's brave book should be cherished by spiritual aspirants of all traditions and paths.

Philip Goldberg, author of *American Veda: From Emerson and the Beatles to Yoga and Meditation, How Indian Spirituality Changed the West*

Pandit Vamadeva Shastri, Vedacharya David Frawley has studied the timeless ancient wisdom of the Vedas. With his beautiful knowledge of Sanskrit, he has put this complex knowledge in a modern scientific way that will help Ayurvedic scholars, Vedic scholars and even those who study quantum physics. He brings us Vedic knowledge in a direct and practical way, so that one can apply this wisdom in his or her daily life.

Vamadeva provides a profound understanding of the play of Agni and Soma. Even students of Ayurveda do not have the complete picture of Ojas, Tejas, and Prana and how Ojas is transformed into Soma. He has beautifully explained the meaning of Agni and Soma and how we can bring about the inner state of enlightenment. This book is an important guide for all those who seek Self-realization.

Vasant Lad, B.A.M.&S., M.A.Sc, Ayurvedic Physician
Author of *Ayurveda: Science of Self-Healing, Textbook of Ayurveda* and Director of the Ayurvedic Institute

Vedic Yoga: The Path of the Rishi is a masterful book that takes the reader back to the earliest original sources of the Yoga tradition and in the process presents unexpected pathways of understanding and self-examination. David Frawley is one of the world's foremost authorities on the Veda and his search for the Vedic roots of Yoga breaks much fresh ground. This new light on Yoga comes at a very good time as practitioners of Yoga around the world are beginning to seek its deeper dimension beyond asanas and meditation to a direct apprehension of reality.

Vedic Yoga is not a mere academic exercise since it is informed by Frawley's own personal spiritual journey, which is described charmingly in the autobiographical sections of the book. Frawley came to know some of the leading masters and scholars of Yoga and the account of these encounters is very instructive. The book will benefit both the scholar and the layperson.

Subhash Kak, Regents Professor at Oklahoma State University and author of *Mind and Self.*

Vedic Yoga is a treasure for every serious practitioner of Yoga. With profound insight, Acharya Vamadeva (Dr. Frawley) reveals the practical yogic secrets hidden within the symbolism of the Vedas, and brings forth the power of the Vedic mantras for developing the cosmic forces of higher awareness within each person. Vedic Yoga is an authoritative, eye-opening journey into the core of this time-honored science for experiencing our true, divine nature.

Gyandev McCord, author of *Spiritual Yoga: Awakening to Higher Awareness*
Co-founder of Yoga Alliance

In this new book on Vedic Yoga, Acharya Vamadeva Shastri David Frawley, a Vedic rishi in his own right, once more goes back to the depths of Vedic knowledge from the Rigveda.

Exploring this largely uncharted territory, he brings to life and makes relevant for our modern yoga times and current environmental crisis the Sadhana of contemplation on the Vedic deities and the world of Nature they represent, and on the Rishis' path itself. Acharya Vamadeva Shastri not only enhances our understanding of the classical paths of Yoga, but also opens us to inspiring hopeful possibilities for a new human consciousness.

Swami Sitaramananda
Acharya, International Sivananda Yoga Vedanta Centers and Ashrams

David Frawley is one of the great exponents of the Vedic philosophy today. This is because he explains it so clearly, both from personal study as well as from his own inner experience. Frawley conclusively draws a connection between classical Yoga and early Vedic teachings, an issue that has been of some controversy in recent years. His book is a necessary reference for all those who are interested in yoga in the deeper sense - to see the Vedic roots of Yoga philosophy.

Stephen Knapp
Author of numerous books on Vedic culture

INDEX

A

B

N

O

P

R

S

W

Y

Endnotes

1. Much like an extension of the tenth book or mandala of the Rigveda that shares many hymns with the *Atharvaveda*.

2. Including rituals involving prana, mantra, and meditation that reflect the older Vedic Yoga.

3. All of what was later called Jnana Yoga, Bhakti Yoga, Karma Yoga, Raja Yoga, and Hatha Yoga.

4. Swami Vivekananda brought Ramakrishna Yoga-Vedanta as the first form of Yoga to the West in 1893. Note that Swami Sivananda of Rishikesh also called his teachings Yoga-Vedanta.

5. Like *Aparokshanubhuti* and *Vivekachudamani*.

6. Atmananda or Ram Alexander wrote a fascinating biographical account of her work with Anandamayi Ma, which she kindly sent me a copy of.

7. Swami Rama Tirtha's writings have been published in India in several volumes under the title of *In Woods of God Realization*.

8. I am in the process of rewriting the book.

9. To Yajnavalkya can be assigned the *Brihadaranyaka*, the longest of the *Upanishads*, the Shatapatha Brahmana, the longest and most esoteric of the *Brahmanas*, *the Shukla Yajurveda*, and the *Brihat Yogi Yajnavalkya*, the most important ancient Yoga text after the *Yoga Sutras*. Yajnavalkya is also prominent in the *Mahabharata* where he gives many teachings in the Moksha Dharma Parva.

10. Note that some later Mother Miras were named after her, though some Miras follow the name of the Hindu devotional poet Mirabai.

11. The *Shukla Yajurveda* is shorter than the *Krishna Yajurveda* as it contains only poetry and no prose sections like the *Krishna Yajurveda*.

12. *Rigveda X.54-56*. Hymns of Brihaduktha Vamadevya

13. *Rigveda IV.26.1 Brihadaranyaka Upanishad I.4.10*

14. This book would later be revised for its American edition as *Wisdom of the Ancient Seers: Selected Mantras of the Rig Veda (1993)*. Yet these translations are overall prior to my discovery of Ganapati Muni.

15. M.P. Pandit, *Adoration of the Divine Mother*, page v.

16. *Collected Works of T.V. Kapali Sastry, Volume Seven, Uma Sahasram of Ganapati Muni.*

17. Vasishtha Kavyakantha Ganapati Muni, *Collected Works, Volume Seven, the Book of Commentaries*. Most of the Muni's Vedic works can be found in this volume, including his translations and commentaries on verses of the *Rigveda*.

18. Vasishtha Kavyakantha Ganapati Muni, *Collected Works, Volume One, the Book of Adoration, Part One, pp. vvi. Editorial by K. Natesan, pp. xvi-xvii.*

19. Vasishtha Kavyakantha Ganapati Muni, *Collected Works, Volume Three, the Book of Adoration, Part Three, Sri Ramana Chatvarimshat.*

20. These letters from Ganapati to Ramana are published under the title, *Epistles of Light* by the Ramanashram.

21. *Bhagavan and Nayana* by S. Shankaranarayanan, for more information on their relationship and Ganapati's role in propagating Ramana's teachings. The book is published by the Ramanashram. For a longer study, note *Glory of Vasishtha Ganapati*, by S.R. Leela, Sri Aurobindo Kapali Sastry Institute of Vedic Culture, Bangalore, India.

22. Vasishtha Kavyakantha Ganapati Muni, *Collected Works, Volume One, the Book of Adoration, Part One, pp. vvi. Editorial by K. Natesan.*

23. Vasishtha Kavyakantha Ganapati Muni, *Collected Works, Volume Five, the Book of Aphorisms, Part One, Rājayogasārasūtram and Yogavyākhyānam.*

24. I followed Ganapati Muni's Shakta and Tantric teachings in my *Tantric Yoga and the Ten Wisdom Goddesses.*

25. *Taittiriya Upanishad, I.13.* The birthplace of Indra, where the skull is opened, sendrayoniḥ yatrāsau keśānto vivartate vyapohya śīrṣakapāle.

26. Vasishtha Kavyakantha Ganapati Muni, *Collected Works, Volume Eight, the Book of Ayurveda and Vedic Astrology.*

27. Vasishtha Kavyakantha Ganapati Muni, *Collective Works, Volume Three, the Book of Adoration, Part Three, Indra Sahasranama.*

28. Vasishtha Kavyakantha Ganapati Muni, *Collected Works, Volume Nine, A Treatise on the Mahabharata*. This is an area where I take a different view than Ganapati Muni. I do not hold that the *Rigveda* reflects actual historical

29. *Mahabharata* events, but that the *Mahabharata* strongly reflects the symbolism of the *Rigveda*.

30. Vasishtha Kavyakantha Ganapati Muni, *Collected Works, Volume Five, the Book of Aphorisms Part One, Mahāvidyāsūtram.*

31. *The Guru and the Disciple: Bhagavan Ramana and Ganapati Muni*, page 10. Published by Ramana Maharshi Center for Learning, Bangalore, India.

32. Vasishtha Kavyakantha Ganapati Muni, *Collected Works, Volume Seven, the Book of Commentaries, Gurmantra Bhashyam.*

33. *Chandogya Upanishad VII.26.2*

34. *Chandogya Upanishad VIII.1*

35. *Rigveda I.65-73*. Hymns of Parashara Shaktya of the Vasishtha line.

36. Sri Aurobindo, *The Life Divine, Chapter 2, The Two Negations: The Refusal of the Ascetic.*

37. Curiously Shankara taught both the Jnana and the Vijnana, the Jnana is highlighted in his works on Advaita Vedanta and the Vijnana in his works on Tantra, Raja Yoga and his many hymns to the Hindu Gods and Goddesses, notably *Saundarya Lahiri*.

38. *Vasishtha Kavyakantha Ganapati Muni, Collected Works, Volume Seven, the Book of Commentaries*, Gṛtsamadasya gaṇānām tve tyādisūkte. Behind all three for me looms the figure of Shankara, who explained not only the pure Advaita Vedanta, but also worship of the Goddess, devotion to the deities, karma yoga, and the upliftment of both India and Sanatana Dharma.

39. I was told by some older TM teachers that Maharishi in fact called Brahmarshi Devrat as "the incarnation of the *Vedas*." However, I have yet to find any documented proof of that statement.

40. Ram Swarup, forewords by David Frawley. *The Word as Revelation: Names of Gods; Meditations: Yogas, Gods, Religions; On Hinduism: Reviews and Reflections; Hinduism and Monotheistic Religions.*

41. I was one of the first westerners to be awarded the titles Jyotish Kovid, Jyotish Vachaspati and Jyotish Medha Prajna by the Indian Council of Astrological Sciences (ICAS).

42. Dr. Raman also rejected the Aryan Invasion theory of India and argued for the Indian origins of Vedic culture.

43. I became the first president of the American Council of Vedic Astrology from 1993-2003. We emphasized the name Vedic astrology, as astrology arose as a limb of the Vedas, Vedanga Jyotish, which most directly translated in English to Vedic astrology.

44. *Rigveda I.155.6.* caturbhiḥ sākam navatim ca nāmabhiś cakram na vṛttam vyatīṁravīvipat

45. David Frawley, *Gods, Sages and Kings: Vedic Secrets of Ancient Civilization*, Vedic Astronomy, the Testimony of the Stars, pp. 147-202.

46. *Yoga of Herbs* by David Frawley and Vasant Lad.

47. David Frawley. *Gods, Sages and Kings, The Image of the Ocean: The Maritime Nature of Vedic Culture*, pp. 45-66.

48. Subhash Kak, *The Astronomical Code of the Rigveda.*

49. With beautiful temples in London, Nairobi, Atlanta, Chicago, Houston, New Jersey, and Los Angeles, as well as Delhi and Ahmdebad in India.

50. David Frawley and N.S. Rajaram. *Hidden Horizons, Unearthing 10,000 Years of Indian Civilization.*

51. S.R. Rao, *Dawn and Devolution of the Indus Civilization.*

52. Graham Hancock, *Underworld: Flooded Kingdoms of the Ice Ages.*

53. Sri Sivananda Murty, *Katha Yoga.*

54. Swami Veda Bharati, *Divo Duhita* or the Daughter of Heaven in Sanskrit, contains several other of Swami Veda's Sanskrit works, including *Chandasi.*

55. *Taittiriya Brahmana III.10.47.* anantā vai vedāḥ

56. It has included Yoga and Vedanta teachers not mentioned in the book as Swami Dayananda of Arshavidya Gurukulam, Amritanandamayi (Ammachi), Swami Muktananda, Swami Chandrashekhar Sarasvati of Kanchipuram, Swami Satchidananda, Swami Yogeshvarananda, Swami Rama of the Himalayan Institute, Amrit Desai, Swami Kriyananda (Ananda), and Roy Eugene Davis. It includes additional texts such as the *Brahma Sutras, Yoga Vasishtha*, Yoga Upanishads, and works of Kashmir Shaivism, particularly relative to the mysticism of the Sanskrit alphabet. Important has also been my chanting of classical Hindu Stotras, particularly those of Shankara like Saundarya Lahiri.

57. *Rigveda III.3.1.* vaiśvanarāya pṛthupājase vipo ratnā vidhanta dharuṇeṣu gātave, agnir hi devān amṛto duvasyatyathā dharmāṇi sanatā no dūduṣat.

58. *Rigveda V.63.1.* ṛtasya gopāvadhi tiṣṭatho ratham satyadharmāṇā parame vyomani, yam atra mitrāvaruṇāvatho yuvam tasmai vṛṣṭir madumat pinvate divaḥ.

59. *Rigveda V.63.7.* dharmaṇā mitrāvaruṇā vipaścitā vratā rakṣethe asurasuya māyayā, ṛtena viśvam bhuvanam vi rājathaḥ sūryam ā dattho divi citryam ratham.

60. There remains some debate as to where the water came for the Sarasvati River and how much derived from Himalayan rivers that had different courses in the early ancient period, or from melting glaciers, or from a larger monsoon. However, the existence of the water in the river necessary for the many settlements along it is not in doubt, which is the main point!

61. *Gods, Sages and Kings, In Search of the Cradle of Civilization, Hidden Horizons, Myth of the Aryan Invasion, and the Rig Veda* and the *History of India.*

62. B.B. Lal, *The Oldest Civilization in South Asia* and *The Homeland of the Aryans: Evidence of Rigvedic Flora and Fauna and Archaeology.*

63. *Rigveda VII.95.2.* sucir yatī giribhya ā samudrāt.

64. *Mahabharata Shalya Parvani Gada Parvani 35-38.*Balarama's pilgrimage down the Sarasvati and his description of the river.

65. *Manu Smriti* II.17, 21

66. B.B. Lal, *The Sarasvati Flows On.*

67. *Vishnu Purana* III.5-20

68. Megasthenes, *Indika*, quoted in *Pliny VI.XXI.4.5, Solinus 52.5, Arrian Indica I.IX.* The complete text is not available.

69. *Rigveda III.17.1.* samidhyamānaḥ prathamānu dharmā samaktubhir ijyate viśvavāraḥ, śociṣkeśo ghṛtanirṇik pāvakaḥ suyajño agnir yajathāya devān.

70. This Manava Dharma is emphasized in the *Manu Smriti* or Manu's Law Code, which though well out of date today, reflects a remarkable ancient attempt to form a society in which spiritual values prevailed.

71. Smriti includes the Epics (*Mahabharata* and *Ramayana*), the *Puranas*, the works of the Six Vedic schools of Philosophy, and other Sutra literature like the *Manu Smriti*. These works contain a variety of opinions on different topics and one need not accept them as the last word on any topic.

72. Paramahansa Yogananda. *Autobiography of a Yogi*.

73. Sri Yukteswar, *The Holy Science*, page 11, relates Manu to Satya Yuga which ended at 6700 BCE.

74. Note Sri Aurobindo's monumental works the *Life Divine, Savitri, and the Synthesis of Yoga*.

75. Helena Petrova Blavatsky, *The Secret Doctrine*.

76. The root ṛ in Sanskrit means to move, specifically to move with truth, inspiration, force, and rhythm. It is this sense of inspiration or internal vibration that is conveyed by the term Rishi.

77. *Rigveda X.97.2*. Purusha Sukta. puruṣa evedam sarvam yad bhụtam yacca bhāvyam, utāmṛtasyeśāno yad annenātirohati.

78. *Yoga Sutras I.3*.

79. *Isha Upanishad 15*.

80. Asura is not a demon as sometimes translated, but a powerful force of the Ignorance.

81. *Chandogya Upanishad VIII.7*, story of Indra and Vairochana, in which Vairochana accepted as true that the Self or soul was the body, Indra probed more deeply.

82. Asura in the *Rigveda* implies power but as a force of Divinity. Only later is it more a negative connotation of power, though there are hints of that in a few Rigvedic verses. It occurs relative to such Vedic deities as Indra, Mitra, Varuna, and Rudra.

83. This was the weapon that Ramana Maharshi had through his power of silence and Self-inquiry that eliminates the root of the ignorance from which all Asuric or negative energies arise.

84. Brahmarshi Daivarata, *Chhandodarshana*, contains many new Vedic style hymns to Brihaspati and to Sarasvati, which is Brihaspati's feminine counterpart.

85. This is a line of thinking I developed in my early book the *Creative Vision of the Early Upanishads* and remains relevant in this context.

86. For example, *Saundarya Lahiri* and *Ananda Lahiri Stotras* of Shankara, but many Hindu hymns to the Goddess do this.

87. *Rigveda IV.54.2*. devebhyo hi prathamam yajñiyebhyo'mṛtatvam suvasi bhāgam uttamam, ādid dāmānam savitar vyūrṇuṣe'nūcīnā jīvitā mānuṣebhyaḥ.

88. *Rigveda III.1.20*. janmañjanman nihito jātavedāḥ.

89. *Bhagavad Gita III.10*. sahayajnāḥ prajāḥ sṛṣṭvā purovāca prajāpatiḥ, anena prasaviṣyadhvam eṣa vo'stviṣṭakāmadhuk.

90. Vasishtha Kavyakantha Ganapati Muni, *Collected Works, Volume Five, the Book of Aphorisms, Part One, Yogavyākhyānam* 2. Tapa upāsanam yogaśceti paryāyāḥ. "Tapas and upsasana are synonymns for Yoga."

91. *Bhagavad Gita IV.25-29.*

92. *Mahabharata Moksha Ashvamedha Parva, Anugita Parvani, 21-25*, discusses the Vedic sacrifice and different hotas or invoking priests, including the mind and senses, along with offerings of thoughts and sensory qualities, specifically mentioning the practice of Yoga as a sacrifice or the *Yoga Yajña 24.14.*

93. *Yoga Sutras I.27-28*

94. *Bhagavad Gita X.25*

95. *Bhagavad Gita IV.24*. brahmārpaṇam brahma havir brahmāgnau brahmaṇā hutam, brahmaiva tena gantavyam brahmakarma samādhinā.

96. The Samkhya system of twenty-four tattvas or cosmic principles as well as a number of additional principles are found in texts like the *Mahabharata* and the *Bhagavad Gita*, going back to the *Upanishads*, notably the *Prashna Upanishad IV*.

97. *Bhagavad Gita IV.1-3*. imam vivasvate yogam proktavān aham avyayam, vivasvān manave prāha manur ikṣvākave'bravīt.

98. *Bhagavad Gita X.37*

99. *Rigveda IX.87.3*. ṛṣir vipraḥ pura etā janānām ṛbhur dhīra uśanā kāvyena, sa cid viveda nihitam yadāsām apīcyam guhyam nāma gonām

100. *Krishna Yajurveda, IV.5* Rudram

101. *Yoga Sutras II.1*, Kriya Yoga

102. *Rigveda X. 190.1*

103. *Taittiriya Upanishad I.17*

104. *Yoga Sutras II.44*

105. *Yoga Sutras I.23*

106. *Yoga Sutras I.27*

107. *Rigveda VIII.62.12*. satyam id vā u tam vayam indram stavāma nānṛtam.

108. *Rigveda IX.108.8*. sahasradhāram vṛṣabham payovṛdham priyam devāya janmane, ṛtena ya ṛtajāto vivāvṛdhe rājā deva ṛtam bṛhat.

109. *Chandogya Upanishad VIII.5*. atha yad yajña ityācaskṣate brahmacaryam eva.

110. David Frawley, *Soma in Yoga and Ayurveda: The Power of Rejuvenation and Immortality*.

111. *Rigveda V.44.14-15*. yo jāgāra tam ṛcaḥ kāmayante yo jāgāra tam u sāmāni yanti, yo jāgāra tam ayam soma āha tavāham asmi sakhye nyokāḥ, agnir jāgāra tam ṛcaḥ kāmayante'gnir jāgāra tamu sāmāni yanti, agnir jāgāra tam ayam soma āha tavāham asmi sakhye nyokāḥ.

112. Vasishtha Kavyakantha Ganapati Muni, *Collected Works Volume Two, Indrani Saptashati* 395, śīrṣe candro hṛdaye bhānur netre vidyut kulakuṇḍe'gni.

113. *Shvetashvatara Upanishad I.3*. te dhyāna yogānugatā apaśyan devātmaśaktim svaguṇair nigūḍām.

114. *Shvetashvatara Upanishad I.1*. tileṣu tailam dadhanīva sarpir āpaḥ srotaḥsu araṇīṣu cāgniḥ, evan ātmā'tmani gṛhyate'sau satyenainam tapasā yo'nupaśyati.

115. *Shvetashvatara Upanishad II.1, Shukla Yajurveda XI.1*, yuñjānaḥ prathamam manas tattvāya savitā dhiyaḥ, agner jyotir nicāyya pṛthivyā adhyābharat. Yoga as yoking the mind or manas and extending the buddhi or dhi.

116. *Rigveda III.22.1* Agni as the digestive fire.

117. *Shvetashvatara Upanishad II.2, Shukla Yajurveda. XI.2*. yuktena manasā vayam devasya savituḥ save suvargyāya śaktyā.

118. *Shvetashvatara Upanishad II.3, Shukla Yajurveda XI.3.* yuktvāya savitā devān svaryato dhiyā divam, bṛhajjyotiḥ kariṣyataḥ savitā pra suvāti tān.

119. *Shvetashvatara Upanishad II.4, Shukla Yajurveda XI.4, Rigveda V.81.1.* yuñjate mana uta yuñjate dhiyo viprā viprasya bṛhato vipaścitaḥ, vi hotrā dadhe vayunāvid eka in mahī devasya savituḥ pariṣṭutiḥ.

120. *Shvetashvatara Upanishad II.5. Shukla Yajurveda XI.5, Rigveda X.13.1.* yuje vām brahma pūrvyam namobhir vi śloka etu pathyeva sūreḥ, śṛṇvantu viśve amṛtasya putrā ā ye dhāmāni divyāni tasthuḥ.

121. *Bhagavad Gita IV.1*

122. *Shvetashvatara Upanishad II.6.* agnir yatrābhimathyate, vāyur yatrādhirudhyate, somo yatrātiricyate, tatra sañjāyate manaḥ.

123. *Shvetashvatara Upanishad II.67.* savitrā prasavena juṣeta brahma pūrvyam tatra yonim kṛṇavase na hi te pūrtam akṣipat.

124. *Shukla Yajurveda XXXII.1.* tadevāgnis tadādityas tadvāyus tadu candramāḥ, tadeva śukram tad brahmā tā āpaḥ sa prajāpatiḥ, sarve nimeṣā jajñire vidyutaḥ puruṣād adhi, nainam ūrdhvam na tiryañcam na madhye pari jagrabhat.

125. Swami Veda Bharati, *Divo Duhita*, page 7. Sanskrit of Swami Vedas Gayatri, dhiyam jinvāya vidmahe, hiraṇyagarbhāya dhīmahi, tan no yogaḥ pracodayāt.

126. *Mahabharata Shanti Parva 349.65*, sāṁkhyasya vaktā kapilaḥ paramarṣiḥ sa ucyate, hiraṇyagarbho yogasya vettā nānyaḥ purātanaḥ.

127. *Mahabharata Shanti Parva 342.95-96.* vidyāsahāyavantam mām ādityastham sanātanam, kapilam prāhur ācāryāḥ sāṁkhyā niścitaniścayāḥ, hiraṇyagarbho dyutimān ya eṣa cchandasi stutaḥ, yogaiḥ sampūjyate nityam sa evāham bhuvi smṛtaḥ.

128. *Mahabharata Shanti Parva 341.8.9.* ṛgvede sayajurvede tathaivātharvasāmasu, purāṇe sopaniṣade tathaiva jyautiṣe-rjuna, sāṁkhye ca yogaśāstre ca āyurvede tathaiva ca, bahūni mama nāmāni kīrtitāni maharṣibhiḥ

129. *Brihadyogi Yajnavalkya Smriti XII.5*

130. *Yoga Sutras I.1.* Vijnana Bhikshu commentary.

131. There is not a single reference to Patanjali that I have found in this literature, though I have not examined all the *Puranas* in detail.

132. *Hatha Yoga Pradipika I.1*

133. *Mahabharata Shanti Parva 300.57.* nānāśāṣtreṣu niṣpannam yogeṣvidam udāhṛtam.

134. *Mahabharata Ashvamedha Parvani Anu Gita Parva 19.15*, yogaśāstram anuttamam and also 18.

135. *Mahabharata Moksha Dharma Parva 316.1.* sāmkhyajñānam mayā proktam yogajñānam nibodha me

136. *Shandilya Upanishad 1*

137. *Yoga Sutras I.1.* atha yogānuśāsanam.

138. *Bhagavad Gita IV.1-3.* imam vivasvate yogam proktavān aham avyayam, vivasvān manave prāha manur ikṣvākave'bravīt, evam paramparāprāptam imam rājarṣayo viduḥ, sa kāleneha mahatā yoga naṣṭaḥ parantapa, sa evāyam mayā te'dya yogaḥ proktaḥ purātanaḥ.

139. *Rigveda X.121. 8.* yo deveṣvadhi deva eka āsīt.

140. *Mahabharata Shanti Parva 339.69.* hiraṇyagarbho bhagavān eṣa cchandasi suṣṭutaḥ, yogaśāṣtreṣu śabditaḥ. "Bhagavan Hiranyagarbha is lauded in the Vedic meters and spoken of in the Yoga Shastras."

141. *Śuklayajurveda Saṁhitā, Uvaṭabhāsya Saṁvalitā*, introduction, so'yam hiraṇyagarbha paramparayābhivyakto nityo vedaḥ, This is the Hiranyagarbha tradition manifested form of the eternal Veda.

142. *Mahabharata Shanti Parva 339.50.* hiraṇyagarbho lokādi caturvaktro'niruktagaḥ, brahmā sanatano devo mam bahvarthacintakaḥ.

143. *Mahabharata Shanti Parva 302.18.* hiraṇyagarbho bhagavān eṣa buddhir iti smṛtaḥ, mahān iti ca yogeṣu viriñciriti cāpyajaḥ.

144. *Mahabharata Shanti Parva 308.45.* hiraṇyagarbhād ṛṣiṇā vasiṣṭena mahātmanā, vasiṣṭād ṛṣiśārdulān narado'vāptavānidam.

145. *Mahabharata Shanti Parva 306.26.* yogadarśanam etāvad uktam te tattvato mayā.

146. *Rigveda VII.33.10-13*, in which Vasishtha takes birth from a pot after Māna (Agastya).

147. Non-dualistic or Advaita Vedanta, for example, teaches Jnana Yoga or the Yoga of Knowledge, while dualistic or Dvaita Vedanta emphasizes Bhakti Yoga or the Yoga of Devotion.

148. *Shukla Yajurveda 20.25.* "Where Brahma and Kshatra (spiritual and princely powers) move together, may I know that pure world where the Gods are together with Agni." Yatra brahma ca kṣatram ca samyañcau carataḥ saha taṁlokam puṇyam prajñeṣam yatra devāḥ sahāgninā.

149. *Rigveda IV.42.8-9*

150. Note the Naina Devi temple in Punjab for Gobind Singh.

151. *Mahabharata* Raja Dharma Parva XV. Arjunena Rājadaṇḍa Mahatvavarṇanam.

152. As conveyed to me by Prof. Lokesh Chandra, a great Buddhist scholar of India.

153. Harappan Yoga Seals

154. *Aitareya Upanishad I.3.3.* parokṣapriyā iva hi devāḥ. Also Taittiriya Brahmana III.12.2.

155. *Rigveda I.164.45.* catvāri vāk parimitā padāni tāni vidur brāhmaṇā ye manīṣiṇaḥ, guhā trīṇi neṅgayanti turīyam vāco manuṣyā vadanti.

156. *Rigveda III.1.6.* sanā atra yuvatayaḥ sayonīr ekam garbham dadhire sapta vāṇīḥ. *Bhagavad Gita VIII.1-4*

157. *Kena Upanishad I.2*

158. *Bhagavad Gita, Chapter IV.25-29*

159. *Rigveda VIII.29.1.* nahi vo astyarbhako devāso na kumārakaḥ viśve satomahānta it.

160. *Rigveda I.164.46.* ekam sad viprā bahudhā vadanti.

161. 3339 is a highly suggestive astronomical number as it reflects the 371 tithis or lunar phases (tithis) in a year multiplied by 9, which are important in Vedic astrology and astronomy.

162. *Brihadaranyaka Upanishad III.9.1-9* A fourth prime deity is Soma, hymns to which are found mainly in one book, the ninth book of the *Rigveda*. It is sometimes related to a fourth world of the Waters, but such a fourfold division is referred to secondarily to the threefold symbolism. We will discuss it later.

163. *Brihaddevata* of Shaunaka

164. *Rigveda IV.1.16*

165. Notably the seven dhatus of Ayurveda, as plasma, blood, muscle, fat, bone, nerve, and reproductive. Indra-Agni: lightning fire or fire of speech, connected to the deity Brihaspati. Indra-Soma: spirit absorbing the mind, the full moon. Indra-Surya: the spiritual light as the ruler of all, the sun at noon. Agni-Surya: union of the individual and universal souls, sun at dawn. Agni-Soma: self and bodily principles, new moon. Surya-Soma: solar and lunar principles. Agni-Krishna: Fire at night. Agni-Arjuna: Fire during the day. Agni-Mitra: Sun at dawn. Indra- Surya or Indra-Vishnu: Sun at noon, summer solstice. Agni-Varuna: Sun at sunset. Agni-Soma: New moon. Indra- Soma: Full moon. Savita: Sun as power of revolution and circulation, rebirth and transformation. Agni-Savita: Hidden power of transformation in the soul.

166. *Shukla Yajur Veda XIX.9*. tejo'si tejo mayi dhehi, vīryam asi vīryam mayi dhehi, balamasi balam mayi dhehi, ojo'si ojo mayi dhehi, manyur asi manyum mayi dhehi, saho'si saho mayi dhehi.

167. *Brihadaranyaka Upanishad VI.7-13*. Describes the primacy of Prana over all our other faculties.

168. *Rigveda III.56.8*. tri uttamā dūṇaśā rocanāni trayo rājantyasurasya vīrāḥ. "Three supreme hard to reach heavens are ruled by three kings, the heroes of the Almighty."

169. *Rigveda I.164.39*. ṛco akṣare parame vyoman yasmin devā adhi viśve niṣeduḥ, yastan na veda kim ṛcā kariṣyati ya ittād vidus ta ime samāsate.

170. Vasishtha Kavyakantha Ganapati Muni, *Collected Works Volume Five, The Book of Aphorisms, Part One, Caturvūhasūtram,* III.8. praṇavānnāparaḥ kālaḥ, and *Siddāntasārasūtram II.6, avyaktaḥ śabdaḥ kālaḥ.*

171. *Chandogya Upanishad VIII.1.3*. eṣo'ntar hṛdaya ākāśa ubhe asmin dyāvāpṛthivī antareva samāhite ubhāvagniśca vāyuśca sūryācandramasāvubhau vidyunnakṣatraṇi yaccāsyehāsti yacca nāsti sarvam tad asmin samāhitam.

172. There are four levels of speech in classical Sanskrit, vaikhari-spoken, madhyama-pranic, pashyanti-perceptive, and para-transcendent. The Vedas take the transcendent level of speech indicated by Oṁ and take it into the other levels, down to vaikhari itself. The Vedas are a para-vaikhari language expressing the Supreme in complex verbal and vibratory sound patterns.

173. For example, the *Chandogya Upanishad I.3,7*, divides up the word Udgītha, which means 'loud chant' into three syllables ud, gī, tha, with ud as Heaven and the Sun, gī as atmosphere and Air, and tha as earth and Fire (dyaur evod antarikṣam gīḥ pṛthivī tham āditya evod vāyur gīr agnistham). This goes against the rules of later Sanskrit etymology. It also associates ud-gītha with the high or loud chant, with ud-gāyati, going upwards or ascending (*Chandogya Upanishad I.3.1*). Here it is equating the root 'ga' or to go, with 'gai' or to sing. This shows that even the Upanishadic era that Vedic Sanskrit was alive and plastic, with the boundaries between words and sounds not as fixed.

174. *Rigveda X.130-4-5*

175. *Bhagavad Gita X.22*

176. *Rigveda III.62.10*

177. *Taittiriya Brahmana III.10.36*

178. *Mahanarayana Upanishad 37*. Aditya Devata Mantra

179. These include the first hymn of the Rigveda of Madhuchchhandas, the Agni immorality mantra of Hiranyastupa Angirasa (Rigveda I. 31.7), the Agni mantra of Vishvamitra (Rigveda III.20.1), the Pushan Gayatri of Vishvamitra (Rigveda III.62.20), the Manu mantra of Vamadeva (Rigveda IV.26.1), the Garbha mantra of Vamadeva (Rigveda IV.27.1), the Hamsa mantra of Vamadeva (Rigveda IV.45.5), the heart ocean mantra of Vamadeva (Rigveda IV.58.11), the Aditi Gayatri of Shyvashva Atreya (Rigveda V.82.2.), the solar rebirth mantra of Vatsa Kanva (Rigveda VIII.6.8.), the Indra protection mantra of Irimbishta Kanva (Rigveda VIII.17.9), the Indra as father and mother mantra of Nrimedha Angirasa (Rigveda VIII. 98.11), and the being and non-being mantra of Trita Aptya (*Rigveda* X.5.7).

180. *Rigveda I.164.41*. gaurī mimāya salilāni takṣatyekapadī dvipadī sā catuṣpadī, aṣṭāpadī navapadī babhūvuṣī sahasrākṣarā parame vyoman.

181. *Rigveda VII.15.9*. upa tvā sātaye naro viprāso yanti dhītibhiḥ upākṣarā sahasriṇī.

182. *Aitareya Aranyaka III.3.2 Aitareya Aranyaka III.6*

183. *Rigveda I.3.7*. Omasas in the plural for the Universal Gods or Viśvedevāḥ.

184. *Rigveda I.164.39*. ṛco akṣare parame vyoman.

185. *Krishna Yajurveda, VII.1,8, 1-2*. Īṃkārāya svāhā, iṃkṛtāya svāhā, reverence to the mantra Īṁ.

186. Brahmarshi Daivarata, *Vak Sudha, Chapter VI*. Guptapraṇavakalā

187. Brahmarshi Daivarata, *Chhandodarshana IV.2*

188. Brahmarshi Daivarata, *Chhandodarshana IV.2.4*. yo akṣaram vācam īm anu svaran, brahma praṇautyanu vācā brahmaṇā, guhyam tam anu praṇavam tapasyan, sendram eva tam vṛṇe śam gamadhyai.

189. Brahmarshi Daivarata, *Chhandodarshana VI.2.4*

190. Brahmarshi Daivarata *Vak Sudha* dedication page and *Chhandodarshana* first page, īm oṁ śrīh, after which he sometimes has the Gayatri Mantra for expressing the essence of the Vedas.

191. Brahmarshi Daivarata, *Chhandodarshana VI.2.1*. Commentary, yaḥ ayam pratyagātmasvarūpaḥ prathamam ādau sṛṣṭer api prāk viśvataḥ sarvatra sīm santataḥ parokṣaḥ babhụva svayam eva, "Who is this inner Self nature at first, before the creation of the universe, everywhere and at all sides in the form of the mantra Sīṁ was continuously existent imperceptible as himself."

192. *Rigveda III.44*. Hari Sukta to Indra.

193. *Aitareya Aranyaka III.2*

194. *Rigveda IV.40.5. Mahanarayana Upanishad*, Dahara Vidya 12. haṁsaḥ śuciṣad vasur antarikṣasad hotā vediṣad atithir duroṇasat, nṛṣad varasad ṛtasad vyomasad abjā gojā ṛtajā adrijā ṛtam. *Mahanarayana Upanishad 12,* Dahara Vidya.

195. *Mahanaranaya Upanishad 34-35*, Gāyatryāvāhana Mantras.

196. Dhī, pronounced dhee, plural dhiyaḥ.

197. This is the view of Brahmarshi Daivarata in his *Chhandodarshana* and *Vak Sudha*, as well as the view of Kavyakantha Ganapati Muni. I am following their line of thought and inspiration here.

198. *Yoga Sutras I.2*, yogaś cittavṛttir nirodhaḥ - requires a development of the Buddhi through inquiry and meditation. It is the Buddhi that is the bridge between the Chitta and the Purusha.

199. *Bhagavad Gita II.39-53*. Buddhi Yoga.

200. Dhyana arises from the root dhyai, which in turn is a diversification of the broader root dhi.

201. What is usually called the manas principle, both in Vedic and later Vedantic thought.

202. *Aitareya Upanishad I.3.3*. parokṣapriyā iva hi devāḥ. Also *Taittiriya Brahmana III.12.2.*

203. *Chandogya Upanishad VIII.7-12*

204. *Aparokshanubhuti* of Shankara, for example.

205. Vasishtha Kavyakantha Ganapati Muni, *Collected Works, Volume Five, The Book of Aphorisms, Part One, Pramāṇa parikṣa IV.4-5.*veda āptavākyād anyaḥ, sa hyaparokṣasyānuvādaḥ. "The Veda is different than the words of those who know, it is an expression of the direct (aparokṣa) knowledge."

206. *Rigveda I.3.12*. maho arṇa sarasvatī pra cetayati ketunā, dhiyo viśvā vi rājati.

207. *Rigveda VI.61.4*. pra ṇo devī sarasvatī vājebhir vājinīvatī dhīnām avitryavatu.

208. *Rigveda VII.34.9*. abhi vo devīm dhiyam dadhidhvam pra vo devatrā vācam kṛṇudhvam.

209. *Rigveda I.40.5*. pra nūnam brahmaṇaspatir mantram vadanti ukthyam, yasminnindro varuṇo mitro aryamạ devā okāṁsi cakrire.

210. *Rigveda IV.50.1*. yas tastambha sahasā vi jmo antān bṛhaspatis triṣadhastho raveṇa, tam pratnāsa ṛṣayo dīdhyānāḥ puro viprā dadhire mandrajihvam.

211. *Rigveda II.25.5*. devānām sumne subhagaḥ sa edhate yamyam yujam kṛṇute brahmaṇaspatiḥ.

212. *Rigveda X.67.1*, imām dhiyam saptaśīrṣṇīm pitā na ṛtaprajātām bṛhatīm avindat, turīyam svij janayad viśvajanyo'yāsya uktham indrāya śaṁsan.

213. *Rigveda X.67.2*. ṛtam śaṁsanta ṛju dīdhyānā divasputraso asurasya vīrāḥ, vipram padam aṅgiraso dadhānā yajñasya dhāma prathamam mananta. Rigveda III.62.10. Tat Savitur vareṇyam bhargo devasya dhīmahi dhiyo yo naḥ pracodayāt.

214. *Rigveda VI.1.1*. tvamhyagne prathamo manotāsyā dhiyo abhavo dasma hotā.

215. *Rigveda VI.1.7*, tvam viśo anayo dīdyāno divo agne bṛhatā rocanena.

216. *Rigveda III.27.9*. dhiyā cakra vareṇyo bhūtānām garbham ā dadhe dakṣasya pitaram tanā.

217. *Rigveda III.27.10.* ni tvā dadhe vareṇyam dakṣasyeḷā sahaskṛtaḥ agne sudītim ṛśijam.

218. *Rigveda III.27.11.* agnim yanturam apturam ṛtasya yoge vanuṣasaḥ viprā vājaiḥ samindhate.

219. *Rigveda I.18.7.* yasmād ṛte sidhyati yajño vipaścitaścana, sa dhīnām yogam invati.

220. *Rigveda VIII.95.5.* indra yas te navīyasim giram mandrām ajījanat, ciktitvan manasam dhiyam pratnām ṛtasya pipyuṣīm.

221. *Rigveda V.81.1.* yuñjate mana uta yuñjate dhiyo viprā viprasya bṛhato vipaścitaḥ, vi hotrā dadhe vayunāvid eka in mahī devasya savituḥ pariṣṭutiḥ.

222. *Rigveda IV.40.5.* haṁsaḥ śuciṣad vasur antarikṣasad hotā vediṣad atithir duroṇasat, nṛṣad varasad ṛtasad vyomasad abjā gojā ṛtajā adrijā ṛtam.

223. *Rigveda IX.100.3.* tvam dhiyam manoyujam sṛjā vṛṣṭim na tanyutaḥ, tvam vasūni pārthivā divyā ca soma puṣyasi.

224. *Rigveda IV.36.1-2.* anásvo jāto anabhīśur ukthyo rathas tri cakraḥ pari vartate rajaḥ, mahat tadvo devyasya pravācanam dyam̐ ṛbhavaḥ pṛthivịm yacca puṣyatha, ratham ya cakruḥ suvṛtam sucetaso'vihvarantam manasas pari dhyayā.

225. *Rigveda I.164.2-3.* sapta yuñjanti ratham ekacakram eko aśvo vahati saptanāmā, trinābhi cakram ajaram anarvam yatremā viśvā bhuvanādhi tasthuḥ, imam ratham adhi ye sapta tasthuḥ saptacakram sapta vahantyaśvāḥ, sapta svasāro abhi saṁ navante yatra gavām nihitā sapta nāma.

226. *Rigveda I.163.4.* trīṇi ta āhur divi bandhanāni trīṇyapsu trīṇyantaḥ samudre, uteva me varuṇaśchantsyarvan yatrā ta āhuḥ paramam janitram. Rigveda VII.69.1-2. ā vām ratho rodasī baddhadhāno hiraṇyayo vṛṣabhir yātyaṣvaiḥ, sa paprathāno abhi pañca bhūmā trivanduro manasā yātu yuktaḥ.

227. *Rigveda VIII.5.2.* nṛvad dasrā manoyujā rathena pṛthupājasā sacethe aśvinoṣasam.

228. *Rigveda VII.67.8.* ekasmin yoge bhuraṇā samane pari vām sapta sravato ratho gāt, na vāyanti subhvo devayuktā ye vām dhūrṣu taraṇayo vahanti.

229. *Brihadaranyaka Upanishad III.2.14.* ayam ātmā sarveṣām bhūtānām madhvasyā-tmanaḥ sarvāṇi bhūtāni madhu, yaścāyam asmin ātmāni tejomayo'mṛtamayaḥ puruṣo yaścāyamātmā tejomayo'mṛtamayaḥ puruṣo'yameva so yo'yam ātedam amṛtam idam brahmedam sarvam.

Brihadaranyaka Upanishad II.5. 14, 16, Rigveda I.116.12. tadvām narā sanaye daṁsa ugram āviṣkṛṇomi tanyatur na vṛṣṭim, dadhyaṅ ha yan madhvātharvaṇo vaṁ aśvasya śīrṣṇā pra yadím uvāceti.

230. *Yoga Sutras I.23 Rigveda VI.51.7-8.* nama id ugram nama ā vivāse namo dādhāra pṛthivīm uta dyām; namo devebhyo nam īśa eṣām kṛtam cid eno namasā vivāse.

231. *Rigveda I.1.7.* upa tvāgne divedive doṣāvastar dhiyā vayam namo bharanta emasi.

232. *Rigveda IV.17.17-18.* trātā no bodhi dadṛśāna āpir abhikhyātā marḍitā somyānām, sakhā pitā pitṛtamaḥ pitṛṇām kartemu lokam uśate vayodhāḥ, sakhīyatām avitā bodhi sakhā gṛṇāna indra stuvate vayo dhāḥ. *Rigveda VI.51.5.* dyauṣpitaḥ pṛthivi mātar adhrug agni bhrātar vasavo mṛḷatā naḥ; viśva ādityā adite sajoṣā asmabhyam śarma bahulam vi yanta.

233. *Rigveda. I.1.9.* sa naḥ piteva sūnave'gne sūpāyano bhava sacasvā naḥ svastaye. Rigveda II.1.9. tvām agne pitaram iṣṭibhir naras tvām bhrātrāya śamyā tanūrucam, tvam putro bhavāsi yastavidhatvam sakhā suśevaḥ pāsyādhṛṣaḥ.

234. *Rigveda VIII.87.11.* tvam hi naḥ pitā vaso tvam mātā śatakrato babhuvitha adhā te sumnam īmahe. *Rigveda VIII.1.6.* yasyām indrāsi me pitur uta bhrātur abhuñjataḥ; mātā ca me chadayathaḥ samā vaso vasutvanāya rādhase.

235. *Rigveda IV.1.16.* te manvata prathamam nāma dhenos triḥ sapta mātuḥ paramāṇi vindan.

236. *Rigveda V.5.10*

237. *Rigveda IX.95.2.* hariḥ sṛjānaḥ pathyām ṛtasyeyarti vācam ariteva nāvam, devo devānām guhyāni nāmāviṣkṛṇoti barhiṣi pravāce.

238. *Rigveda I.24.1* kasya nūnam katamasyāmṛtānām manāmahe cāru devasya nāma.

239. *Rigveda I.68.2.* bhajanta viśve devatvam nāma ṛtam sapanto aṃrtam evaiḥ.

240. *Rigveda VIII.11.5.* martā amartyasya te bhūri nāma mañamahe viprāso jātavedasaḥ.

241. *Rigveda III.20.3.* agne bhūrīṇi tava jātavedo deva svadhāvo'mṛtasya nāma, yāśca māyā māyinām viśvaminva tve pūrvīḥ saṁdadhuḥ pṛṣṭabandho. *Rigveda VI.1.5.* padam devasya namasā vyantaḥ śravasyavaḥ śrava āpannamṛktam; nāmāni ciddīdhire yajñiyāni bhadrāyām te raṇayanta samdṛṣṭau.

242. *Rigveda V.30.5*. paro yattvam parama ājaniṣṭḥāḥ parāvati śrutyam nāma bibhrat.

243. *Rigveda III.37.3*. nāmāni te śatakrato viśvābhir gīrbhir īmahe indrābhimātiṣāhye.

244. *Rigveda VII.22.5*. sadā te nāma svayaśo vivakmi.

245. Vasishtha Kavyakantha Ganapati Muni, *Collected Works, Volume Seven, the Book of Commentaries, Gurmantra Bhashyam*.

246. *Rigveda VII.20.5*. Hymn to Indra

247. The Karma Khanda and Jnana Khanda idea that the Vedas contained a book of works or ritual represented by the earlier Vedic texts and a book of knowledge represented by the *Upanishads*.

248. *Rigveda IV.26.1*. aham manur abhavam sūryaśca. *Rigveda II.1.1*. tvam agne dyubhis tvam āśuśukṣaṇis tvam adbhyas tvam aśmanaspari; tvam vanebhyas tvam oṣadhībhyas tvam nṛnām nṛpate jāyase śuciḥ.

249. *Rigveda VII.52.1*. ādityāso aditayaḥ syāma pūr devatrā vasavo martyatrā, sanema mitrāvaruṇā sananto bhavema dyāvāpṛthivī bhavantaḥ.

250. *Chandogya Upanishad IV.11-13*. ya ȩsa āditye puruṣo dṛṣyate so'ham asmi sa evāhamasmi, yo eṣa candramasi puruṣo dṛṣyate so'ham asmi sa evāhamasmi, ya eṣa vidyuti puruṣo dṛṣyate so'ham asmi sa evāhamasmi.

251. Ganapati Muni made a special booklet of Parashara's Rigvedic hymns only.

252. *Rigveda I.65.1*. paśvā na tāyum guhā catantam namo yujānam namo vahantam, sajoṣā dhīrāḥ padair anu gmannupa tvā sīdan viśve yajatrāḥ.

253. *Rigveda I.65.2*. ṛtasya devā anu vratā gur bhuvat pariṣṭir dyaur na bhụma, vardantīm āpaḥ panvā suśiśvam ṛtasya yonā garbhe sujātam.

254. *Rigveda I.67.2*. haste dadhāno nṛmṇā viśvānyame devān dhād guhā niṣīdan, vidantīm atra naro dhiyaṁdhā hṛdāyattaṣṭān mantrām aśaṁsan.

255. *Rigveda I.67.3*. ajo na kṣām dādhāra pṛthivīm tastambha dyām mantrebhiḥ satyaiḥ, priyā padāni paśvo ni pāhi vísvayur agne guhā guham gāḥ.

256. *Rigveda I.67.4*. ya īm ciketa guhā bhavantam ā yaḥ sasāda dhārām ṛtasya vi ye cṛtantyṛtā sapanta ādid vasūni pra vavācāsmai.

257. *Rigveda VII.23.3.* yuje ratham gaveṣaṇam haribhyām upa brahmāṇi jujuṣānṇam asthuḥ, vi bādhiṣṭa sya rodasī mahitvendro vṛtrāṇyapratī jaghanvān.

258. *Rigveda IV.26.1.* aham manur abhavam sūryaścāham kakṣīvān ṛṣirasmi vipraḥ, aham kutsam ārjuneyam nyṛñje'ham kavir uśanā paśyatā mā.

259. *Rigveda IV.27.1* garbhe nu sannanvẹsām avedam aham devānām janimāni viśvā, śatam mā pura āyasīr arakṣannadha śyenau javasā niradīyan.

260. *Aitareya Upanishad III.1 Rigveda III.26.7.* agnir asmi janmanā jātavedā ghṛtam me cakṣur amṛtam ma ạsañ; arkas tridhātū rajaso vimāno'jasro gharmo havir asmi nāma. *Rigveda III.26.8.* tribhiḥ pavitrair apupodvyarkam hṛdā matim jyotiranu prajānam; varṣiṣṭhạm ratnam akṛta svadhābhir ādid dyāvāpṛthivī paryapaśyan.

261. *Rigveda I.164.4-5.* ko dadarśa prathamam jāyamānam asthanvantam ya anasthā bibharti, bhūmyā asur asṛg ātmā kva svit ko vidvāṁsam up gāt praṣṭum etat, pākaḥ pṛcchāmi manasāvijānan devānām enā nihitā padāni.

262. *Rigveda I.164.31.* apaśyam gopām anipadyamānam ā ca parā ca pathibhiścarantam, sa sadhrīcīḥ sa viṣūcīr vasāna ā varīvarti bhuvaneṣvantaḥ.

263. *Rigveda VIII.6.10.* aham iddhi pituṣpari medhām ṛtasya jagrabha, aham sūrya ivājani.

264. *Rigveda V.62.1.* ṛtena ṛtam apihitam dhruvam vām sūryasya yatra vimucantyaśvān, daśa śatā saha tasthus tad ekam devānām śreṣṭam vapuṣām apaśyam. *Rigveda V.15.1.* pra vedhase kavaye vedyāya giram bhare yaśase pūrvyāya, ghṛta prasatto suśevo rāyo dhartā dharuṇo vasvo agniḥ.

265. *Rigveda V.15.2.* ṛtena ṛtam dharuṇam dhārayanta yajñasya śāke parame vyoman, divo dharman dharuṇe seduṣo nṛñjātair ajātām abhi ye nanakṣuḥ.

266. *Rigveda VIII.44.23, 29.* yad agne syām aham tvam tvam vā ghā syā aham syuṣṭe satyā ihāśiṣaḥ, dhīro hyasyadmasad vipro na jāgṛviḥ sadā agne dīdayasi dyavi.

267. *Taittiriya Upanishad III.10.* aham annam annam adantam ādmi, aham viśva bhuvanam abhyabhavām survar na jyotīh. *Rigveda VI.61.11-12.* āpapruṣī pārthivānyuru rajo antarikṣam sarasvatī nidaspātu, triṣdhasthā saptadhātuḥ pañca jātā vardhayantī vājevāje havyā bhūt.

268. *Brihadaranyaka Upanishad V.2.1*

269. *Rigveda IV.58.11*. dhāmante viśvam bhuvanam adhi śritam antaḥ samudre hṛdy'ntarāyuṣi, apām anīke samithe ya ābhṛitas tam aśyāma madhumantam ta ūrmim.

270. *Taittiriya Aranyaka Aruna Prashna 78-8*.

271. *Mahanarayana Upanishad 34-35, Gayatri Avahana Mantras*, oṁ āpo jyotīraso'mṛtam brahma bhūr bhuvas suvar oṁ.

272. This is called majjana in Sanskrit. Ramana Maharshi emphasizes this diving into the heart in his teachings.

273. *Rigveda X.45.1*. divaspari prathamam jajñe angir asmad dvitīyam pari jātavedāḥ, tritīyam apsu nṛmaṇā ajasram indhāna enam jarate svādhīḥ.

274. *Rigveda X.45.2*. vidmā te agne tredhā trayāṇi vidmā te dhāma vibhṛitā purutrā, vidmā te nāma paramama guhā yad vidmā tam utsam yata ājagantha.

275. *Rigveda X.45.3*. samudre tvā nṛmaṇā āpsvamtar nṛcakṣā īdhe divo agna ūdhan, tṛtīye tvā rajasi tasthivāṁsam apāmupasthe mahiṣā avardhan.

276. The avarana shakti or veiling power of the ignorance (avidya) mentioned in Advaita Vedanta.

277. *Mahanarayana Upanishad 1*. A very important ancient *Upanishad* found in the *Taittiriya Aranyaka* along with the *Taittiriya Upanishad*

278. *Brihadyogi Yajnavalkya Smriti X*, chapter on Snana.

279. *Rigveda VII.34.2*. viduḥ pṛthivyā divo janitram śṛṇvantyāpo adha kṣarantīḥ.

280. David Frawley, *Yoga and the Sacred Fire*.

281. Vasishtha Kavyakantha Ganapati Muni, *Collected Works, Volume Seven, the Book of Commentaries*, Agneḥ catasro vibhuṭayaḥ

282. Vasishtha Kavyakantha Ganapati Muni, *Collected Works, Volume Seven, the Book of Commentaries*, page 96.

283. Prana, Vak, and Manas in Vedic terminology.

284. Mātari-śvā, meaning the breath, śvā, which grows in the mother, mātari.

285. A fact emphasized in Sri Aurobindo's Yoga.

286. *Rigveda II.3.11*

287. *Rigveda III.1.20.* etā te agne janimā sanāni pra pūrvyāya nūtanāni vocam, mahānti vṛṣṇe savanā kṛtemā janmañjanman nihito jātavedāḥ.

288. *Rigveda III.1.21.* janmañjanman nihito jātavedāḥ viśvāmitrebhir idhyate ajasraḥ, tasya vayam sumatau yajñiyasyāpi bhadre saumanase syāma.

289. *Rigveda VII.4.4.* ayam kavir akaviṣu pracetā marteṣvagnir amṛto ni dāyi, sa mā no atra juhuraḥ sahasvaḥ sadā tve sumanasaḥ syāma.

290. *Rigveda VI.9. 5.* dhruvam jyotir nihitam dṛśaye kam mano javiṣṭham patantvantaḥ, viśve devāḥ samanasaḥ saketā ekam kratum abhi vi yanti sādhu.

291. *Rigveda VI.9.6.* vi me karṇā patayato vi cakṣur vīdam jyotir hṛdaya āhitam yat, vi me manaścarati dūrādhīḥ kim svid vakṣyāmi kim u nū maniṣye.

292. *Rigveda VI.7.9* viśve devā anamasyan bhiyānās tvām agne tamasi tasthivāmsam, vaiśvānaro'vatūtaye no'martyo'vatūtaye naḥ.

293. *Rigveda I.98.1.* vaiśvānarasya sumatau syāma rājā hi kam bhuvanānām abhiśriḥ, ito jāto viśvam idam vi caṣṭe vaiśvānaro yatate sūryeṇa.

294. *Rigveda I.98.2.* pṛṣṭo divi pṛṣṭo agniḥ pṛthivyām pṛṣṭo viśvā oṣadhīr ā viveśa, vaiśvānaraḥ sahasā pṛṣṭo agniḥ sa no divā sa riṣaḥ pātu naktam.

295. As in the several Apri Suktas of the *Rigveda.*

296. *Mahabharata Vanaparva 125*

297. *Rigveda III.11.3.* agnir dhiyā sa cetati ketur yajñasya pūrvyaḥ artham hyasya taraṇi.

298. *Rigveda IV.1.10.* sa tū no agir nayatu prajānannacchā ratnam deva bhaktam yadasya, dhiyā yad viśve amṛtā akṛṇvan dyauṣpitā janitā satyam ukṣan.

299. *Rigveda I.31.1.* tvam agne prathamo aṅgirā ṛṣir devo devānām abhavaḥ śivā sakhā.

300. *Rigveda I.31.7.* tvam tam agne amṛtattva uttame martam dadhāsi śravase divedive, yas tātṛṣāṇa ubhayāya janmane mayaḥ kṛṇoṣi pray ā ca sūraye.

301. *Rigveda X.5.7.* asacca sacca parame vyoman dakṣasya janmannaditer upasthe, agnir ha naḥ prathamajā ṛtasya pūrva āyuni vṛṣabhaśca dhenuḥ.

302. *Rigveda VI.16.13.* tvām hi agne puṣkarād adhyatharvā niramanthata mūrdhno viśvasya vāghataḥ.

303. David Frawley, *Soma in Yoga and Ayurveda*

304. Vasishtha Kavyakantha Ganapati Muni, *Collected Works Volume 2, Indrani Saptashati 395*, śīrṣe candro hṛdaye bhānur netre viyut kulakuṇḍe'gni.

305. *Rigveda IX.74.2*. divo yaḥ skambho dharuṇaḥ svātata āpūrṇo aṁśuḥ pareyeti viṣvataḥ, seme mahī rodasī yakṣad āvṛtā samīcīne dādhāra samiṣaḥ kaviḥ.

306. *Rigveda IX.33.4-5*. abhi brahmīr anūṣata yahvīr ṛtasya mātaraḥ marmṛjyante divaḥ śiśum, rāyaḥ samudraṁścaturo'smbhyam soma viśvataḥ ā pavasva sahasriṇaḥ.

307. *Rigveda IX.107.1*. soma ya uttamam haviḥ.

308. *Rigveda IX.9.4*. sa sap̄ta dhītibhir hito nadyo ajinvad adruhaḥ, yā ekam askṣi vāvṛdhuḥ.

309. *Rigveda IX.44.2*. matī juṣṭo dhiyā hitaḥ somo hinve parāvati, viprasya dhārayā kaviḥ.

310. *Yoga Sutras III.4*

311. *Rigveda IX. 42.2*. eṣa pratnena manmanā devo devebhyaspari, dhārayā pavate sutaḥ.

312. *Rigveda IX.68.5*. sam dakṣeṇa manasā jāyate kavir ṛtasya garbho nihito yamā paraḥ. *Rigveda IX.75.2*. ṛtasya jihvā pavate madhu priyam vaktā patir dhiyo asyā adābhyaḥ, dadhāti putraḥ pitror apīcyam nāma tṛtīyam adhi rocane divaḥ.

313. *Rigveda IX.113.11*. yatrānandāśca modāśca mudaḥ pramudaḥ āsate, kāmasya yatrāptāḥ kāmās tatra māmṛtam kṛdhīdrāyendo pāri srava.

314. *Rigveda IX.96.5*. somaḥ pavate janitā matīnām janitā divo janitā pṛthivyāḥ, janitāgner janitā sūryasya janitendrasya janitota viṣṇoḥ, ṛṣimanā ya ṛṣikṛt svarṣāḥ sahasraṇīthaḥ padavīḥ kavīnām.

315. *Rigveda IX.107.24*. pavasva vājasātaye'bhi viśvāni kāvyā, tvam samudram prathamo vi dhārayo devebhyaḥ soma matsaraḥ, sa tū pavasva pari pārthivam rajo divyā ca soma dharmabhiḥ, tvām viprāso matibhir vicakṣaṇa śubhram hinvanti dhītibhiḥ.

316. *Rigveda IX.76.4*. viśvasya rājā pavate svardṛśa ṛtasya dhītim ṛṣiṣaḷavīviśat, yaḥ sūryasyāsireṇa mṛjyate pitā matīnām asamaṣṭakāvyaḥ.

317. *Rigveda I.115.1*. citram devānām udagād anīkam cakṣur mitrasya varuṇasyāgneḥ, āprā dyāvāpṛthivī antarikṣam sūya ātmā jagatastasthuṣaśca.

318. Subhash Kak. *The Astronomical Code of the Rigveda.*

319. *Rigveda III.62.10.* tat savitur vareṇyam bhargo devasya dhīmahi dhiyo yo naḥ pracodayāt.

320. *Rigveda III.62.9.* yo viśvābhi vipaśyati bhuvanā sam ca paśyati sa naḥ pūṣāvitā bhuvat.

321. *Rigveda V.82.6.* anāgaso aditaye devasya savituḥ save viśvā vāmāni dhīmahi.

322. *Shukla Yajurveda XXXI.18.* vedāham etam puruṣam mahāntam ādityavarṇam tamasaḥ parastāt, tam eva viditvāti mṛtyum eti nānyaḥ panthā vidyate'yanāya.

323. *Rigveda I.50.10.* udvyam tamasapari jyotiṣpaśyanta uttaram, devam devatrā sūryam aganma jyotir uttamam.

324. *Rigveda VIII.6.10.* aham iddhi pituṣpari medhām ṛtasya jagrabha, aham surya ivājani.

325. *Isha Upanishad XVI.* Pūṣannekarṣe yama sūrya prājāpatya vyūha raśmīn samūha tejo yatte rūpam kalyāṇatamam tatte paśyami, yo'sāvasau puruṣaḥ so'ham asmi.

326. *Chandogya Upanishad I.5.1.* atha khalu ya udgīthaḥ sa praṇavo yaḥ praṇavaḥ sa udgītha ityasau vā āditya udgītha eṣa praṇava omiti hyeṣa svaranneti.

327. *Brihadaranyaka Upanishad I.IV.10*

328. *Rigveda IV.26.1.* aham manur abhavam sūryasca.

329. *Bhagavad Gita IV.1-3.* imam vivasvate yogam proktavān aham avyayam, vivasvān manave prāha manur ikṣvākave-bravīt

330. *Mahabharata Shanti Parva 342.95-96.* vidyāsahāyavantam mām ādityastham sanātanam, kapilam prāhur ācāryāḥ sāṁkhyā niścitaniścayāḥ, hiraṇyagarbho dyutimān ya eṣa cchandasi stutaḥ, yogaiḥ sampūjyate nityam sa evāham bhuvi smṛtaḥ.

331. *Brihad Yogi Yajnavalkya Smriti IX.88.* sūrya ātmā jagataḥ prāṇākhyo hṛdi saṁsthitaḥ.

332. *Maitrayani Upanishad VI. 1-3.* dvidhā vā eṣa ātmānam bibharti, ayam yaḥ prāṇo yaścāsāvādityaḥ, atha dvau vā etā asya panthānā antar bahiścāhorātreṇaitau vyāvartete, asau vá ādityo bahir ātmā'antarātmā prāṇo'to bahirātmakyā gatyā'antarātmano'numiyate gatirityevam hyāha.

333. *Shatapatha Brahmana XII.3.2.8*

334. *Rigveda V.81.1* yuñjate mana uta yuñjate dhiyo viprā viprasya bṛhato vipaścitaḥ, vi hotrā dadhe vayunāvid eka in mahī devasya savituḥ pariṣṭutiḥ.

335. *Rigveda I.89.5.* tam iśānām jagatas tasthuṣaspatim dhiyamjinvan avase hūmahe vayam, pūṣā no yathā vedasām asad vṛdhe rakṣitā pāyur adabdhaḥ svastaye.

336. *Rigveda II.27.4.* dhārayanta ādityāso jagatsthā devā viśvasya bhuvanasya gopāḥ, dīrghādhiyo rakṣamāṇā asuryam ṛtāvānaścayamānā ṛṇāni.

337. *Rigveda VII.60.1.* yadadya sūrya bravo'nāgā udyan mitrāya varuṇāya satyam, vayam devatrādite syāma tava priyāso aryaman gṛṇantaḥ.

338. *Rigveda I.164.39.* ṛco akṣare parame vyoman.

339. *Rigveda X.136.7*

340. *Taittiriya Aranyaka Aruna Prashna 91* connects these Vatarashana Rishis to other Vedic Rishi groups like the Arunaketavas and the Vaikhanasas.

341. *Rigveda X.136.2.* munayo vātaraśanāḥ piśaṅgā vasate malā, vātasyānu dhrājim yanti yad devāso avikṣata, unmaditā mauneyena vātām ā tasthivān vayam, śarīredsmākam yūyam martāso abhi paśyata.

342. *Rigveda I.89.7.* pṛṣadaśvạ marutaḥ pṛśnimātaraḥ śubhyāvāno vidatheṣu jagmayaḥ, agnijihvā manavaḥ sūracakṣaso viśve no devā avasā gamaniha.

343. *Rigveda VII.59.12.* tryambakam yajāmahe sugandhim puṣṭivardhanam, urvārukam iva bandhanān mṛtyor mukṣīya māmṛtāt.

344. *Krishna Yajurveda, IV.5.8.* Rudram

345. This includes such *Atharvaveda* forms as Bhava, Sarva, Manyu, and the Vratya.

346. *Rigveda II.33.4.* bhiṣaktamam tvā bhiṣajām.

347. *Rigveda VI.74.3.* Somārudrā yuvam etānyasme viśvā tanūṣu bheṣajāni dhattam, ava syatam muñcatam yanno astri tanūṣu baddham kṛtam eno asmat.

348. *Rigveda IV.3.1.* ā vo rājānam adhvarasya rudram hotāram satyayajam rodasyoḥ, agnim purā taniyitnor acittād hiraṇyarūpam avase kṛṇudhvam.

349. *Shatapatha Brāhmana IV.1.3.10-18.* Names of Agni as Rudra, Śarva, Paśupati, Ugra, Aśani, Bhava, Mahadeva, Īśāna, Kumāra.

350. *Mahabharata Anushasana Parvani Dana Parvani 14, 287-288*

351. Vasishtha Kavyakantha Ganapati Muni, *Collected Works, Volume Five, The Book of Aphorisms, Part One, Indreśvarābheda Sūtram.*

352. *Aitareya Brahmana III.33*

353. *Rigveda X.8.7-9*

354. *Rigveda IV.18.12-13*

355. *Rigveda VIII.24.9,12*

356. *Rigveda I.10.11*

357. *Chandogya Upanishad II.22.3.* sarve svarā indrāsyātmānaḥ.

358. *Rigveda III.53.1*, Indra-Parvata.

359. *Rigveda VI.61.5*

360. *Rigveda VIII.13.20.* tad id rudrasya cetati yahvam pratneṣu dhāmasu mano yatrā vi tad dadhur vicetasaḥ

361. *Aitareya Upanishad I.3. Shvetashvatara Upanishad IV.10*

362. *Kaushitaki Upanishad III.2*

363. *Mahabharata Vanaparva 125*

364. *Rigveda II.23.1*

365. *Mahanarayana Upanishad 12, Dahara Vidya*, last verse. yo vedādau svaraḥ prokto vedānte ca pratiṣṭitaḥ tasya prakṛtilīnasya yaḥ parasya maheśvaraḥ.

366. *Rigveda VII.59.12.* Tryambakam mantra of Vasishtha.

367. *Rigveda VII.33.1.* Vasishthas as Kapardas.

368. *Kena Upanishad III.12.* Uma Haimavati.

369. *Shvetashvatara Upanishad III.2.* There is only one Rudra not a second, who rules over these worlds with his ruling powers. eko hi rudro na dvitīyāya tasthur ya imam̐llokā īśata īśanībhiḥ.

370. *Mahabharata Anushasana Parvani Dana Parvani 17, Shiva Sahasranama.* Note this and the previous sections for more information on Shiva 14-17.

371. *Brihadaranyaka Upanishad II.4.10*

372. *Taittiriya Upanishad I.1.* namaste vāyo tvam eva pratyakṣam brahmāsi, tvām eve pratyakṣam brahma vadiṣyāmi

373. *Brihat Yogi Yajnavaykya Smriti IX.5.* hṛdyāgniścaiva vāyuśca jīveṣaḥ samudāhṛtaḥ

374. *Chandogya Upanishad IV.3.*

375. *Brihadaranyaka Upanishad III.7.2.* vāyur ve gautama tat sūtram vāyuna vai gautama sūtreṇayam ca lokaḥ sarvāni ca bhụtani saddṛbdhāni bhavanti

376. Time is Kāla in Sanskrit, whereas division or art is Kalā. While these two often end up spelled the same in English, we should remember that they are different words.

377. *Rigveda II.1̤.1.* vāyavā yāhi darśateme somā araṁkṛtāḥ teṣām pāhi śrudhī havam

378. *Rigveda VII.61.1.* kuvidaṅga namasā ye vṛdhāsaḥ purā devā anavadyāsa āsan, te vāyave manave bādhitāyāvāsayannuṣasam sūryẹna

379. *Rigveda I.11.1.* indram viśvā avīvṛdhan samudravyacasam giraḥ, rathītamam rathīnām vājānām satpatim patim.

380. *Rigveda III.32.8.* indrasya karma sukṛtā purūṇi vratāni devā na minanti viśve, dādhāra yaḥ pṛthivīm dhyām utemām jajāna sūryam uṣāsam sudaṁsāḥ.

381. *Rigveda III.32.9.* adrogha satyam tava tan mahitvam sadyo yajjāto apibo ha somam, na dhyāva indra tavatasas ta ojo nāhā na māsāḥ śarado varanta.

382. *Rigveda III.32.10.* tvam sadyo apibo jāta indra madāya somam parame vyoman, yaddha dyāvāpṛthivī āviveśīr athābhavaḥ pūrvyaḥ kārudhāyāḥ.

383. *Rigveda II.15.1, 2.* pra ghā nvasya mahato mahāni satyā satyasya karaṇāni vocam, avaṁśe dyām astabhāyad bṛhantam ā rodasī apṛṇad antārikṣam, sa dhārayat pṛthivīm paprathacca somasya tā mada indraścakara.

384. Vasishtha Kavyakantha Ganapati Muni, *Collected Works Volume Five, The Book of Adoration, Part One*, Siddāntasārasūtram.̤1-3. Indro viśvasya rājā, saguṇo nabhaḥ śarīraḥ, nirguṇo viśvasmād uttaraḥ.

385. *Rigveda VI.30.1,4,5.* pra ririce diva indraḥ pṛthivyā ardham id asya prati rodasī ubhe, satyam ittana tvāvān anyo astīndra devo na martyo jyāyān, rājābhavo jagataścarṣaṇīnām sākam sūryam janayan dyām uṣāsam.

386. *Rigveda I.52.11.* yad indra pṛthivī daśabhujir ahāni viśvā tatananta kṛṣṭyaḥ, atrāha te maghavan viśrutam saho dyām anu śavasā barhaṇā bhuvat.

387. *Rigveda I.52.12.* tvam asya pāre rajaso vyomanaḥ svabhūtyojā avase dhṛṣan manaḥ, cakṛṣe bhūmīm pratimānam ojaso'paḥ svaḥ paribhūreṣyā divam.

388. *Rigveda I.52.13.* tvam bhuvaḥ pratimānam pṛthivyā ṛṣva vīrasya bṛhataḥ patir bhūḥ, viśvam āprā antarikṣam mahitvā satyam addhā nakir anyas tvāvān. *Rigveda VI.47.18.* Brihadaranyaka Upanishad I.V.19. rūpam rūpam pratirūpo babhūva tad asya rūpam praticakṣaṇāya; Indro māyābhiḥ pururūpa īyate yuktā hyasya harayaḥ śatā daśa.

389. *Brihadaranyaka Upanishad II.5.19.* ayam vai harayo'yam vai daśa ca sahasrāṇi bahūni cānantāni ca tad etad brahmāpūrvam aparam anantaram abāhyam ayam ātmā brahma sarvānubhūr.

390. *Rigveda V.44.2.* sugopā asi na dabhāya sukrato paro māyābhir ṛta āsa nāma te.

391. *Rigveda VIII.100.3.* pra su stomam bharata vājayanta indrāya satyam yadi satyam asti, nendro astīti nema u tva āha ka īm dadarśa kam abhi ṣṭavāma.

392. *Rigveda VIII.100.4.* ayam asmi jaritaḥ paśya meha vīśvā jātānyabhyasmi mahnā, ṛtasya mā pradiśo vardayantādardiro bhuvanā dardarīmi.

393. *Rigveda III.54.17.* mahat tad vaḥ kavayaścāru nāma yadva devā bhavatha viśva indre, sakha ṛbhubhiḥ puruhūta priyebhir imām dhiyam sātaye takṣatā naḥ.

394. *Rigveda VII.90.5* te satyena manasā dīdhyānāḥ svena yuktāsaḥ kratunā vahanti, Indravāyū vīravāham ratham vāmīśānayor abhi pṛkṣaḥ sacante.

395. *Rigveda VI.61.5.* yas tvā devi sarasvatyupabrūte dhane hite indram na vṛtratūrye.

396. *Vasishtha Kavyakantha Ganapati Muni, Collected Works, Volume Five, the Book of Aphorisms Part One, caturvyūhasūtram I.4,* ākāśa kāla sūrya vaidyutāgni bhedād indraścaturdhā.

397. *Aitareya Upanishad I.3.3.* sa etam eva puruṣam brahma tatam apaśyad idam adarśamitī, tasmād idandro nāmedandro ha vai nāma tamidandram santam idra ityācakṣate parokṣeṇa parokṣapriyā iva hi devāḥ.

398. *Taittiriya Upanishad I.7.* yaśchandasām ṛṣbho viśvarūpaḥ chandobhyo'dhyamṛtāthsaṁbabhūva sa mendro medhayā spṛṇotu.

399. *Kaushitaki Upanishad III.2.* sa hovāca prāṇo'smi prajñātmā tam mām āyur amṛtam ityupāssva.

400. *Rigveda I.61.2.* indrāya hṛdā manasā manīṣā pratnāya patye dhiyo marjayanta. *Rigveda I.18.6-7.* sadaspatim adbhutam priyam indrasya kāmyam, sanim medhām ayāsiṣam; yasmād ṛte sidhyati yajño vipascitaścana, sa dhīnām yogam invati.

401. *Rigveda VIII.13.26.* indra tvam avitedasītthā stuvato adrivaḥ, ṛtādiyarmi te dhiyam manoyujam.

402. *Rigveda II.12.1.* yo jāta eva prathamo manasvān.

403. *Rigveda I.3.23.* indravāyū manojuvā viprā havanta ūtaye, sahasrākṣā dhiyaspatī.

404. Note author's *Ayurveda and the Mind, and Yoga and Ayurveda.*

405. Vasishtha Kavyakantha Ganapati Muni, *Collected Works, Collected Works Volume Five*, Gotrapravaranirṇayaḥ.

406. *Aitareya Brahmana, III.33-34*

407. The famous astrological Bhrigu readers are well known for their great accuracy in telling the events of a person's life.

408. Vasishtha Kavyakantha Ganapati Muni, *Collected Works, Volume Seven, the Book of Commentaries, page 126.* Brahmaṇaspatireva tāntriko gaṇapatiḥ.

409. For example, *Vishnu Purana IV.4, 6-19*

410. Of the five Vedic peoples, Turvashas and Yadus, were born of Devayani, the daughter of Bhrigu. The other three Anus, Druhyus and Purus were born of Sharmishta, daughter of Vrisha Parva, the king of the Asuras. This shows the Asuric blood in humanity.

411. *Aitareya Brahmana VII.34*, has a list of a number of great Vedic kings and their Purohits.

412. *Matsya Purana I.1.13.* The Malaya Mountains mentioned here are those of Kerala. Manu is stated as a king who achieved the highest Yoga (yogam uttamam). *Jaiminiya Brahmana II.219.* athākāmayātātrir bhūyiṣṭḥāma ṛṣayaḥ prajāyām ājāyerann iti, sa etam triṇavam stomam apaśyat; tam āharat; tenāyajata; tejo vai triṇava stomānām, tato vai tasya bhūhiṣṭḥā ṛṣayaḥ prajāyām ājāyanta, parasahasrā hāsya prajāyām mantrakṛta āsur, api hāsya striyo mantrakṛta āsuḥ, tasmād yo'py ātreyīm striyam hanti, tam paryeva caḳsate, tejasvi bahvati ya evam veda.

413. David Frawley, *Wisdom of the Ancient Seers: Selected Mantras of the Rig Veda*, Chapter 7, The Goddess, the Power of the Divine Word pp. 225-252.

414. *Manu Samhita 1.21*

415. *Brihadaranyaka Upanishad II.4.10*

416. *Taittiriya Brahmana III.10.47*. anantā vai vedāḥ meaning "*Vedas* are endless."

417. Rudolph Steiner, *Anthroposophy, An Introduction*, H. Collison, London, 1931, page 64.

418. The writer's own translation from the Hindi version of Sri Aurobindo's *Secret of the Vedas*. He wrote a commentary on the Rigveda, a decisive work on the meaning of all the Vedas. See Bhandarkar's Report on Sanskrit MSS. in Bombay Presidency 1882-1883, Grantha Malika Stotra, verse 7. H.P. Blavatsky, *From the Caves and Jungles of Hindustan*, trans. from the Russian 1892, Theosophical Publishing Society, London. page 19.

419. Aravinda Ghosha (Sri Aurobindo), Dayananda, the Man and His Works, Reprint form Vedic Magazine, Lucknow, 1935, page 21.

420. Op. cit.

421. H.P. Blavatsky, *The Secret Doctrine*, Vol. 1, Third Edition 1905. Theosophical Publishing Society: London. Page 21.

422. Ibid, Page 291.

423. Sri Aurobindo, see footnote 2.

424. Arthur Anthony Macdonell, The *Brhad Devata*, Attributed to Saunaka, A Summary of the Deities and Myths of the Rig-Veda, Part II Publ. Harvard Univ. Cambridge, Mass. 1904.

425. *Bhagavad Gita* 15.14,

426. *Chandogya Upanishad* 5.11-24

427. *Shatapatha Brahmana* 10.6.1.11

428. *Brahma Sutras* of Vyasa 1.2.24

429. Herman Oldenberg. *Selections of Hymns and Verses of the Rig-Veda*. Sacred Books of the East Series, Mandala III, Hymn 2, 2,3To Agni Vaisvanara, 1897, Claredon Press, Oxford.

430. House of Clay, metaphorically the material body; called also the House of Dust and the Insubstantial House. Compare this with Matthew 7:24

431. *Rigveda* X.151 Ralph T.H. Griffith. *The Hymns of the Rigveda*. Preface to the First Edition, Vol. I, page x., 1896-7.

432. *Rigveda* I.22.16-22.

433. These include: The Wheel of Time (*Rigveda* 1.164.48), *Atman* (*Rigveda* II.26.7-8), Knowledge (*Rigveda* X. 191.2-4), *Bhāva-vṛtta*, History of Being (*Rigveda* X.129), and *Śraddhā* (*Rigveda* X.151).

434. *Rigveda* I.3.11. codayitrī sūnṛtānām cetantī sumatīnām

435. *Rigveda* I.21 and in other Apri Suktas as the three feminine counterparts of Agni.

436. *Jabala Upanishad* 2

437. *Rigveda* III.33

438. *Rigveda* X.75.5

439. *a-yudh*: in which there ought to be no conflict or friction. *Atharvaveda* X.2.31. aṣṭacakrā nava-dvārā devānām pūr ayodhyā, tasyām hiraṇyayạ koṣaḥ svaryo jyotṣāvṛtaḥ.

440. *Mundaka Upanishad* 2.2.9

441. *Brahma Sutras* 1.1.30 Herman Oldenberg, *Selections of Hymns and Verses of the Rigveda*, page 449.

442. For a more spiritual translation of what this ashva is, go to *Brihadaranyaka Upanishad* 1.1.1-2. It begins with "Dawn is the head of the sacrificial horse" and explains the entire universe as its manifestation. This horse is indicative of the Life-force or Prana that is to be sacrificed to the divinity within. This becomes the vehicle that takes us to the Gods or the higher reality.

443. *Atharvaveda* X.8.32

444. *Shandilya Upanishad* 2.2

445. Sa meaning "with," and kha meaning "space."

446. See *Yoga Sutras* 1.21, 22